NEUROPHYSIOLOGIC STUDIES
IN
TISSUE CULTURE

Neurophysiologic Studies
in
Tissue Culture

Stanley M. Crain
Departments of Neuroscience and Physiology
and
Rose F. Kennedy Center for Research in Mental Retardation
and Human Development
Albert Einstein College of Medicine
Yeshiva University
Bronx, New York

Raven Press ▪ New York

Raven Press, 1140 Avenue of the Americas, New York, New York 10036

Made in the United States of America

International Standard Book Number 0–89004–048–6
Library of Congress Catalog Card Number 75–14567

To Bea, Steven, and Michael—
with gratitude for their
love, inspiration, and
patience through the years

Preface

This monograph reviews the progress made during the past two decades in developing tissue culture models which demonstrate a remarkable mimicry of many important structures and functions of the mammalian central nervous system (CNS) and related peripheral sensory and motor elements. Emphasis is placed on correlative electrophysiologic, pharmacologic, and electron microscopic analyses, which have provided a firm foundation for critically evaluating the integrity of a wide variety of cultured neural tissues—both intact explants and arrays of dissociated neurons. Systematic applications of sophisticated biophysical and biochemical techniques are becoming increasingly attractive and fruitful as confidence develops in the reliability of these neural cultures as a faithful model system.

Electrophysiologic studies of mammalian cerebral and spinal cord cultures during long-term maturation *in vitro* have demonstrated the intrinsic capacity of CNS tissues to organize complex "organotypic" neural networks after complete isolation from the fetal or neonatal animal. Generation of patterned synaptically mediated bioelectric discharges, including significant electroencephalogram (EEG)-like components, in such small cultured fragments of CNS tissue (<1 mm^3) sets limits to hypotheses regarding the anatomic organization and the functional networks required to account for similar bioelectric activities when recorded from the CNS *in situ*.

Organotypic features of CNS tissues developing in culture have been shown to include formation of specialized synaptic junctions between nerve cells; these have characteristic pharmacologic sensitivities and functionally connect specific groups of neurons into regionally organized networks that lead to transmission of nerve impulses along preferential pathways. Arrays of CNS neurons growing in a culture chamber on a thin coverglass therefore provide a remarkable "window" to facilitate not only direct microscopic observation but also flexible experimental manipulation of some of the intricate cellular networks characteristic of the mammalian brain.

Organized neural tissue cultures are being utilized for basic studies in developmental neurobiology—including mechanisms of synaptogenesis; formation of connections between specific types of target neurons; neurotrophic as well as bioelectric interactions; direct effects of neurotransmitters, hormones, and other metabolic agents; and even early stages of embryonic behavior. These cultures also provide valuable model systems for studies of cellular mechanisms underlying complex cerebral functions, e.g., EEG activities and neural plasticity in relation to memory and learning; they also supplement *in situ* investigations of neurologic disorders, e.g., epilepsy and multiple sclerosis, and problems in CNS regeneration.

Highlights of earlier physiologic studies of cultured neural tissues are assembled here for correlative analyses; they are integrated with exciting new experiments from the author's laboratory as well as those by many other neuroscientists working in this rapidly expanding field of research. It is hoped that this book will provide a useful guide and further stimulus to investigators seeking insights into some of the many intricate neural functions that may be clarified by viewing them through the tissue culture "window" to the brain.

Stanley M. Crain

Acknowledgments

This book is dedicated to Edith R. Peterson and Murray B. Bornstein who skillfully prepared, faithfully nurtured, and critically evaluated — by serial light-microscopic observations — the neural tissue cultures used for our coordinated cytologic and electrophysiologic studies during the past two decades. These fruitful collaborative experiments were initiated in the stimulating milieu generated at Columbia University during the early 1950s by Drs. Margaret R. Murray, Fred A. Mettler, and Harry Grundfest, and they have continued to flourish during the past decade following transfer of our laboratories to the Albert Einstein College of Medicine. Development of this research program has been greatly facilitated by the strong support and encouragement provided by the former and present directors of the Rose F. Kennedy Center for Research in Mental Retardation and Human Development at Albert Einstein College of Medicine, Drs. Harry H. Gordon and Dominick P. Purpura.

Thanks are also due to the National Institute of Neurological and Communicative Disorders and Stroke, which has generously supported our neural tissue culture research efforts during the past two decades, and to the following organizations, which have provided additional funds at critical stages along the way: Joseph P. Kennedy Foundation for Mental Retardation, Alfred P. Sloan Foundation, National Science Foundation, National Multiple Sclerosis Society, and the Epilepsy Foundation of America.

I want to express grateful appreciation to my faithful secretary, Debbie Cahn, who has been of great help in preparing this monograph, and who skillfully and patiently traversed my zigzag mazes of often barely legible notes and transformed them into elegantly ordered arrays of type.

Finally, I wish to thank Dr. Alan Edelson for initially stimulating me to prepare this monograph and for his valuable advice and warm encouragement during the course of its development.

Stanley M. Crain

Contents

I. Tissue Culture Models of Neural Functions...................... 1
   A. General Strategies 1
   B. Initial Experiments 5

II. Tissue Culture and Bioelectric Techniques 13
   A. Preparation of Tissue Cultures................................. 13
   B. Bioelectric Recording Systems................................. 18

III. Action Potentials in Peripheral Ganglion Explants 31
   A. Dorsal Root Ganglia... 31
   B. Sympathetic Ganglia 40

IV. Development of Organotypic Synaptic Networks in CNS
   Explants 43
   A. Spinal Cord and Innervation of Muscle 43
   B. Spinal Cord Innervation by Dorsal Root Ganglia........... 69
   C. Brainstem: Specific and Nonspecific Networks 79
   D. Cerebral Neocortex, Hippocampus, and Limbic
      Regions... 92
   E. Cerebellum... 124
   F. Invertebrate CNS... 128

V. Formation of Functional Synaptic Networks in Cultures
   of Dissociated Neurons 131
   A. Peripheral Ganglia 131
   B. Spinal Cord and Brainstem...................................... 141
   C. Cerebral Cortex and Cerebellum 149

VI. Characteristic Sensitivities of CNS Explant Discharge
   Patterns to Selective Pharmacologic and Metabolic Agents... 153
   A. Strychnine versus Glycine.. 153
   B. Bicuculline versus GABA.. 157
   C. d-Tubocurarine versus Acetylcholine 162
   D. Chloride-free Media 164
   E. Caffeine and Cyclic AMP versus Mg^{++} and Low Ca^{++} ... 166
   F. Serum Depressant Factors 177

VII.   Spontaneous Patterned Discharges in CNS Explants in
       Relation to Embryonic Motility, EEG, and Inhibitory
       Control Systems 183
       A. Spontaneous Discharges and Embryonic Motility 183
       B. EEG Models 186
       C. Cerebral Hyperexcitability and Collateral Sprouting 197
       D. Role of Inhibitory Systems in Masking Early "Behav-
          ioral Repertoire" of CNS Cultures and Embryos 198

VIII. Tissue Culture Models for Studies of CNS Plasticity,
       Trophic Factors, and Regeneration 209
       A. CNS Plasticity 209
       B. CNS Neurotrophic Factors 215
       C. CNS Regeneration 228

  IX. Overview 231
       A. Limitations of CNS Culture Models 231
       B. Potentialities 233

       References 237

       Index 267

I

Tissue Culture Models of Neural Functions

A. GENERAL STRATEGIES

In view of the complexity of the mammalian brain, many attempts have been made to study some of the fundamental mechanisms underlying cerebral functions by utilizing simpler model systems. Electrophysiologic studies of surgically isolated slabs of cerebral cortex have been carried out in adult mammals by Burns (1958) and others; this technique has been combined with ontogenetic parameters by Purpura and Housepian (1961) in studies of neuronally isolated cerebral slabs in the neonatal kitten. Libet and Gerard's (1939) pioneering electrophysiologic experiments with much smaller fragments of adult frog cerebrum, which continued to generate rhythmic electroencephalogram (EEG)-like activity for hours after complete isolation in a dish of Ringer's solution, demonstrated the potentialities of studying cerebral function in a phylogenetically as well as surgically simplified system. McIllwain (1963) and others developed a still more radical dissection of brain tissue which permits experimental study of thin (300 μm) slices of adult mammalian cerebral cortex for at least several hours after isolation *in vitro*. Yamamoto and McIllwain (1966) demonstrated that these brain slices can generate characteristic cerebral evoked potentials, indicating the maintenance of complex synaptic functions in this freshly isolated tissue (Yamamoto and Kawai, 1967).

Application of tissue culture techniques greatly enhances these surgical isolation methods. Not only can small cerebral fragments (ca. 1 mm³) be maintained in sterile glass vessels for long periods of study under direct microscopic observation, but the tissues may be explanted from early embryos and grown under culture conditions that permit sequential development *in vitro* of characteristic organized structures and functions of the central nervous system (CNS). Capillary circulation is no longer essential in such small pieces of brain tissue — simple diffusion of nutrients from the supernatant culture medium permits metabolic activities to proceed normally, and catabolites within the tissue can similarly diffuse out into the bathing fluid.

Electrophysiologic studies of mammalian cerebral and spinal cord explants during maturation *in vitro* demonstrated the intrinsic capacity of these CNS tissues to organize complex "organotypic" neural networks after complete isolation from the fetal or neonatal animal (Crain, 1966)

(Chap. IV). Generation of complex patterned synaptically mediated bioelectric discharges in such small cultured fragments of CNS tissue sets limits to hypotheses regarding the anatomic organization and the critical functional components required to account for similar bioelectric activities when recorded from the CNS *in situ*.

Maximow (1925) classified cultured tissues—including those of the CNS —in terms of their pattern of growth, using the term "histiotypic" to describe the diffuse outwandering of cells from a cut surface, and reserving "organotypic" for more organized growth which involved progressive histologic as well as cytologic differentiation. The orderly development in the latter case is based on maintenance of significant intercellular relationships, so that "the tissue largely retains its characteristic architecture, remains functional and if derived from undifferentiated material, it may develop in culture in a surprisingly normal way" (Fell, 1951). A small endocrine gland (e.g., parathyroid) explanted *in toto* at an embryonic stage (Gaillard, 1955; Gaillard and Schaberg, 1965) provides an excellent example of an organotypic culture in which the basic structure and function of the entire organ develops in an organized fashion. Many organs, on the other hand, especially the CNS, must be surgically subdivided in order to obtain fragments small enough for standard tissue culture procedures (Chap. II). To the extent that these isolated portions of an organ show progressive histologic differentiation in culture, the term organotypic can still be meaningfully employed to emphasize maintenance of specialized, characteristic properties unique to tissue from that organ.

It is in this sense that organotypic is used to describe cultured neural tissues that differentiate in a "surprisingly normal way" after isolation from the organism. In the case of an embryonic spinal sensory ganglion, for example, organotypic development in culture involves primarily the orderly establishment of intercellular relationships between the neurons and the Schwann (and other supporting) cells. On this basis axons mature *in vitro*, develop the capacity for normal propagation of action potentials (Crain, 1956) (Chaps. I-B, III), and may show progressive myelination (Peterson and Murray, 1955).

Organotypic development of tissues explanted from the CNS, on the other hand, involves far more complex processes. In addition to orderly relationships between neurons and a variety of glial cells, specialized synaptic junctions form between nerve cells, functionally connecting particular groups of neurons into organized networks and permitting transmission of nerve impulses along preferential pathways. Such organotypic arrays of CNS neurons growing in a culture chamber on a thin coverglass provide, therefore, a remarkable "window" to facilitate not only direct observation but also flexible experimental manipulation of some of the intricate cellular networks characteristic of the mammalian brain.

Similar organotypic synaptically mediated bioelectric activities also develop in small clusters of neurons which reaggregate *in vitro* after complete dissociation and random dispersion of fetal mouse cerebral cortex, cerebellum, brainstem, or spinal cord cells (Crain and Bornstein, 1972; Nelson and Peacock, 1973; Nelson, 1973, 1975; Ransom and Nelson, 1975) (Chap. V). Abundant synaptic junctions form in these dissociated CNS cultures (Bornstein and Model, 1972) as in cord and brain explants isolated at "presynaptic" stages (Bunge et al., 1967a; Model et al., 1971). Techniques are therefore now available for preparation of neuronal arrays in cultures of varying complexity, ranging from intact explants containing a few thousand closely packed neurons and glial cells, to monolayers of completely separated neurons. Synaptogenesis can occur in all of these types of cultures derived from embryonic CNS tissues, but intact explants have so far been more reliable as model systems for studying mature synaptic networks with reproducible organotypic bioelectric activities and characteristic pharmacologic sensitivities. Emphasis has therefore been placed on analyses of mechanisms underlying development of the functional integrity of CNS explants as a foundation for systematic correlative cytologic and electrophysiologic studies of various types of simpler neuronal arrays. The latter preparations facilitate direct microscopic observation, microelectrode manipulations, and other biophysical analyses (Chap. V), but some of the uniquely interesting cerebral functions related to memory and learning, and perhaps also mechanisms underlying rhythmic behavior patterns (Chaps. VII, VIII) may require more complex cellular assemblies. Intact 1 mm^3 CNS explants provide a drastically simplified neuronal array relative to the overwhelming complexities of the whole mammalian brain, and they are at least 1,000 times smaller than the usual neuronally isolated cerebral slab preparations *in situ* which have been utilized in many neurophysiologic studies (Burns, 1958; Purpura and Housepian, 1961).

Pharmacologic analyses of the complex bioelectric activities of intact CNS explants provide, moreover, a powerful tool for linking selective neuropharmacologic effects in the whole organism and direct molecular actions on individual cells. This volume therefore includes recent evidence demonstrating the remarkable degree to which characteristic pharmacologic sensitivities can develop and be maintained in identified regions within mammalian CNS explants in relation to their capacity to generate specific synaptically mediated organotypic bioelectric network discharges (Chaps. IV, VI).

The term "neural tissue culture" is used in this volume in its literal sense, i.e., the culture of neural tissues. In microbiology a culture generally refers to a system in which bacteria or cells are growing—or are at least being maintained in a state of dynamic metabolic equilibrium—in a nutrient medium. This view of neural tissue cultures helps to distinguish these preparations from freshly isolated portions of the nervous system maintained in simple balanced solutions for a few hours or even a few days. Much of traditional experimental neurophysiology has been carried out on isolated frog nerves, ganglia, spinal cord strips, brain slices, etc., which may retain characteristic functions for short periods in Ringer-type solutions, but to refer to these preparations as tissue or organ cultures (e.g., Nelson, 1975) obscures the significant differences between cultured tissues and merely isolated tissues. All neural tissue and organ cultures obviously consist of isolated portions of the nervous system, but the reverse is not true since most freshly isolated neural tissues or organs are rapidly degenerating, structurally and functionally, unless special procedures are introduced to prevent these trends. These "special procedures" are incorporated into the techniques of "tissue culture" which permit long-term development of many types of embryonic neurons, as well as maintenance or regeneration of at least some mature neural tissues, after isolation *in vitro* (Chap. II-A). The distinction between freshly isolated neural tissues and neural tissue cultures is of course not a sharp one, since many freshly isolated preparations, especially embryonic ones, may continue to metabolize relatively normally for experimentally useful periods *in vitro* without introduction of special nutrient media. They could just as well be characterized as short-term tissue or organ cultures incubating "in their own juice" — e.g., neonatal rat spinal cord (Otsuka and Konishi, 1974) or adult frog cerebellum (Hackett, 1972). This terminology, however, should be applied judiciously (see also Chap. IV-A3).

Emphasis on the culture of neural *tissues* serves to distinguish these preparations from *cell* cultures. The latter generally involve histiotypic growth of dissociated cells without maintenance of organized intercellular relationships characteristic of the tissue of origin. Cell cultures of neurons, neuroblastoma cells, glial cells, etc. provide valuable preparations for analyses of basic cellular properties, but they are often less suitable for studies of specialized cellular interrelationships of the nervous system, e.g., synaptic and trophic interactions between specific types of neurons, myelination, etc. Recent improvements in cell dissociation techniques indicate, however, that arrays of thinly dispersed neurons can indeed develop significant synaptic connections under appropriate culture conditions, thereby providing the basis for valuable new experimental model systems that facilitate sophisticated biophysical and biochemical analyses at the single cell level (Chap. V).

It is also useful to distinguish between neural tissues explanted into nutrient media *in vitro* versus those isolated in special compartments *in situ,* e.g., anterior eye chamber, amphibian tail, chick chorioallantoic membrane. Weiss (1950) suggested using the term "deplants" to refer to transplants of neural tissues into relatively indifferent surroundings in the host animal, thereby permitting the "deplant" to grow *in situ* under conditions analogous to an "explant" growing *in vitro*. These experimental preparations are less readily available for direct cytologic and physiologic analyses, but they may provide a more natural metabolic environment for optimal development of neuronally isolated tissues, especially if they become vascularized by the host animal. Correlative physiologic and histologic studies have been carried out on several types of CNS deplants.

The pioneering studies carried out by Weiss (1941*a*, 1950) using deplants of larval newt spinal cord in the transparent amphibian dorsal fin provided an elegant demonstration of the self-organizing properties of isolated amphibian CNS tissues (Weiss, 1941*b*). They certainly constituted a powerful stimulus to our own extension of these experiments to mammalian CNS explants, and further analyses of amphibian cord deplants were carried out by Székely and Szentagothai (1962) (Chap. VII-D). This experimental method was recently extended to deplants of mammalian CNS tissues in a series of elegant studies by Olson and Seiger (1972, 1973, 1974) on fetal rat brain tissues in the rat anterior eye chamber (Chap. IV-C). Effects of subsequent innervation by the nervous system of the host animal provide an additional parameter for analysis of neural deplants [e.g., ingrowth of host adrenergic nerves into deplants of fetal cerebellar cortex (Hoffer et al. 1975*a*) and into deplants of fetal cerebral cortex (Seiger and Olson, 1975)], but this factor may also be a source of ambiguity unless precautions are taken to preclude such innervation during attempts to study neuronally isolated deplants. Seiger and Olson (1975) emphasize that their "recent studies dealing with cerebellar cortex transplants (Hoffer et al. 1974, 1975*a*) or hippocampal cortex transplants . . . (Hoffer et al., 1975*b*, 1976; Olson et al., 1976) show that not only histologically but also electrophysiologically do the transplants [from fetal and neonatal rats] mimic adult brain tissue from the corresponding regions. It is therefore possible that cortex cerebri transplants also possess a series of normal or near-normal electrophysiological features" (although bioelectric tests of cerebral neocortex deplants have not yet been made). This new series of deplantation studies provides, therefore, excellent confirmation of our electrophysiologic analyses of the development of organotypic activities in fetal mouse cerebral explants in culture (Crain, 1966) (Chap. IV-D). Correlative studies of the same CNS tissue growing as a deplant *in situ* and an explant *in vitro* may provide further insight into the role of circulating factors *in situ* during critical stages of neural maturation [Chap. IV-C; see also more complex interactions during development of embryonic rat cerebellar and cerebral neocortex tissue transplanted into the cerebellum of neonatal rats (Das and Altman, 1972; Das, 1975), in contrast to deplantation into "neutral" regions of the host animal].

B. INITIAL EXPERIMENTS

The first attempt to utilize organotypic CNS cultures as a model system to supplement functional neurobiologic studies *in situ* was made approximately 70 years ago by Harrison in the course of his pioneering development of neural tissue culture techniques for analysis of basic mechanisms underlying the outgrowth of nerve fibers (Harrison, 1907, 1910; see also

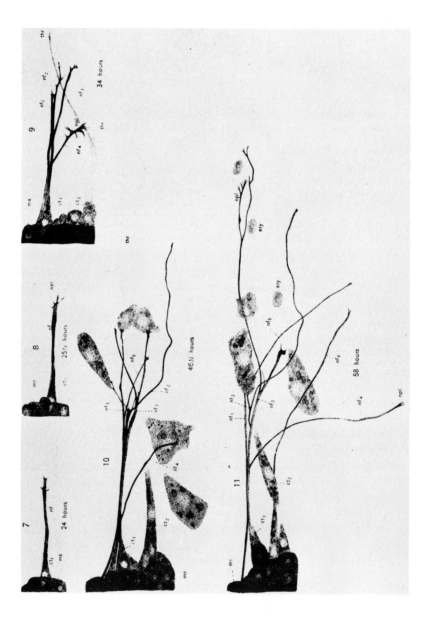

Harrison, 1969). His simple, elegant demonstration of the individuality of the nerve cell, by direct observation of the outgrowth of nerve fibers from a fragment of frog embryo spinal cord embedded in a drop of clotted lymph (Fig. I-1), set sharp limits to earlier speculations and hypotheses regarding nerve formation by complex multicellular fusion processes. Harrison (1910) concluded that:

> . . . neuroblasts are competent to form primitive nerve fibers within a foreign unorganized medium simply by the amoeboid outgrowth of their protoplasm. By eliminating from the periphery all formed structures which have heretofore been supposed to transform themselves into nerve fibers and leaving only the neuroblasts in the field, it is demonstrated that the latter are the sole elements essential to the formation of nerves. The concepts of both Hensen and Held are rendered untenable.

In addition to establishing this basic principle (see also review by Hughes, 1968), Harrison obtained indirect evidence that functional neuromuscular transmission had probably developed in cultures of frog embryo spinal cord and myotomes. This was based on observations of spontaneous muscle contractions that occurred only when the explants included spinal cord components (Harrison, 1907, 1910). These initial experiments were extended by Szepsenwol (1941, 1946, 1947) in a larger series of investigations of chick embryo spinal cord and myotomes in culture. He reported, moreover, that these spontaneous muscle twitches could be "completely inhibited after slight curarization of the explant" (for review see Fell, 1951; Crain, 1965a, 1966). In view of the common occurrence of various types of spontaneous muscle contractions in completely isolated muscle explants (Murray, 1965a), interpretations regarding innervation based solely on visual observations may not be reliable. Direct electrophysiologic experiments were clearly required in order to evaluate the degree to which neuromuscular transmission could develop under isolated conditions in culture. It was not until 1964, however, that direct electrophysiologic recordings demonstrated the capacity of spinal cord neurons to establish functional connections with skeletal muscle fibers in cultures (prepared by Bornstein and Breitbart, 1964) of fetal mouse myotomes attached to the cord explant (Crain, 1964b) (Chap. IV-A). These preliminary cord-myotome experiments were subsequently extended to studies of the innervation

---

FIG. I-1. *First* demonstration of the outgrowth of nerve fibers in tissue culture. "All figures were drawn from camera lucida sketches of living specimens of [frog] embryonic tissue isolated in clotted lymph. **7–11:** Five views of the same group of nerve fibers made at different times; medullary cord tissue from *R. palustris*, 3.3 mm long; lymph from *R. pipiens* (the interval between the first and last figure represents 34 hours). **7:** Apparently single fiber (nf) growing out from a pointed cell (ct₁), which projects from a mass of cells (ms) one day after isolation of tissue. April 28, 1908, 12:25 P.M. **8:** Same fiber, 2 P.M. Fiber is now clearly double. **9:** Same group of fibers, 10:25 P.M. Four distinct fibers (nf₁–nf₄) are now visible. The fibrin filaments (thr) shown in this figure were present in the earlier stages but were omitted from the original sketches. **10:** Same group, April 29, 11 A.M. nf₅ possibly a branch of nf₁. **11:** Same group, 10:30 P.M. Continuation of nf₁ and upper branch of nf₂ unfortunately left out of sketch. Note migration of cell (ct₂). Identity of other isolated cells in **10** and **11** is uncertain." (From Harrison, 1910.)

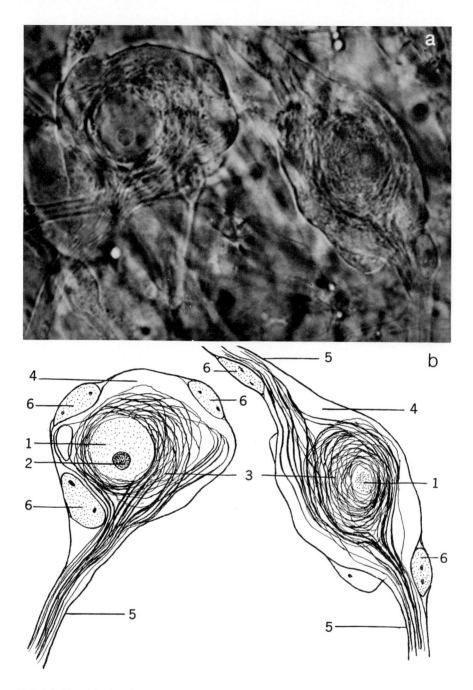

FIG. I-2. Two bipolar dorsal root ganglion cells from an 8-day chick embryo, cultivated *in vitro* for 7 days. **a:** The living cells. (×1,650). **(b):** Diagram of same, to show the main course of the neurofibrils (3), which can be observed in the living cell as discrete and continuous microscopic threads. 1, nucleus. 2, nucleolus. 3, fibrillar basket. 4, peripheral hyaloplasm. 5, axon. 6, nucleus of sheath or satellite cell. (See lower-power views of typical ganglion explants in Figs. I-3 and III-1; see also details of neuritic arborizations in Figs. III-5,8.) (From Weiss and Wang, 1936.)

in vitro of completely separate explants of fetal and even adult rodent and human muscle fibers by fetal rodent cord neurons (Crain, 1968, 1970*a;* Crain et al., 1970; Crain and Peterson, 1974*a;* morphologic correlates in Peterson and Crain, 1970, 1972).

The 1964 experiments on neuromuscular transmission in culture were made possible by technical developments during the preceding decade both in methods of preparing organotypic neural tissue cultures and in carrying out microelectrode analyses of the bioelectric activities of the explanted neurons (Chap. II). These techniques were applied initially to explants of chick embryo spinal ganglia in the tissue culture laboratory of Dr. Margaret Murray at the College of Physicians and Surgeons, Columbia University. Edith Peterson was the first to demonstrate that myelin sheaths could form *de novo* in long-term ganglion cultures (Peterson, 1950); cytologic studies during the maturation of these ganglion cells *in vitro* were carried out during the next few years (Peterson and Murray, 1955) and then extended to cultures of fetal rat dorsal root ganglia (Fig. I-3; see also Figs.

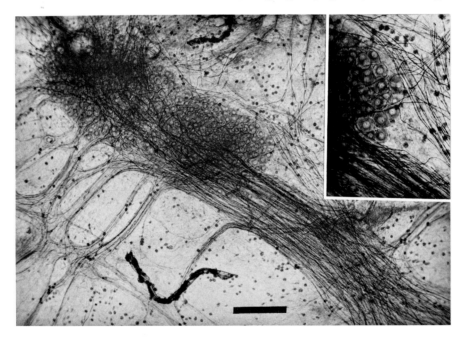

FIG. I-3. Dorsal root ganglion explant from a 16-day rat fetus, 49 days *in vitro* (stained with Sudan black). Note the abundant array of neuron perikarya that survived and matured in normal culture medium (no nerve growth factor added — cf. Fig. IV-17; see also Chap. IV-B) and the well-developed fascicles of selectively blackened myelinated axons extending for long distances away from the ganglion explant. **Inset:** Higher-power view of right edge of explant; note small group of neuron perikarya showing well-stained cytoplasm (primarily mitochondria) and a characteristic large, centrally located nucleus with prominent nucleolus (see still higher-power views in Figs. I-2 and III-1). Scale: 200 μm in low-power view and 100 μm in inset. [Photomicrograph, *ca.* 1960, by Edith R. Peterson; see also related illustrations in Bunge et al., 1967*b*.]

II-1, III-1, IV-20). Earlier pioneering neurocytologic studies of chick embryo dorsal root ganglia in short-term cultures by Levi and co-workers (e.g., Levi, 1915–1916; Levi and Meyer, 1937, 1945) (Fig. III-5), Weiss and Wang (1936) (Fig. I-2), and others were well reviewed by Murray (1965*b*). It was still a moot question as to whether neurons in culture, isolated from their normal sources of stimulation, would retain their characteristic excitability properties or undergo "atrophy" as in denervated muscle (Chap. VIII-B). In the absence of direct electrophysiologic data from cultured neurons, Lumsden's comments in 1951 reflect the speculative approach which was still necessary at that stage, based on morphologic studies of ganglion cells *in vitro:*

> Since the neuroblast of the embryonic nerve tissue . . . manifests in tissue culture a degree of morphological differentiation which is indeed unique for all tissues *in vitro* then it would seem a logical assumption that, biochemically, the neuron is no less advanced in differentiation than it is in structure in these respective instances. If the problem is viewed in this way, therefore, it would seem not at all improbable that even the neuroblast in the explant of the posterior spinal root ganglion of the 9-day chick embryo is already an electrically functioning unit.

My own studies of the bioelectric properties of these cultured ganglion cells began in 1952 (in collaboration with Peterson and Murray), and led to the first demonstration that neurons isolated in long-term cultures could indeed maintain their characteristic membrane excitability properties, including the capacity to generate propagated action potentials in response to local electric stimuli (Crain et al., 1953; Crain, 1954*a,b,* 1956) (Chap. III-A).[1] These experiments utilized intracellular microelectrode recordings to measure resting and action potentials of the ganglion cells following preliminary intracellular studies on cultured cardiac and skeletal muscle fibers (Mettler et al., 1952; further details in Crain, 1954*a,* 1965*a,* 1973*a;* morphologic correlates in Peterson and Murray, 1955; Murray, 1965*a,b*).

Concomitant with bioelectric studies of nerve and muscle cells in culture,

---

[1] The introductory paragraph of this first paper on bioelectric activity of neurons in culture (Crain, 1956) is of interest in view of the fruitful developments during the past two decades: "Tissue cultures of nerve cells provide a powerful new tool for the study of neural function. In the first place, such neurons can often be directly observed under the highest powers of the optical microscope simultaneously with the detailed investigation of various aspects of their functioning. Moreover the possibility arises for maintaining these experimental conditions with respect to a particular cell, or group of cells, not merely for a few hours—as is the case in the usual freshly isolated tissue preparations—but for days or even weeks. The potentialities are, therefore, quite favorable for significant correlations of neurocytic structure and function, not only during short-term, 'steady-state' conditions, but also during such dynamic periods as embryological development and regeneration. Since a search of the literature has failed to reveal any conclusive evidence—obtained by direct experimental methods—that nerve cells could actually retain their characteristic functions after cultivation *in vitro,* the object of this paper is to describe various types of electrical activity observed in cultures of chick embryo spinal ganglia." After quoting Lumsden's remarks of 1951 regarding the probability that ganglion cells in culture are "electrically functioning units" (see above) the Introduction ends with: "As will be shown below, this prediction has now been fully confirmed by direct electrical measurements."

attempts were begun in 1955, after the initial promising results with spinal ganglia, to apply this method to CNS tissues. Pomerat and co-workers had already made substantial progress in developing techniques for long-term cultures of neonatal kitten cerebellum explants (e.g., Pomerat and Costero, 1956). Demonstration of myelin formation in explants of newborn kitten and rat cerebellum (Hild, 1957; Bornstein and Murray, 1958) raised hopes that CNS functions might also become available for direct study *in vitro*. Initial microelectrode studies by Hild and Tasaki (1962) were disappointing in regard to evidence of synaptic interactions, but they nevertheless obtained valuable bioelectric data demonstrating propagation of nerve impulses along dendritic branches of cerebellar neurons. The dendrites could be visualized simultaneously at high magnification in thinly spread explants (Chap. IV-E). No signs of neuronal interactions characteristic of CNS *in situ* were detected, and it was concluded [rather prematurely (!)] that "a neuron *in vivo* is always part of a neural network, whereas a neuron in tissue culture no longer has synaptic connections with other neurons" (Hild and Tasaki, 1962). Explants of fetal spinal cord (rat, chick, and human) proved to be far more fruitful for studies of synaptic activities, and in 1963 we reported the first clear-cut electrophysiologic data demonstrating that "nerve cells in cultures may maintain, for months *in vitro*, not only the capacity to propagate impulses along their neurites but also a remarkable degree of functional organization resembling the activity of synaptic networks of the central nervous system" (Crain and Peterson, 1963, 1964). This work paved the way for collaborative experiments with Dr. Murray Bornstein (after he had set up his own neural tissue culture laboratory at New York's Mt. Sinai Hospital following several years of training and fruitful research at Columbia) on the cord-myotome cultures noted above and on explants of cerebral cortex (*vide infra*).

Electrophysiologic studies of cerebral cultures had been the original goal of my doctoral research project, as formulated in 1951, together with Drs. Fred A. Mettler, Margaret R. Murray, and Harry Grundfest. It was with this plan in mind that I studied the onset and development of electrical activity in rat cerebral cortex *in situ* (Crain, 1952) to provide background data for more direct investigation of these dynamic events after isolation of "prefunctional" cerebral tissue in culture (Chap. IV-D). Development of the culture techniques prerequisite for such *in vitro* studies did not, however, become feasible until 1963 when Bornstein's efforts to obtain healthy cerebral explants finally began to succeed (Bornstein, 1963, 1964). The evoked and spontaneous bioelectric discharges recorded from these embryonic cerebral tissues during maturation *in vitro* (Crain, 1963, 1964*a;* Crain and Bornstein, 1964) demonstrated that fragments as small as 1 mm³ have the intrinsic capacity to organize neural networks that can generate long-lasting rhythmic activities resembling some of the important patterns of the EEG (Crain, 1966; see also discussion by Crain in Robertson, 1966). These exciting collaborative experiments involved many carefully executed auto-mobile trips to transport the cerebral cultures from Bornstein's laboratory at Mt. Sinai Hospital through hectic city traffic to my electrophysiology laboratory at Columbia (with great care taken to avoid spilling the precious "drop" of nutrient medium from its required confinement to the culture coverglass within the Maximow depression-slide chambers (Chap. II-A-1). These logistic problems were finally eliminated in 1966 when we both trans-ferred our laboratories to much more spacious, as well as conveniently located, facilities at the Albert Einstein College of Medicine, where trans-portation of cultures was reduced to brief strolls through quiet corridors.

Electrophysiologic studies of neural tissue cultures have thus developed from the "pipe-dream stage" in 1950 to a well-established experimental method that has recently begun to be applied in many laboratories through-out the world. Although the experimental techniques utilized during most of our studies of cultured CNS tissues have been limited to relatively crude extracellular recordings of summated population discharges (see, however, Chap. IV-D), they have facilitated demonstration of—in broad brush-stroke fashion (Crain, 1969; see also Purpura, 1969)—the remarkable degree to which small fragments explanted from a wide variety of immature CNS tis-sues can develop sufficient cellular interrelationships to permit generation of complex organotypic synaptic network activities during long periods of isolation in culture. These dramatic demonstrations of the functional ca-pacities of CNS explants as they develop *in vitro* have undoubtedly played a significant role in stimulating serious interest in utilizing neural tissue culture models for studies of cellular mechanisms underlying normal and abnormal functions of the nervous system. Systematic application of sophis-ticated multidisciplinary techniques to these neural cultures is becoming in-creasingly attractive as confidence develops in their reliability as faithful model systems. Many of the earlier nerve tissue culture studies, which were limited to microscopic observations of the living cells, were fraught with ambiguities and misinterpretations (Murray, 1965b; Crain, 1966). Cor-relative electrophysiologic and electron microscopic analyses have now provided a firm foundation for critically evaluating the integrity of neural tissue culture preparations, and they will undoubtedly encourage serious studies of the molecular mechanisms underlying development of these spe-cialized neuronal structures and functions *in vitro* (see reviews of biochemi-cal aspects by Schrier et al. 1974; Richelson, 1975).

Valuable general reviews of the neural tissue culture field have been pub-lished by Murray (1965a,b, 1971), Lumsden (1968), Silberberg (1972), Bornstein (1973c), Herschman (1974), Bunge (1975), Nelson (1975), and Varon (1975). More specialized reviews are noted in other chapters of this volume. (See also the extensive tissue culture bibliography by Murray and Kopech, 1953.)

II

Tissue Culture and Bioelectric Techniques

A. PREPARATION OF TISSUE CULTURES

1. Slab Explants

The procedure that has produced the most highly differentiated central nervous system (CNS) cultures involves explantation of small fragments (ca. 1 mm³) of embryonic tissue (e.g., fetal rodent spinal cord: Figs. II-1, IV-17) onto collagen-coated coverglasses[1] with their subsequent incubation at 34°–35°C in Maximow depression-slide chambers as "lying-drop" preparations (Peterson et al., 1965; Peterson and Crain, 1970; Bornstein, 1973a; for more general details and references regarding culture techniques see also Moscona et al., 1965; Murray, 1965b, 1971). The explants are cut so that one dimension is well under 1 mm in order to facilitate diffusion of metabolites to and from the cells within the central region of the tissue. Dissection of embryonic CNS tissues and slicing to appropriate explant size require considerable skill to minimize surgical trauma to the extremely fragile structures. The culture medium is changed twice a week and generally contains mammalian serum in a balanced salt solution (BSS) with embryo extract or other special nutrients. A medium often used for culturing mammalian CNS explants consists of human placental serum (25–40%), Eagle's synthetic medium (25%), and Simms' BSS[2] supplemented with glucose

---

[1] Collagen gel reconstituted from dialyzed acetic acid extracts of rat tail tendon has been found to be an excellent substrate for long-term cultivation of neural and other tissues (Bornstein, 1958). Recent experimental procedures requiring a more resilient, porous collagen substrate to accommodate to actively contracting skeletal muscle *in vitro* (Chaps. IV-D, VIII-B) prompted development of a relatively rapid and innocuous photochemical procedure for forming such collagen gel substrates (Masurovsky and Peterson, 1973). Although muscle, connective tissue, and neural outgrowth is most abundant along the substrate surface, nerve fibers may work their way into and move along the matrix fibrils where they can develop and become myelinated. Furthermore, the greater porosity of these gels provides an additional substrate-permeated reservoir of culture medium which may effectively nourish deeper regions of thick explants. In this regard, neural tissue explants may not flatten out as much on this collagen substrate as on ammoniated collagen gels, possibly favoring more organotypic culture organization, e.g., mouse cord-muscle explants maintained for more than 1 year *in vitro* (Chap. VIII-B). Engraved Aclar plastic film reticles can readily be incorporated into these collagen substrates for precise, reproducible cell localization from light through electron microscope levels (Masurovsky et al., 1971; see also Masurovsky and Bunge, 1968).

[2] Simms' BSS contains the following salt concentrations in millimoles per liter of glass-distilled water: NaCl (137), KCl (2.7), $CaCl_2$ (1.0), $MgCl_2$ (1.0), Na_2HPO_4 (1.36), NaH_2PO_4 (0.15), $NaHCO_3$ (6.0), glucose (5.5).

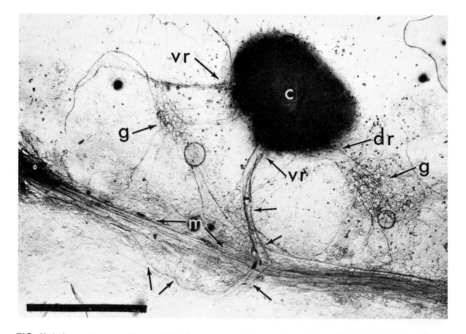

FIG. II-1. Long-term culture of fetal mouse spinal cord explant, with attached dorsal root ganglia (Chap. IV-A,B), after innervation of mouse skeletal muscle (2 months *in vitro;* muscle added to 4-day cord culture). Low-power view of living culture. The spinal cord cross section (c) shows distinct dorsal (dr) and ventral root (vr) fibers emerging from the explant. Note well-organized, myelinated motor nerve fascicle (*arrows*) penetrating the central region of the long muscle strip. Muscle fibers (m) in central region have regenerated *in vitro* after contact with cord neuritic outgrowth (residual "parent" muscle fibers are present toward the ends of the strip). Note the clusters of dorsal root ganglion perikarya (g) and their myelinated peripheral branches arborizing diffusely throughout the area. (Dorsal root ganglion on left is located in aberrant position due to slight asymmetry of original hand-sliced cord cross section.) Scale: 1 mm. (From Crain and Peterson, 1974*a*.)

(600 mg%), rat or chick embryo extract, and insulin. The total volume of medium in the Maximow chamber is approximately 0.1 ml and the overlying air space about 2 ml. Care must be taken to ensure sterility during all of the experimental manipulations, especially since antibiotics are generally omitted to avoid possible noxious side effects of these agents on neural tissues. Meticulous technique is also necessary to minimize chemical impurities in the culture chamber components and in the nutrient media since CNS tissues are particularly sensitive to many chemical contaminants.

The relatively small volume (ca. 0.1 ml) of nutrient fluid used in the Maximow slide assembly has been considered useful in facilitating automatic "conditioning" of the culture medium. Cellular exudates favorable to neuronal maturation might thereby be maintained at significantly higher concentrations in the vicinity of the explant. This stratagem, however, involves the risk that noxious catabolites might not be adequately diluted away from the neurons. The small volume of nutrient also requires frequent replenishment, depending on the rate of metabolic activity of the tissue. Alternatively, a thin dialysis membrane can be laid over the explant to restrict leaching away of macromolecular exudates while permitting small molecules to be diluted into a relatively large volume of supernatant BSS on the other side of the membrane (Rose et al., 1958). In cases where it is necessary to culture large numbers of explants together (or where long strips or large slices of tissue are used), the collagen-coated culture coverglass is submerged in a larger volume of nutrient medium in a Petri dish, test tube, or flask (e.g., Bunge and Wood, 1973). Small plastic Petri dishes (sterile, disposable types) are being used more and more extensively, and are generally incubated in a moist atmosphere containing approximately 5% CO_2-air mixtures (Fischbach, 1972; Peacock et al., 1973). This also ensures more stable pH and CO_2 levels than in the sealed Maximow slide chamber. Inverted microscopes facilitate observation of cells growing on the floor of these dishes with minimal disturbance of the culture (see section B1a).

Methods for culture of CNS tissues from *adult* mammals have not yet been satisfactorily developed (Crain, 1966). Explants of adult rat spinal cord (Kiernan and Pettit, 1971) and adult rat cerebellum (Drayton and Kiernan, 1973) appeared to maintain significant histologic organization after 1 week *in vitro*, but no correlative electrophysiology or electron microscopy was carried out. An alternative method for tissue culture studies of the regenerative properties of adult CNS tissues utilizes *in vitro*-matured mammalian CNS explants (Chap. VIII-C). Explants of adult frog and fish nerve tissue, on the other hand, may adapt more easily to culture conditions. Explants or dissociated neurons from the CNS of the adult teleost *Carassus auratus* show extensive neurite outgrowth in culture (De Boni et al., 1975, 1976), and on the basis of histologic, electrophysiologic, and autoradiographic data, De Boni et al. suggest that electrically active neurons arise by differentiation of immature cells localized in matrix zones in the brain of these fishes. Explants of sympathetic[3] and dorsal root ganglia from adult bullfrogs (*Rana catesbiana*) also show neuritic outgrowth during months in

---

[3] The ability of neurons in adult mammalian sympathetic ganglion explants to maintain their integrity and to develop extensive neuritic outgrowth in culture has been well demonstrated in human tissues by Murray and Stout (1947) and in rat tissues by Silberstein et al. (1971). No correlative electrophysiologic data were obtained, however, from these types of adult ganglion cells.

An extensive cytologic and histochemical study has also been recently carried out on adult frog sympathetic ganglia (Hill and Burnstock, 1975) under improved culture conditions which provided a clearcut demonstration that these adult neurons could begin to regenerate nerve fibers within 1–2 days after explantation (comparable to the onset of neuritic outgrowth from many embryonic neural explants in culture). The neurons showed characteristic growth sensitivity to nerve growth factor (NGF), and monoamine fluorescence in the outgrowing neurites and nerve terminals was greatly enhanced by NGF (see also fluorescent histochemical studies of cultured mammalian and chick sympathetic ganglion cells in Chap. III-B).

culture (Padjen et al., 1975). Normal resting and action potentials—and depolarizing responses to microiontophoresis of acetylcholine or γ-aminobutyric acid (GABA) (Chap. V-A)—have been recorded intracellularly from these sympathetic ganglion cells after 4–6 weeks *in vitro* (see also data on spinal cord cultures from bullfrog tadpoles in Chap. IV-A).

2. Dissociated Cells

Methods have also been developed to dissociate embryonic tissues into suspensions of completely isolated cells using various combinations of enzymatic and mechanical agitation procedures (Moscona, 1965). These techniques have been successfully applied to CNS tissues so as to permit neuritic growth and synaptogenesis in cultures of dissociated neurons (Meller et al., 1969; Shimada et al., 1969). In some cases the suspensions of cells were cultured in flasks mounted on a rotating-shaker apparatus, which appears to facilitate more systematic reaggregation of the dissociated cells into organotypic arrays (ca. 0.1–1 mm^3) sometimes resembling laminated cortex *in situ* (DeLong, 1970; Seeds, 1971, 1973; Seeds and Vatter, 1971; Garber and Moscona, 1972; Levitt et al., 1975; Palacios et al., 1975). In other cases the dissociated cells were explanted onto collagen-coated coverglasses and cultured in stationary chambers to produce low-density cellular arrays (Fischbach, 1970, 1972) or to permit formation of a more graded series of two-dimensional reaggregates varying from two to dozens of neurons per cluster (Bornstein and Model, 1971, 1972). In the latter experiments 18-day fetal mouse cerebral neocortex or 13- to 14-day spinal cord and brainstem were dissociated by enzymatic treatment in 0.25% trypsin (in a Ca^{++}- and Mg^{++}-free physiologic salt solution) and repeated pipetting. Suspensions of cells in concentrations of approximately 10^6 cells per milliliter of standard culture medium were then explanted onto collagen films, using 0.05–0.1 ml per coverglass (22 mm diameter), and were grown in Maximow slide chambers. This procedure produced cultures containing many widely dispersed, small clusters of neurons and glial cells connected by neuritic bridges and organized into complex synaptic networks (Crain and Bornstein, 1971, 1972) (Chap. V-B,C).

Introduction of antimitotic agents at critical periods during the first 2 weeks *in vitro* greatly reduces overgrowth of the neurons by non-neuronal cells. Cytosine arabinoside or aminopterin, for example, were used successfully in cultures of dissociated spinal cord and cerebellar neurons (Fischbach, 1972; Nelson and Peacock, 1973) and rendered the neurons far more accessible for microelectrode impalements or focal iontophoretic applications (Chap. V-B). Introduction of fluorodeoxyuridine (FdU; 20 μg/ml) during the period from 7–11 days *in vitro* was also effective in producing "naked," functional neurons in dissociated fetal rat cerebral cultures (Godfrey, et al., 1975). Under the culture conditions used in this study, no signs of electrical excitability could be detected in cerebral neurons that were *not* treated with FdU. Godfrey et al. (1975) used a mechanical dissociation technique with a nylon mesh sieve so as to avoid exposure of the cerebral tissue to proteolytic enzymes (see also Bray, 1970; Bird and James, 1973; and below). After optimal FdU treatment many cerebral neurons showed good cytologic and bioelectric integrity even after 1–2 months *in vitro* (Chap. V-C; see also Bunge et al., 1974; Chap. V-A2).

Attempts have also been made to develop techniques for separation of dissociated peripheral nervous system (PNS) and CNS neurons into specific cell types. Okun (1972) utilized differential adhesion to glass of dorsal root ganglion (DRG) neurons versus Schwann and supporting cells, and obtained relatively "pure" cultures of chick embryo DRG neurons by allowing non-neuronal cells to adhere to glass beads prior to plating the neurons (Okun et al., 1972). More elaborate velocity sedimentation techniques were developed by Barkley et al. (1973) to separate different types of dissociated neonatal cerebellar neurons prior to culture. Fischbach (1976) applied similar techniques to dissociated chick embryo spinal cord and obtained significantly enriched large-neuron fractions, containing what appeared to be relatively high concentrations of motor neurons. When cultures of the latter cell fractions are mixed with muscle fibers (Chap. V-B), as many as 30–50% of the neurons develop functional neuromuscular junctions whereas only approximately 10% do so in routine cultures of dissociated spinal cord neurons. These techniques may be extremely valuable for more systematic analyses of the specific role of different types of PNS and CNS neurons and glia in neural networks (see also Capps-Covey and McIlwain, 1975).

Techniques for mechanical dissociation of neonatal rat sympathetic ganglia have been particularly well developed (Bray, 1970; Mains and Patterson, 1973), involving vortexing forceps-teased tissues with a mixture of swirling and vibratory motions for 2–3 min. Elegant intracellular microelectrode studies have been carried out on these dissociated neurons (Bunge et al., 1974; O'Lague et al., 1974) (Chap. V-A2). Neural (DRG) tissues were also dissociated by free-hand dissection with microneedles (e.g., Hintzsche, 1954). Shahar et al. (1975) used this technique to facilitate preparation of relatively isolated neonatal mouse DRG neurons which developed myelinated axons and other mature cytologic (and bioelectric) features during months in culture.

Techniques have also been developed to culture neurons dissociated from larval lobster ventral nerve cord (Kravitz et al., 1973). These large lobster neurons (ranging up to 50 μm) have been observed to grow processes in culture at a rate of 0.1 mm/day. Electrophysiologic studies on these cultured lobster neurons have not yet been reported, but this preparation will undoubtedly provide a valuable model system, especially in relation to the elaborate neurochemical analyses that have been carried out on identified neurons in these ganglia (e.g., Otsuka et al., 1967). Similar techniques should be feasible and fruitful with leech and *Aplysia* ganglion cells, as an extension of the electrophysiologic studies that have already been successful in long-term organ cultures of these invertebrate ganglia (Chap. IV-F).

B. BIOELECTRIC RECORDING SYSTEMS

1. Recording Chambers and Micromanipulators

The methods described below are oriented on the application of micrurgical techniques — i.e., micromanipulation at high magnification (Chambers and Kopac, 1950) — to electrophysiologic studies of neural tissue cultures. They are designed to permit correlative bioelectric and cytologic studies of the unique, relatively two-dimensional organotypic arrays of various types of neurons and related cells as described above (Crain, 1973*a*).

A. Conventional Open System

(1) With upright microscope
  (*i*) *Shallow dish.* The simplest chamber for electrophysiologic studies of neural tissue cultures consists of a shallow dish attached to the mechanical stage of a standard upright microscope. The culture coverglass is attached to the floor of the dish with clamps (or silicone grease), and the tissue is bathed in a volume of approximately 1 ml. In some cases the tissue can be grown directly on the floor of the dish, e.g., small glass or plastic Petri dishes (ca. 3 cm diameter and 4 mm height). This completely open dish permits maximum flexibility in the positioning of microelectrodes with respect to the tissue. The major restriction depends on the working distance of the microscope objective lens. If, for example, a high-powered water-immersion objective is required, the microelectrodes must enter the narrow space between the objective and the tissue at a critical angle. For low-power studies, however, a working distance of 5–10 mm may be available, permitting more convenient approaches with straight or bent electrodes (see section B2). Microscope focusing controls should be independent of the stage plate; otherwise the cells are displaced with respect to the fixed microelectrodes during vertical scanning. This type of focusing system also permits complete removal of the stage plate so that the microscope can be mounted on a sliding pedestal independent of the rigidly fixed chamber-micromanipulator array (see below). These same principles apply when *inverted* microscopes are used with conventional micromanipulators (see below), but this restriction becomes unnecessary when the micromanipulators are incorporated directly into the culture chamber (section B).
  Temperature can be conveniently maintained at 34°–37°C by infrared lamps positioned approximately 2 feet from the chamber (and connected to

variable-voltage regulators for intensity control). Thermistor (or thermo-couple) probes in the chamber can be used with monitoring or thermoregu-lating circuits. Evaporation of the culture bath is minimized by various per-fusion or infusion techniques, or by covering the culture medium with a layer of oil (Commandon and deFonbrune, 1938; Kopac, 1959; Lieberman, 1967). The pH of bicarbonate-buffered culture media (e.g., Simms' BSS; see section A1) is controlled by flowing suitable CO_2-air mixtures over the chamber.

(*ii*) *Hanging drop.* Micrurgical procedures requiring high magnification can often be carried out more conveniently by the use of the hanging-drop method (Chambers and Kopac, 1950; Crain, 1956). The culture coverglass is mounted so as to form the roof of a moist chamber (Fig. II-2), and the explant (firmly adherent to the collagen-coated glass) is bathed in a hanging

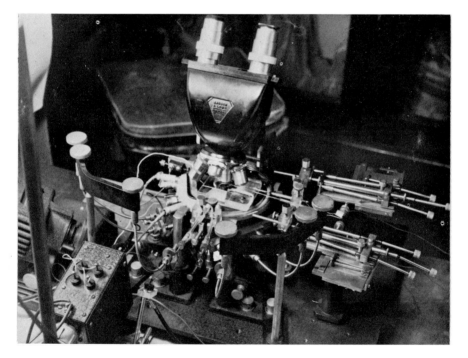

FIG. II-2. Simple micrurgical moist chamber used in initial electrophysiologic studies of cultured dorsal root ganglion cells (Chap. III-A). Culture is mounted as a hanging-drop preparation (coverglass forms roof of chamber). Chamber is clamped to the mechanical stage of an upright microscope with a built-in thermostatically controlled heating unit. Two recording (microsaltbridge) electrodes entering the chamber via the front tunnel are controlled by Chambers micromanipulators; two stimulating electrodes entering via the side tunnel are controlled by Fitz micromanipulators. All four manipulators, as well as the microscope, are firmly clamped to a common, heavy steel baseplate, which is isolated from the workbench by shock mountings. (From Crain, 1956.)

drop (0.1–0.2 ml). This permits unrestricted observations with oil-immersion objectives even though the chamber height may be quite large (e.g., 5–10 mm) for easy access with microelectrodes (tips bent upward several milli-meters from the tip). A long working distance condenser lens is required in this case. Precautions must be taken in these hanging-drop arrangements to avoid excessive evaporation of the small volume of liquid, especially when its temperature is kept at 37°C [see Crain (1973a) for further technical de-tails]. The optical resolution can be improved by decreasing the height of the chamber to approximately 3–4 mm so that the air space in the optical axis can be completely filled with liquid, without spilling out at the openings in the side walls (Hild and Tasaki, 1962, 1964; see also deFonbrune, 1949, Kopac, 1959). These inverted coverglass methods depend on firm attach-ment of the cultured tissue to the collagen film (or other mechanical sub-strate) so that there is no gradual sagging of the cells with respect to the elec-trodes. Furthermore, perfusion of the liquid in these hanging cultures is also more difficult to control, in contrast to the simplicity and stability of fluid covering tissue lying on the floor of a dish.

  (iii) *Micromanipulators.* A wide variety of conventional, massive micro-manipulators can be used with open chambers, e.g., lever-controlled ball-bearing slides (Leitz), greased sliding plates and differential screws (Zeiss), pneumatic drives (deFonbrune), and various micrometer-actuated ball-bearing slides as used in fine-focusing microscope mechanisms (see reviews by Chambers and Kopac, 1950; El-Badry, 1963; Kopac, 1964). The micro-scope and manipulators are firmly clamped to a common, rigid metal base-plate shock-mounted from the worktable. Microelectrodes are positioned into the chamber with coarse micromanipulator controls and adjusted so that all electrode tips are in the optical axis of the microscope. The tissue to be studied is centered in the microscope field by means of the mechanical stage. The electrodes are then positioned critically near or inside the tissue with the fine controls of the micromanipulators.

  (iv) *Sliding microscope and fixed chamber.* Instead of attaching the cham-ber to the movable mechanical stage of the microscope, it can be clamped to a rigid platform erected on the same heavy baseplate that supports the micro-manipulators. Rigid coupling between the cells and microelectrodes is there-by greatly improved, and the microscope becomes an auxiliary to, rather than a central component of, the mechanical system. The optical axis of the microscope can then be easily and accurately positioned with respect to the tissue and electrodes by sliding the entire microscope on a large greased plate fixed to the table top (Cechner et al., 1970; Crain, 1970a). (If the microscope is very heavy, it can be mounted on small ball-bearing casters to reduce friction sufficiently so that smooth sliding movements can be made manually.) Magnetic blocks (with push-button control) can be incor-porated into the sliding pedestal to permit convenient clamping of the micro-scope to a greased steel plate at any desired location. The entire stage plate of the microscope is removed, and the objective and condenser lenses are focused with the usual rack and pinion controls. This system has the further advantage that large areas of the culture can be readily scanned at high magnification without removing microelectrodes inserted into the tissue. When the chamber is attached to the mechanical stage of the microscope, on the other hand, the field of view cannot be changed without prior removal of all microelectrodes, which could otherwise tear the tissue. This introduces considerable restraints on the maneuvers required during electrophysiologic experiments, especially in cultures containing complex arrays of electrodes and cells over relatively large areas of the coverglass.

(2) *With inverted microscope*

Similar dishes can be used with inverted as with upright microscopes, and by attaching a thin coverglass over a hole in the floor of the dish it becomes possible to observe the cells and microelectrodes with oil-immersion objectives independent of the volume of liquid overlying the culture (Fig. II-3). Use of a long working distance condenser permits clearance of 10–20 mm over the culture for much easier access with microelectrodes (and also less optical interference than with dishes in upright setups where the electrode must pass *between* the objective lens and the cells, thereby producing image distortions).

When large numbers of microelectrodes are used simultaneously, it is generally awkward to change culture dishes without tediously raising and lowering all electrodes so that the tips clear the wall of the dish. A more convenient technique is to construct a socket in the floor of the chamber, so that the culture dish can be plugged into position from below (Fig. II-4). This permits rapid insertion or removal of cultures with minimal disturbance of complex microelectrode arrays (Crain, 1970a) but requires a large cutout in the mechanical stage of the microscope. Alternatively, the stage plate of the microscope can be completely removed and the chamber mounted independently on a rigid platform designed to provide better access to the underside of the chamber floor. The microscope is then mounted on a sliding pedestal (see above).

Even when the culture bath contains more than a milliliter, problems of excessive evaporation may occur, especially when maintained at 37°C for long periods of time. In cases where perfusion of the bath or an oil overlay are undesirable, a moist chamber similar to the type used for hanging-drop preparations can be constructed, with openings in the side walls for inserting electrodes (Crain, 1970a, 1973a).

A much more elegant solution to this problem is to enclose the culture bath completely in a moist chamber with no holes at all for entrance of microelectrodes. Instead, mobile electrodes are sealed within the micrurgical chamber and then positioned into or out of the tissue by "remote control" (see below).

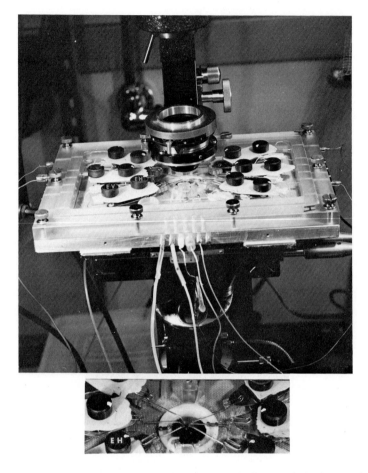

FIG. II-3. Sealed micrurgy chamber with six magnetically coupled micromanipulators suspended from a greased glass roof (see sketches in Fig. II-4). Front view (top) shows that entire array is easily supported on the mechanical stage of an inverted microscope (stage is positioned in three dimensions by standard rack and pinion controls). Note the pairs of external control magnets (EH and EV) used to position micropipette electrodes manually into the central culture dish (seen more clearly in bottom figure, through the glass roof after removal of microscope condenser-lens housing and illuminator). Flexible insulated silver wires connect electrodes with sockets sealed into the chamber wall. These sockets can then be coupled to external recording and stimulating circuits. Teflon tubes for perfusion of the culture dish, leads for bath electrodes, thermistor probes, etc. are all sealed into the floor of the chamber (entering through gasketed holes in the front edge of the metal base plate) and are mounted over the peripheral region of the culture dish. (From Crain, 1972a, 1973a.)

B. Closed Miniaturized System

In order to provide rigorous control of the physicochemical environment of a culture during electrophysiologic study, it would be desirable to carry out the micrurgical procedures in a closed chamber that is really suitable

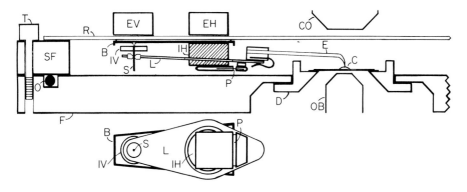

FIG. II-4. Cross-sectional side view of a portion of a sealed micrurgy chamber (F, O, SF, T, R) with a miniature magnetically coupled micromanipulator (B, IV, S, L, IH, P) suspended from the glass roof (R). Top view of micromanipulator is shown alone in lower portion of the figure. The micromanipulator consists of just three moving parts: (1) the base plate (B) and attached internal horizontal magnet (IH); (2) the lever (L) attached to the base plate assembly by a leaf-spring pivot (P); (3) a rotor consisting of a screw (S) concentrically attached to the internal vertical magnet (IV). Both internal magnets (IH, IV) are disks polarized along a diameter, as are the external control magnets (EH, EV). The microelectrode (E; bent at a right angle near the tip) is mounted in a plastic block which is firmly attached to the lever (L) by a steel spring clip. Manual displacement of the magnet (EH) from its equilibrium position directly above the other magnet (IH) produces movement of the entire manipulator (and electrode) in the horizontal plane (layer of fluorosilicone grease between the baseplate (B) and glass roof (R) facilitates controlled movements as small as a few micrometers). Manual rotation of magnet EV causes magnet IV and screw S (000–120) to rotate in the threaded Teflon plug in the lever (L) and thus causes the lever to pivot about the spring-pivot (P), thereby raising or lowering the electrode (E) (200 μm per rotation). The chamber is constructed of a glass roof (R; 1.3 mm thick) glued to the rectangular plastic (polycarbonate) side frame (SF; 1 cm thick), and the aluminum floor (F; 1 cm thick) with a central hole for inserting the culture dish (D). The frame of the roof assembly is clamped to the floor by thumbscrews (T) around its edge; and an O-ring (O) makes a gastight seal between the frame and floor, producing interior chamber dimensions of 10 × 16 × 1 cm. The glass-bottomed dish (D) containing the tissue culture (C) permits observation of the cells and electrodes with a high-powered objective lens (OB), using a long working distance condenser (CO). Six micromanipulators are suspended from the glass roof, three on each side of the chamber (Fig. II-3). (From Baer and Crain, 1971.)

for long-term maintenance of the tissue *in vitro*. Most long-term bioelectric recordings in closed chambers have been limited to the use of relatively large, immovable wire electrodes sealed into the culture chamber during explantation of the neural tissue (Cunningham, 1962; Shtark et al., 1974) (Chaps. IV-D, VII-B). This technique precludes recording from individual cells or changing electrode positions during the course of an experiment (see below). Many attempts have been made to provide special seals over holes in micrurgy chambers in which microelectrodes or microtools operated by conventional, large micromanipulators located outside the chamber gain access to the chamber interior through ball-and-socket arrangements, flexible sleeves, or oil barriers (Reyniers, 1933; Chambers and Kopac, 1950; Kopac, 1959, 1964). These sealing techniques, however, either compromise the quality or ease of micromanipulation, or they fail to maintain long-term environmental constancy.

A radically new system was recently developed which combines the advantages of previous open-manipulatable and closed-embedded micro-electrode arrangements. This is achieved by incorporating a group of micro-manipulators as well as microelectrodes inside a gastight chamber under conditions that still permit convenient external control of the manipulators for precise positioning in three dimensions at high magnification (Crain and Baer, 1969; Baer and Crain, 1971). A group of miniaturized magnetically coupled micromanipulators are suspended from the rigid glass roof of a closed chamber, and microelectrodes can be accurately positioned by man-ually controlling small magnets located on the external surface of the glass sheet (Figs. II-3;4). The magnetic manipulator is moved by a "joy-stick" control for horizontal movements, and a separate rotating control produces vertical movements. With practice, the operating ease, precision, and stabil-ity of this miniature magnetic manipulator is comparable to conventional large micromanipulators. Six miniature micromanipulators can be sealed into a culture chamber with interior dimensions as small as $10 \times 16 \times 1$ cm so that the entire assembly can be easily supported on the mechanical stage of a microscope (Fig. II-3).

A socket in the floor of the chamber permits insertion of a glass-bottomed culture dish from below (Fig. II-4), just as in the open dish chamber de-scribed above. Similarly, Teflon tubes for perfusion of the culture dish, leads for bath electrodes, thermistor, probes, etc. are all sealed into the floor of the chamber, and their tips are mounted over (but independent of) the cul-ture dish (Fig. II-3). The dish is therefore readily transferable from one assembled micrurgy chamber to another or between a micrurgy chamber and a small "satellite" chamber without manipulators for incubation be-tween periods of electrophysiologic study (Crain, 1970c). Moreover, in-corporation of the manipulators into the micrurgy chamber permits free movement of the culture relative to the microscope objective lens without disturbing the critical relations between the microelectrodes and the cells under study, even when the sliding-microscope scanning technique is not used. Vibration problems are also reduced by eliminating the long lever arms generally required between remotely positioned massive manipulators and the cells in a micrurgy chamber that has restricted openings for intro-ducting microelectrode shafts.

The microelectrodes are mounted on small plastic blocks attached to the micromanipulator lever (Figs. II-3;4). The shafts of the microelectrodes are bent at right angles near their tips (Fig. II-4). The dimensions of this bend are critical because of the limited vertical travel of the manipulator. The length of the microelectrode assembly is kept under 3 cm to conserve space in the chamber. Connections from the electrodes to sockets sealed in the chamber wall (Fig. II-3) are made with flexible, insulated silver wire. These sockets can then easily be electrically coupled to external stimulating and recording circuits. All components of the magnetic micromanipulators and the sealed chamber are constructed of stainless steel, Teflon, polycarbonate, and other autoclavable, noncorrodible materials to facilitate use of this system for long-term electrophysiologic studies of neural cultures under sterile conditions.

Initial construction and standardization of the miniaturized magnetically coupled micromanipulators so as to permit reliable positioning of microelectrodes under the critical geometric conditions in these sealed chambers have been time-consuming and required meticulous control of a large number of technical details. Nevertheless, routine preparation and assembly for acute unsterile electrophysiologic experiments are now comparable to the procedures involved in preparing for conventional open-chamber experiments. Furthermore, *sterile* assembly of the sealed chamber array permits prolonged use of a particular setup by eliminating the need for frequent dismantling and cleaning due to bacterial contamination of the microelectrodes and chamber components. The miniaturized magnetically coupled micromanipulators are simpler and less expensive to construct than their conventional counterparts (Baer and Crain, 1971), but our current models are still quite fragile and require a relatively greater degree of mechanical servicing and adjustment.

An alternative technique for carrying out chronic recordings in sterile culture chambers has been developed by etching thin metal films deposited on glass coverslips so as to produce a grid of 10–30 metal electrodes (ca. 10 μm width, 100 μm spacings, and suitably insulated) on which the tissue is placed at explantation (Thomas et al., 1972; Shtark et al., 1974). This method has great potential for application of the elegant fabrication techniques developed by the microelectronics industry. Problems were noted, however, in ensuring good contact between the electrodes and the excitable cells (e.g., Thomas et al., 1972). Nevertheless, electrocardiogram (ECG)-like potentials have been recorded from heart muscle tissue growing on this type of multielectrode array (Thomas et al., 1972), and EEG-like potentials from cerebral explants (Shtark et al., 1974) (Chap. VII-B). With improved design it may be possible to obtain better contacts between these electrodes and the overlying neurons so that single-unit recordings may be feasible. Problems of toxicity introduced by these metal electrodes in close contact with the neural tissue may also complicate long-term recordings.

Another interesting alternative mode of recording bioelectric activities of neural explants, developed by Walker and Hild (1972), eliminated the conventional positioning of electrodes in contact with the tissue. Instead, a small hole (ca. 100–200 μm) was drilled in a glass coverslip and the neural explant positioned over the hole. The tissue was embedded in a plasma clot to ensure good adhesion to the coverslip and to facilitate growth of neurites and other cellular elements to plug the small hole. The coverslip was then placed in a special chamber which permitted the addition of BSS above and below the tissue with contiguity of the fluid only at the hole. Salt-agar bridges carrying silver-silver chloride (Ag-AgCl) electrodes (see section 2) were immersed in the fluid above and below the tissue; thus no perturbation of the tissue occurred from manipulation of the electrodes. "The tissue was grown, so to speak, in the tip of the recording electrode" (Walker, 1975). One electrode was at ground and the other recorded neuronal activity between upper and lower chambers. In addition the preparation was made to form one arm of an alternating current bridge from which impedance imbalance was recorded and over which shocks to the preparation were delivered. This unusual recording method has been used to study aspects of "spreading depression" (Walker and Hild, 1972) and rhythmic discharges of various CNS explants during recordings over periods of approximately an hour (Walker, 1975); it should also be useful for long-term recordings under sterile conditions (Chaps. IV-D, VII-B).

2. Extracellular Microelectrode Recordings

Bioelectric activities of single neurons or small groups can be effectively recorded extracellularly with microelectrodes having 1–5 μm tip diameters. The electrode tips must be carefully positioned near or in the neural tissue so they are located sufficiently close to the active cells without damaging the excitable membranes. Distances of a few micrometers are often critical, especially when the neurons are covered by connective tissue or other short-circuiting membranes. This requirement has impeded application of metallic multielectrode matrices rigidly embedded in the culture chamber (see above) and was a major factor in encouraging our development of miniaturized micromanipulators that could be sealed into a sterile culture chamber and yet permit accurate positioning of microelectrodes with external controls to critical sites in the neural tissue (as described above).

Micropipettes filled with isotonic saline (or a more complete physiologic salt solution) provide a reliable means of contacting the cultured cells. Use of these micro salt bridges avoids possible toxic effects of direct cell contacts with electrode metals, and stable electrode potentials can be obtained by inserting a chloridized silver (i.e., Ag-AgCl) wire into the pipette shaft (see reviews by Kennard, 1958; Frank and Becker, 1964). Pyrex glass capillary tubing with an outer diameter of 0.8 mm and inner diameter of 0.6 mm has been convenient for constructing sharply tapered micropipettes with tip orifices ranging from 1 to 10 μm. Smooth tips of desired diameter can be made automatically by carefully controlling the heat and weight applied to the glass tubing mounted in a simple vertical micropipette puller (with provision for application of relatively small weights). The shafts of the pipettes are bent at right angles approximately 4 mm from their tips (Fig.

II-4); this is done by softening the glass with a small heating coil under a dissecting microscope and then applying gentle manual pressure to the shaftlet with a needle suitably mounted with respect to the axis of the pipette. The pipettes are then filled with saline by injection through a fine hypodermic needle (No. 31) inserted into the tapered region of the pipette. The silver electrode (0.25 mm diameter) is sealed into the pipette at the rear end to prevent evaporation of the saline bridge between the wire and the pipette tip. The resistance of these saline-filled micropipettes can be kept in the range of 1–5 Megohms (MΩ) (for 5- and 1-μm tips, respectively) by careful control of the taper near the pipette tip. Similar pipettes with 5- to 10-μm tips are often used for applying local electric stimuli to the cultured neurons (with resistances of 0.8–1.5 MΩ). The pipettes can also be filled with a saline-agar gel (ca. 2%) to minimize diffusion of fluid from the orifice, which may be injurious to the neurons, especially when filled with concentrated salt solutions, e.g., 3 M KCl (Li et al., 1959; Provine et al., 1970). Higher electrolyte concentrations are of course desirable to reduce microsaltbridge resistance and thereby minimize recording noise levels. An analogous reduction in effective electrode impedance can also be produced by using insulated metallic electrodes. Chloridized silver-core micropipettes with 25-μm tips have been useful for recording both slow waves and spike potentials in CNS cultures (Crain and Bornstein, 1964; Crain and Peterson, 1964), but these microelectrodes generally are not as stable and reliable as microsaltbridge pipettes (Frank and Becker, 1964). Platinum-black electrodes with still smaller tips (1–10 μm) have also been used with moderate success, especially for single-unit spike potentials, and they may be particularly convenient for long-term recordings under sterile conditions.

Pairs of electrodes are generally positioned (under direct visual control — at 100–400×) one against (or inside) the tissue and the other in the fluid nearby. A large chloridized silver wire in the periphery of the culture bath serves as a ground electrode. Bioelectric signals are recorded with differential, high-input-impedance preamplifiers and a four-channel oscilloscope (passband generally from 0.2 Hz to 10 kHz) (for technical details see Thompson and Patterson, 1973). Small unity-gain probes, utilizing a field-effect transistor (FET) circuit as an impedance-lowering device, can be mounted close to the recording electrodes. The output from these FET units can then be fed into conventional high-gain preamplifiers which need not have high input-impedance. Single-ended, rather than differential, recording is often adequate in cases where shielding from extraneous electric fields is optimal. Electric (square wave) stimuli, from 0.1 to 0.5 msec in duration and up to 100 μA in strength, are applied locally through pairs of saline-filled pipettes with 10-μm tips. Radio-frequency stimulus-isolation circuits are used to minimize shock artifacts. The stimulating current can be well localized to individual neurons or small groups of cells. Slight withdrawal of the stimulating electrode from contact with the excitable tissue results in sharp attenuation of all bioelectric responses mediated by neural pathways (e.g., Fig. IV-15).

Methods for computer analysis of tape-recorded bioelectric activities obtained with extracellular microelectrodes in cultured neural tissues (e.g., interspike-interval and "cross-interval" histograms) have been described (Cechner et al., 1970; Cunningham et al., 1970; Schlapfer, 1970; Schlapfer et al., 1972; Gähwiler, 1975, 1976; Shtark et al., 1976). These quantitative methods should be particularly valuable for analyses of organotypic CNS networks during long-term recordings with microelectrodes sealed into the culture chamber (Chaps. IV-D, VII-B, VIII-A).

3. Intracellular Microelectrode Recordings

For intracellular recordings the tips of the microsaltbridges are simply "sharpened" to approximately 0.1 μm so that they can impale neurons with minimal damage to the cell membrane. Pyrex capillary tubing with a thicker wall (0.8 mm O.D.; 0.5 mm I.D.) is convenient for producing these ultra-fine micropipettes, and a standard two-stage magnetic pipette-puller is used (Frank and Becker, 1964). The shafts of the pipettes are bent at right angles near their tips (see above) if they are to be used in a restricted micrurgy chamber. They are then filled with concentrated electrolyte solutions (e.g., 3 M potassium chloride or citrate) by capillary action. Introduction of distilled water into the shaft of the pipette accelerates the rate of filling by automatic transfer of water into the concentrated solution in the pipette tip owing to the large vapor-pressure gradient between the two liquid compartments (Caldwell and Downing, 1955; Chowdhury, 1969). Adequate filling of the shaftlet with water may take 1–2 days if left at room temperature, but this transfer can be greatly accelerated by increasing the temperature of the water in the shaft relative to the fluid in the pipette tip. With suitable temperature gradients, satisfactory water transfer from shaft to tip can be produced even if distilled water is used in the tip instead of a salt solution. This is desirable to avoid possible etching of fine pipette tips by concentrated salt solutions. The water in the shaft is then replaced with the desired electrolyte solution (using a No. 31 hypodermic needle on the day of the experiment. The resistance of 3 M KCl- or 3 M potassium citrate-filled pipettes that have produced successful impalements of cultured ganglion and brain cells ranged from 30 to 100 MΩ (Chaps. III-A, IV-D, V). More sharply tapered pipettes with slightly larger tips (10–20 MΩ) have generally led to rapid deterioration of the impaled neurons within a few minutes, whereas stable intracellular recordings could often be maintained for several hours when finer-tipped pipettes were used.

A serious obstacle to systematic intracellular studies of neurons in cultured tissues has been the frequent growth of thin layers of tough connective tissue over the explants (Crain, 1956; Hild and Tasaki, 1962). Mechanical barriers often lead to tip breakage or to crude impalements by a pipette tip covered with fibrous tissue debris. In some cases these fibrous layers can be selectively softened with proteolytic enzymes (e.g., trypsin or pronase), but this procedure involves the risk of seriously disrupting the entire tissue culture array and its becoming detached from the collagen-coated cover-glass. This problem appears to be less serious in meninges-free CNS explants (Chap. IV-D) and is still more favorably resolved in dissociated cell cultures where much of the connective tissue is digested away prior to explantation (Scott et al., 1969; Fischbach, 1970) or prevented from growing *in vitro* by antimitotic agents (see section A2; Chap. V). Piezoelectric or electromagnetic devices can be used to produce microelectrode thrusts more suitable for reliable impalements of these cultured neurons.

Successful intracellular recordings of cultured neurons have so far been limited to microelectrodes positioned with conventional massive micromanipulators during short-term experiments in open chambers (Chaps. III-A, IV-D, V). Attempts are now in progress to carry out similar intracellular studies in CNS cultures concomitant with, or at least directly following, long-term extracellular recordings in closed chambers with sealed-in magnetically coupled micromanipulators. This combined approach should facilitate analysis of the role of different types of neuronal and glial cells in the generation of the complex organotypic discharge patterns of many cultured CNS tissues.

Neutralized input-capacity preamplifiers, with high input resistance and low grid current, facilitate reliable intracellular recordings of membrane resting and action potentials (Frank and Becker, 1964). Special bridge circuits are used for simultaneous recording and stimulation through a single micropipette (Araki and Otani, 1955; Peacock and Nelson, 1973; Peacock et al., 1973; see also review by Dichter, 1973). Other components of the experimental setup are the same as for extracellular recording.

III

Action Potentials in Peripheral Ganglion Explants

A. DORSAL ROOT GANGLIA

The first bioelectric recordings from neurons in tissue culture were carried out on dorsal root ganglion (DRG) cells (Fig. III-1; see also Fig. I-2) explanted from chick embryos (Crain, 1954a,b, 1956). The major results of this study were summarized as follows (Crain, 1956):

1. Action potentials in response to electrical stimulation were observed in chick embryo spinal ganglion cells [Figs. III-2;3] which had been cultured by the Maximow slide method for as long as 7 weeks (without transferral). Intracellular as well as extracellular recordings were made, via micro-salt-bridge leads, under direct visual control.

2. The amplitude of the membrane action potentials of many of the ganglion cells reached 80–95 mV, involving overshoots of 30–40 mV above a resting potential range of 50–65 mV [Figs. III-2;3]. The spikes, which occurred after latencies varying from less than a few tenths of a millisecond up to 12 msec, often had rising phases of 0.2–0.4 msec and falling phases of 2–3 msec. They were frequently preceded by a more slowly rising "prepotential" and followed by a phase of hyperpolarization during which a peak amplitude of 3–10 mV was reached within 1–4 msec after crossing the resting level—the final return to that level occurring much more slowly [Fig. III-3].

3. In some cases the response pattern indicated that the perikaryon had probably been excited directly by the applied stimulus. At low-stimulus intensities small, graded subthreshold responses appeared, but above a critical depolarization level (ranging from 10 to 30 mV) "all-or-none" spikes were evoked—the latency of the spike with respect to the prepotential varying from the stimulus strength [Fig. III-3]. In some cases the data were more readily accounted for in terms of impulse propagation from a peripherally excited neurite to its impaled soma (i.e., perikaryon).

4. Postspike soma refractoriness was demonstrated by means of pairs of supraliminal stimuli, while repetitive stimuli resulted in soma block after three or four spikes at 100/sec, intermittent failure at 20–50/sec, and faithful responses at 10/sec. Temporal summation of subliminal stimuli was observed at stimulus intervals as long as 0.4–1.0 msec.

5. Comparison of the recordings from the cultured ganglion cells with those from various types of neurons *in situ* or shortly after isolation revealed important similarities, demonstrating that the cultured cells could retain at least many of their characteristic functions when properly maintained *in vitro*. Where deviations were observed the evidence indicated that these were probably due more to peculiarities in cell morphology and in recording technique than to significant alteration *in vitro* of the basic pattern characteristic of neurons in general.

In addition to showing normal membrane resting and action potentials, intracellular recordings from cultured chick embryo spinal sensory DRG cells also demonstrated several interesting types of repetitive spike patterns. Immediately after impalement, "injury discharges" were often recorded (before the membrane sealed up around the shaft of the impaling micro-

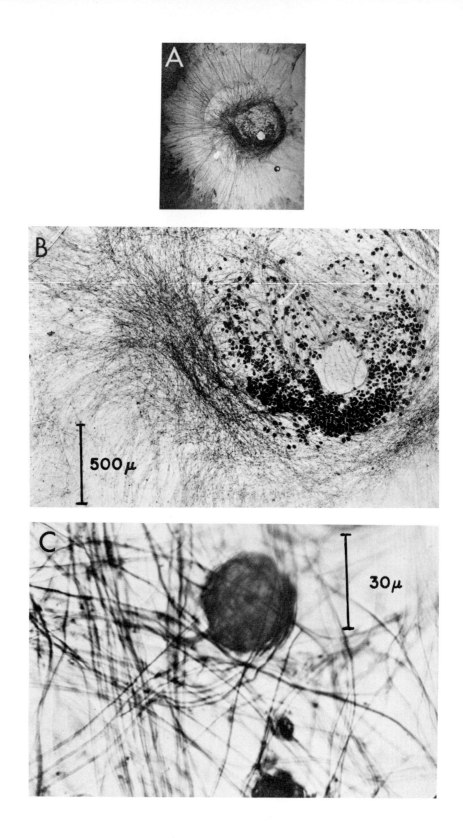

FIG. III-1. Dorsal root ganglion (DRG) culture, explanted from 9-day chick embryo, 7 weeks *in vitro* (silver-impregnated, Bodian method). Low-power **(A)** and medium-power **(B)** views of the culture. Note the concentration of DRG perikarya in the lower portion of the explant and the thinly spread array in the upper region. The network of neurites is most dense and complex at the periphery of the explant; the fibers then proceed radially outward into the surrounding growth zone (see also rat DRG array in Fig. I-3). Many DRG neurons near the hole in the explant (lower right) were destroyed by microelectrode impalements during several hours of experimentation in a moist chamber prior to fixation (as evidenced by the poorer staining capacity of such cells). **C:** DRG neuron marked with arrow in B is shown at higher magnification. The perikaryon of this cell had been impaled for 15 min (Fig. III-3A), after which no response could be elicited, although the membrane resting potential had decreased only slightly. (The stimulating electrodes had been located approximately 100 μm to the right of this perikaryon.) Note the relatively thick neurite arising at the lower left region of the perikaryon and the many thinner neurites traveling past the cell in all directions (see living DRG neurons in Fig. I-2 and tracing of complex neuritic arborizations within an explant in Fig. III-5). (From Crain, 1956.)

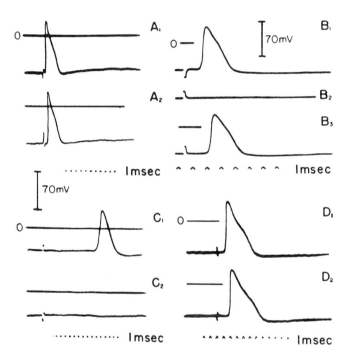

FIG. III-2. Intracellularly recorded membrane resting and action potentials evoked in cultured chick embryo DRG cells. In each of the four cases, the stimulating electrodes were located approximately 200–300 μm from the impaled soma. Note the relatively abrupt onset of the spikes, their rapid rising phase, and the "hump" **(A, B, and D)** during their falling phase. The second record in each sequence shows the effect of reversing the stimulus polarity (B_3 resulting from an increase in the stimulus intensity at the polarity used in B_2). Responses could be evoked from the cell in **B** for 30 min. The ages for **A** through **D,** respectively, were: 19, 42, 21, and 27 days *in vitro*, from 7- to 9-day embryos. [*Note:* In Figs. III-2–7, the upper sweep in each record indicates the baseline potential obtained before impalement (0). In these intracellular recordings, and all others in subsequent figures, upward deflection indicates positivity at the microelectrode with respect to the reference electrode. Unless otherwise specified, all recordings illustrated in this volume were made after dilution or replacement of the long-term culture medium with Simms' balanced salt solution (BSS); see Chap. II-A_1 for composition.] (From Crain, 1956.)

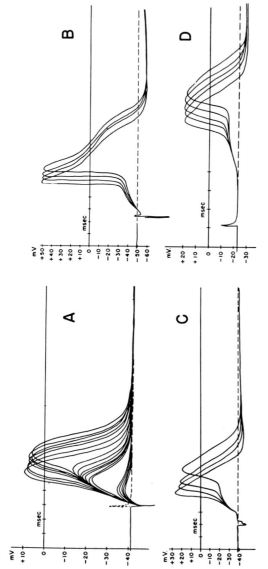

FIG. III-3. Changes in the response pattern recorded from impaled DRG cells following progressive changes in the stimulus intensity in the vicinity of the spike threshold. In each of the four sequences (superimposed tracings) the stimulating electrodes were located approximately 100–200 μm from the impaled perikaryon (records in **A** were obtained from the neuron shown in Fig. III-1, at arrow). Note the abrupt onset of the spike on the rising phase of the well-defined prepotential; the progressive increase in spike latency and the frequently concomitant, slight attenuation in spike amplitude with decreasing stimulus strength; and the graded, subthreshold responses which appeared alone at lower stimulus intensities (**A**) and which seemed to form two discrete groups (the smaller amplitudes being evoked by shock strengths approximately 0.8 of threshold and the larger ones by strengths of 0.9–1.0). The dashed curve in **A** represents the response to a reversal of the stimulus polarity, and the dashed line in **B–D** the resting potential level. (Note the absence of postspike hyperpolarization in **A**, in contrast to **B–D**.) The ages in **A–D**, respectively, were: 49, 20, 20, and 42 days *in vitro*, from 7- to 9-day embryos. (From Crain, 1956.)

electrode). The repetitive spike bursts that occur during such periods involve gradual membrane depolarization following each spike, leading to triggering of the next one (Fig. III-4C$_1$); this pattern is similar to those recorded from spontaneously contracting cardiac and skeletal muscle fibers *in vitro* (Fig. III-4A,B), except for the large differences in time scale. Aside from these transient injury discharges, the membrane potential of cultured spinal sensory DRG cells generally remained stable unless excited by electric stimuli (Crain, 1956; Scott et al., 1969).

Many of the ganglion cells in explants of whole chick spinal ganglia develop extraordinarily complex arborizing neurites in culture (Fig. III-5) (Levi and Meyer, 1938). Gross electrical stimulation of such neuritic arborizations may lead to sequential propagated invasions of the impaled perikaryon by impulses arriving from several neurites with substantially different conduction times from the sites of impulse origin (Fig. III-4C$_2$). These repetitive spikes arise abruptly from the resting potential level, in contrast to the gradual depolarization preceding each spike when the impulse is generated directly in the soma region (Fig. III-4C$_1$ and III-4C$_2$). The injury-discharge spike pattern can also be systematically produced by passing small depolarizing currents across the ganglion cell membrane

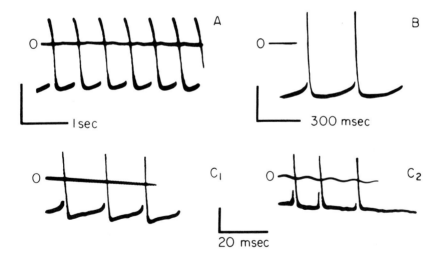

FIG. III-4. Membrane resting and action potentials of spontaneously contracting, cultured chick embryo cardiac **(A)** and fetal rat skeletal **(B)** muscle fibers compared with repetitive activity of cultured chick embryo DRG neuron recorded immediately following injury associated with microelectrode impalement **(C$_1$)**. Note the similarity in the basic pattern — involving gradual depolarization following each spike, which leads to triggering of the next one — in spite of large differences in the time scale. Record **C$_2$** shows the absence of depolarizing prepotential between repetitive spikes in another ganglion cell where impulses are propagating toward the recording site from a peripherally excited neurite, rather than being generated directly in the soma region (cf. Fig. III-6). Amplitude calibrations: 50 mV. (From Crain, 1954a, 1965a.)

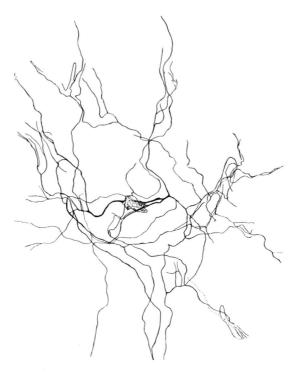

FIG. III-5. Complex neuritic arborization traced to a single large bipolar neuron within a thinly spread DRG explant (10-day chick embryo, 20 days *in vitro*); drawn from photomicrographs after silver impregnation. ×168. (From Levi and Meyer, 1938.)

(cf. Fig. III-6 and III-4C$_1$). The frequency of these repetitive spike responses can be graded from under 100/sec to more than 300/sec by careful control of the depolarizing current intensity, at least during intervals up to 20 msec.

It is ironic that the first attempt to record intracellularly from cultured central nervous system (CNS) neurons failed to demonstrate any evidence of synaptic potentials (Hild and Tasaki, 1962) (Chaps. I, IV-E), whereas long-lasting depolarizing potentials resembling excitatory postsynaptic potentials (EPSPs) have actually been detected in explants of spinal sensory ganglia where synapses are not ordinarily encountered *in situ*. A complex discharge sequence was evoked in some cultured chick embryo DRG neurons (Crain, 1971*a*) consisting of an early spike potential followed by a long-duration depolarization (Fig. III-7A$_1$,B$_1$); often a second or third spike occurred during the rising phase of this depolarization, with latencies of 8–20 msec (Fig. III-7A$_2$–A$_4$,B$_2$). The duration of these post-spike depolarizing potentials ranged from approximately 50 to several hundred milliseconds, and they were graded in amplitude (Fig. III-7B). This complex pattern

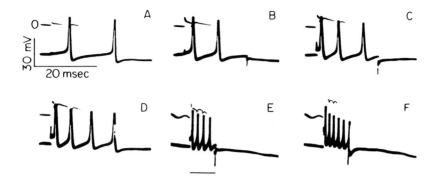

FIG. III-6. Repetitive activity of cultured chick embryo DRG neuron evoked during passage of a depolarizing current (20 msec duration) across the soma membrane by direct application through the intracellular recording electrode. The upper sweep in each record indicates the onset and magnitude of the stimulating current during these membrane potential measurements, increasing from less than 10^{-10} to approximately 3×10^{-9} ampere in records **A** to **E**. Termination of the 20-msec stimulus is indicated by the shock artifact in the lower sweep of records **B, C, E,** and **F,** and by the gap during the final spike in records **A** and **D**. A bridge circuit was used to balance out most of the artifact produced in the voltage recording by this mode of stimulation. Note the increase in frequency of spike discharges from less than 100 to approximately 300/sec. Gradual depolarization occurs preceding each spike (except for initial spike bursts elicited at high-current intensity). Note the similarity to soma injury-discharge patterns (Fig. III-4C$_1$), in contrast to the effect of sequential invasion of propagated impulses (Fig. III-4C$_2$). (From Crain, 1973a.)

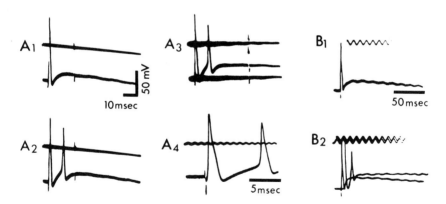

FIG. III-7. Long-duration depolarizing potential (resembling EPSP) following the early spike response evoked by a single stimulus in cultured DRG neurons (from a 9-day chick embryo; 1 month *in vitro*). **A**$_1$ and **B**$_1$ are intracellular recordings from DRG neurons in different cultures. Note the second spike which occurs during the rising phase of this depolarizing potential (**A**$_{2-4}$ and **B**$_2$). **A**$_3$ shows a response similar to that in **A**$_2$ but superimposed on a control record obtained by reversing the polarity of the stimulating electrodes. The **B**$_2$ response is similar to that in **B**$_1$ but superimposed on a repetitive response, similar to **A**$_2$. Note the increased amplitude of postspike depolarization following the latter response. The stimulating electrodes were located 200–300 μm from the impaled perikaryon. (A 1-msec calibrating square pulse follows the spike in records **A**$_1$–**A**$_3$. (From Crain, 1971a.)

of repetitive-spike and slow-wave responses following a single brief electric stimulus is in sharp contrast to the pattern observed in cells where peripherally initiated propagated impulses sequentially invade the soma (cf. Figs. III-7 and III-4C$_2$).

It is tempting to interpret this long-lasting postspike depolarizing potential recorded in some cultured sensory DRG cells as an EPSP generated in the impaled perikaryon after an impulse, initially evoked in the cell body, propagates through recurrent collateral pathways leading back to junctions on the same perikaryon.[1] This simple interpretation is based on Nakai's (1956) direct cinematographic observations of the growth of recurrent collaterals in dissociated ganglion cells in culture (Chap. V-A), where some neuritic branches are seen to loop back (over distances of hundreds of micrometers) and to terminate on their perikarya of origin (Fig. III-8). Recent electron microscopic demonstrations of axosomatic synaptic junctions in cultures of dissociated chick embryo spinal sensory DRG cells (Miller et al., 1970) may indeed provide the ultrastructural basis for the above interpretations, but the evidence is still only circumstantial and needs to be proved by correlative cytologic and electrophysiologic analyses of the same identified cells in culture.

Although synapses have not been detected in ultrastructural studies of mammalian sensory DRGs *in situ* (Andres, 1961; Tennyson, 1970) and *in vitro* (Bunge et al., 1967*b*), light-microscopic evidence has demonstrated that recurrent collaterals from ganglion cell axons often appear to fuse with their own perikarya in normal sensory ganglia *in situ*, i.e., *Paraphytenbildung* or *Fensterapparat* (Scharf, 1958). The bioelectric discharge patterns of cultured sensory DRG cells described above suggest, then, that these recurrent collaterals may be functionally significant, and under certain conditions may lead to excitatory axosomatic synaptic feedback within individual neurons of this type. Alternatively, functional synapses may form *between* DRG neurons under certain conditions *in vitro*, as suggested by intracellular microelectrode analyses in cultures of dissociated chick DRG cells (Peacock et al., 1973; Fischbach and Dichter, 1974) (Chap. V-A). Contamination of DRG cultures by sympathetic ganglion cells could provide still another source of synaptic junctions in all of these experiments.

---

[1] Similar post-spike depolarizing potentials were recorded intracellularly in dissociated chick embryo DRG neurons (Dichter, 1975; Dichter and Fischbach, *in preparation*). These depolarizing potentials could still be evoked even after removal of extracellular Na$^+$ or addition of tetrodotoxin (TTX) (see Chaps. IV-A and V-A) at concentrations which blocked generation of action potentials in the DRG axons. Removal of extracellular Ca^{++} on the other hand, abolished this depolarizing potential. Dichter (1975) concludes that although "the exact origin of this potential is now known . . . it does not appear to be a synaptic potential." The preliminary data reported by Dichter (1975) do not, however, preclude synaptic mediation of these large depolarizing potentials since their Ca^{++}-dependence and their insensitivity to TTX are quite compatible with properties of synaptic potentials (see Chap. V-B and Fig. V-5D). More detailed analyses are required to clarify these ambiguities (e.g., Dichter and Fischbach, *in preparation*).

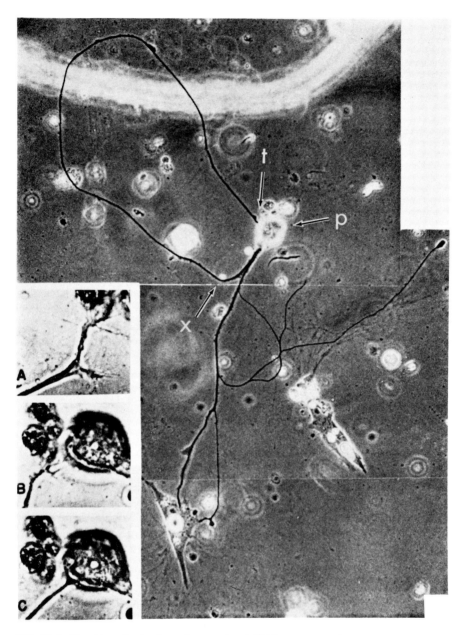

FIG. III-8. Neuritic arborization of an isolated DRG neuron 6 days after explantation (from an 11-day chick embryo) as a completely dissociated perikaryon, with original neurites torn off during an enzymatic-mechanical dissociation procedure (Chaps. II-A2, V-A). The photomicrograph was prepared after making a cine record. ×310. Note collateral neurite which bends sharply (at x), close to its perikaryon (p), and then makes a wide loop prior to terminating on another region (t) of the *same* perikaryon. (The major neuritic branches of this cell have been retouched for clarity.) **Insets A, B,** and **C** are selected cine film frames showing successive stages in the establishment of contact between the growth cone of the uppermost recurrent process and the perikaryon of the same neuron. ×700. (From Nakai, 1956.)

B. SYMPATHETIC GANGLIA

Preliminary electrophysiologic recordings have been made on vertebral sympathetic ganglion neurons[2] explanted in chains of two to six ganglia from 2- to 3-day-old mice (Crain et al., 1964a). Action potentials initiated by electric stimuli in one ganglion could propagate for much longer distances in explants that had matured during chronic exposure to high concentrations of nerve growth factor (NGF; 400 units/ml) (Chap. IV-B). Some of the nerve impulses initiated in the rostral portion of the stellate ganglion could propagate through that ganglion as well as the adjoining two thoracic ganglia, whereas in control chains action potentials were detected only when the recording electrodes were within the same ganglion as the stimulating electrodes (and even these responses were seldom obtained). The poor maturation of the control ganglia may have been due to general suboptimal culture conditions, or it may indicate a strict dependence of mouse sympathetic ganglia on sustained exogenous NGF (in contrast to the critical period during early development when DRG neurons require exogenous NGF) (Chap. IV-B). At any rate, the presence of NGF in the culture medium appeared to have a marked stimulating effect on the growth and development of these cultured sympathetic ganglion cells, either by permitting more "normal" maturation of cultured sympathetic neurons under adverse environmental conditions (Levi-Montalcini and Angeletti, 1963) or by promoting a true hypertrophy of these cells *in vitro* as occurs *in situ* (Levi-Montalcini and Booker, 1960; Levi-Montalcini and Angeletti, 1968a,b).

Although no bioelectric analyses of interneuronal synaptic connections were made during the course of these preliminary studies, O'Lague et al. (1974) demonstrated the formation of cholinergic synapses between neurons in cultures of dissociated sympathetic ganglia (Chap. V-A). Evidence was obtained in our study, however, suggesting that fetal mouse sympathetic ganglia can establish adrenergic synaptic functions with separate explants of cardiac muscle (both tissues obtained from 15-day fetal mice). After 2 weeks in culture, brief volleys of stimuli (5–10/sec) to sympathetic ganglion neurons elicited marked increases in the usual 1–2/sec rate of spontaneous cardiac contractions to more than 5/sec (Crain, 1968). The enhanced heart

---

[2] These bioelectric and cytologic experiments on long-term cultures of newborn mouse sympathetic ganglia were carried out in 1959–1961, at Abbott Laboratories (North Chicago, Ill.), during the course of a 4-year period as director of the neural tissue culture laboratory in their Cell Physiology Dept. (along with related studies of catecholamine levels in neonatal mouse sympathetic ganglia *in situ* after NGF-hypertrophy: see Crain and Wiegand, 1961). The mouse culture studies were extended, after my return to Columbia University (Chap. I-B), to chick sympathetic ganglion explants (in collaboration with Ms. H. Benitez in Margaret Murray's laboratory) (see Crain et al., 1964a).

Action potentials were recently recorded intracellularly from neurons in long-term explants of adult bullfrog sympathetic ganglia (Padjen et al., 1975) (Chap. II-A1; see also similar recordings from dissociated fetal rat and chick embryo sympathetic ganglion cells in Chap. V-A).

rate occurred after a latency of approximately 1 sec and continued for up to 10 sec after cessation of stimulation. Correlative electron microscopy in similar types of cultures revealed evidence of close proximity of sympathetic nerve terminals to cardiac muscle fibers (Masurovsky and Benitez, 1967). Although no definitive synaptic junctions were detected, nerve endings near cardiac fibers were often packed with dense-core vesicles (see also Chamley et al., 1972; Benitez et al., 1973; Cook and Peterson, 1974). These cytologic features are consonant with the observed excitatory, adrenergic effects of sympathetic ganglion volleys on cardiac contractions in our cultures (see also Coté et al., 1975).

Purves et al. (1974) observed similar increases in the rate of spontaneous contraction of trypsin-dissociated cardiac muscle cells in response to sympathetic ganglion volleys in cultures prepared from neonatal rat tissues. On the other hand, some myocardial clumps showed a *decreased* rate of contractions, suggesting mediation by cholinergic nerve terminals. The latter view was supported by the marked effects of anticholinergic agents on sympathetic-evoked contractile responses in some of the cardiac and in several types of smooth-muscle explants (Purves et al., 1974; see also Chamley et al., 1972, 1973). The data are also consistent with our own unexpected observations of short-latency contractions in some skeletal muscle fibers evoked by single stimuli to nearby fetal mouse sympathetic ganglia which could be blocked by *d*-tubocurarine (Crain and Peterson, 1974*a*) (Chaps. IV-A, V-A, and VIII-B). These experiments have now been more elegantly confirmed with intracellular recordings demonstrating formation of clear-cut cholinergic synapses between dissociated rat sympathetic ganglion cells and skeletal myotubes in culture (Nurse and O'Lague, 1975) (Chap. V-A).

Cultures of adult rat superior cervical ganglia have been utilized for studies of mechanisms regulating reinnervation of iris tissue. Although no electrophysiologic analyses were made, fluorescence histochemical techniques demonstrated that noradrenergic nerve fibers grew profusely into nearby iris tissue, so that after 1 week *in vitro* a dense plexus of fluorescent fibers formed in close relation to the iris muscles and showed characteristic patterns as observed *in situ* (Silberstein et al., 1971; Johnson et al., 1972*a*). Introduction of NGF (100 units/ml) into the culture enhanced the rate and extent of ganglion reinnervation of the iris tissue. This model system should be valuable for analyses of sympathetic innervation of target tissues, and it is of further interest in relation to recent evidence that injured adult brainstem catecholaminergic neurons also sprout neurites which form characteristic patterned networks in iris tissue implanted into the brainstem lesion and which are also sensitive to NGF (Chap. IV-C).

Fluorescence histochemical techniques have also been effectively utilized in systematic analyses of the cytology and catecholaminergic properties of the specialized types of neurons in explants of chick embryo and neonatal rat sympathetic ganglia (Benitez et al., 1973, 1974; Coté et al., 1975). Correlative electron microscopy has demonstrated significant synaptic and other close relationships between the principal neurons of the ganglion and the small intensely fluorescent (SIF), monoamine-containing inter-neurons with characteristic large dense-core vesicles (Benitez et al., 1974). Correlative electrophysiologic studies on the catecholaminergic inter-neurons in these ganglion explants have not yet been reported, but elegant intracellular analyses of the principal neurons have been carried out in cultures of dissociated superior cervical ganglion cells (Bunge et al., 1974; O'Lague et al., 1974) (Chap. V-A).

IV

Development of Organotypic Synaptic Networks in CNS Explants

A. SPINAL CORD AND INNERVATION OF MUSCLE

1. Spinal Cord

Cross sections (0.5–1 mm thick) of spinal cord from 13- to 14-day rat and mouse fetuses and from smaller groups of human (6-week) and chick (9-day) embryos have been explanted for various developmental neurobiology studies [see Peterson et al. (1965) for details of the spinal cord culture technique and morphologic development; see also Chap. II-A1]. The cord segment is frequently explanted together with its attached dorsal root ganglia (DRGs) and associated meningeal tissues (Fig. IV-17). A large number of cord neurons survive and mature *in vitro*. Many of the axons become myelinated in both the explant and the outgrowth zones (Figs. II-1; IV-6;7;20). Although the neuronal somas generally remain thickly invested in a framework of neurites and glia, the explants may become thin enough (100–300 μm) to permit at least some of the perikarya to be visible in the living state at high magnification (Peterson et al., 1965) (Fig. IV-9B; see also Figs. IV-8;9A). A dense neuropil (ca. 100 μm thick) containing fine arborizing neurites (and glial cells) often covers the main body of the explant (Bunge et al., 1965) and extends irregularly outward onto the collagen gel as the clearly visible "neuritic growth zone" (see also Guillery et al., 1968). The term "neurite" is used here to refer to branches of neurons that cannot be definitely identified as "dendrites" or axons. Only in the vicinity of the neuron perikarya can this distinction be clearly made on the basis of structural characteristics (Fig. IV-9B) (Peterson et al., 1965), and even there it is often difficult to evaluate. The profuse sprouting of collaterals in these neuronally isolated central nervous system (CNS) explants tends to simulate the appearance of dendritic arborizations. Myelination is probably the only clear-cut feature by which we can differentiate with the light microscope between peripheral branches of axons and dendrites. After silver impregnation (Bodian or Holmes) the neurofibrillar arrays in many of the dendrites and axons, and in some of the perikarya, become selectively blackened (Figs. IV-8;9A;26) (Peterson et al., 1965; Guillery et al., 1968; Sobkowicz et al., 1968).

Histologic analyses have been difficult to carry out on these relatively

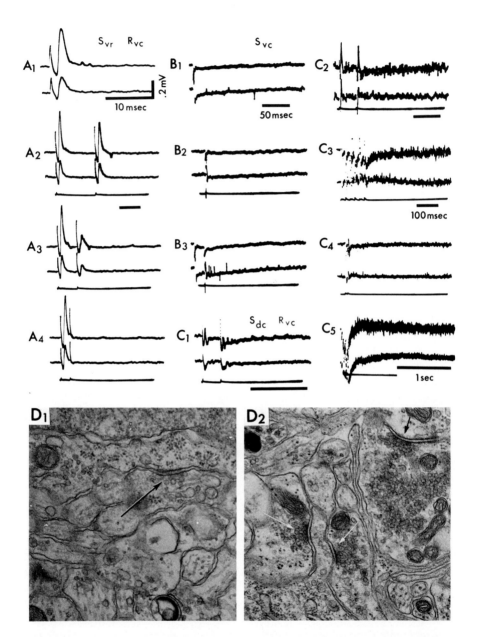

FIG. IV-1. Transition from simple to complex bioelectric responses in spinal cord tissue cultured for 2–4 days after explantation from a 14-day fetal rat. **A** and **B:** Two days *in vitro*. **A₁**: Simultaneous extracellular recordings of simple spike potentials evoked in two sites of ventral cord (300 μm apart) by a stimulus applied to ventral root (400 μm from edge of explant). Application of paired stimuli demonstrates relative (**A₂,₃**) and absolute (**A₄**) refractoriness to test stimulus. (Responses to dorsal cord, or root, stimulus were much smaller in amplitude, in both dorsal and ventral cord.) **B₁,₂**: Similar simple spike potentials evoked in another region of ventral cord by stimulus applied nearby, within the cord explant. **B₃**: Paired stimuli, at a 15-msec test interval, elicit a multiple spike burst of small amplitude lasting more than 35 msec (barely detectable in most explants at 2 days *in vitro*, even with tetanic stimuli and strychnine). **C:** Four days *in vitro*. **C:** Longer lasting after-

thick cord explants, since application of the standard Nissl and silver techniques to whole-mount preparations generally results in excessively dense staining. Systematic analyses of sectioned explants at the light microscopic level have unfortunately not yet been carried out. Morphologic studies have focused instead on electron microscopic analyses of representative local regions within the cord explants (see below and Figs. IV-1D;3). However, in a series of cord explants (cross sections) where meninges and DRGs were removed at explantation, the originally thick (ca. 1 mm) explants thinned out during maturation in culture to approximately 30–70 μm so that fruitful analyses of whole mounts could be made with Nissl and silver stains (Guillery et al., 1968; Sobkowicz et al., 1968). These analyses demonstrated that many of the major groups of neuron perikarya present in immature spinal cord were maintained with good regional localization in the long-term cross-sectional explants. Dorsal and ventral horn regions could be clearly characterized, and the former could be subdivided into zones resembling substantia gelatinosa; a dorsomedial zone seemed to correspond to Clarke's column (Sobkowicz et al., 1968). Silver impregnation of the cord neurons showed, moreover, that well-organized axon tracts had developed both within the explant and in the surrounding growth zone (see below and Figs. IV-8;9).

During the first 2 days after explantation of 13- to 14-day fetal rodent spinal cord (Fig. IV-17A) at essentially "presynaptic" stages (see below), generally only simple spike potentials are detected in response to single or tetanic electric stimuli applied to these immature cord explants. The spikes (Fig. IV-1A$_1$) are similar to those observed in neurons of cultured DRGs (Chap. III-A), where impulses can propagate along the conductile portions of the neurons, but no bioelectric evidence of transmission from one neuron to another has been detected. Application of paired stimuli reveals only

---

discharge (small amplitude) in ventral cord evoked by paired stimuli to dorsal cord. C_2: Strychnine (10 μg/ml) now enhances barrage response even at test intervals of 30 msec. C_{3-5}: Brief tetanic stimulation (20/sec) produces a further increase in duration and amplitude of afterdischarges.

[*Note:* In these extracellular recordings and all others in subsequent figures, upward deflection indicates negativity at active recording electrode. Time and amplitude calibrations, and specification of recording and stimulating sites, apply to all succeeding records, *until otherwise noted.* Onset of stimuli is indicated, where necessary, by a sharp pulse (or arrow) or a break in the baseline of the third sweep (see also Note in Fig. III-2).]

D_1: Electron micrograph of cultured spinal cord tissue approximately 4 days after explanation as a "synapse-free" slice from a 14.5-day fetal rat. Note the typical, newly formed synapse (at arrow) with moderate synaptic membrane density and intervening cleft substance. A few synaptic vesicles are clustered on the presynaptic side of this axosomatic junction (near *arrowhead*) ×32,500. Compare with Fig. IV-3a,b. D_2: Similarly prepared electron micrograph of fetal rat cord explant after 10 weeks *in vitro*. Synaptic membrane density and cleft substance are more pronounced at the axodendritic (*black arrow*) and the two axosomatic (*white arrows*) synapses. Many more synaptic vesicles have accumulated at the presynaptic side of all three junctions ×28,500. Compare with Fig. IV-3c. (**A–C** from Crain and Peterson, 1967. **D** from Bunge et al., 1965, 1967a.)

refractory properties characteristic of electrically excitable, conductile membranes (Fig. IV-1A$_{2-4}$). Both unit and summated spike potentials can be recorded depending on the size of the recording electrode tips and their location relative to the active neurons (see also Fig. IV-29A and section D), as well as other features of the volume-conductor recording conditions (Crain, 1954a, 1956).

On the other hand, by 2–3 days in vitro facilitation effects can be demonstrated in the cord explants with paired stimuli at long test intervals, and long-lasting spike barrages and "slow-wave" potentials may be evoked with single or brief tetanic stimuli at critical thresholds (Fig. IV-1B,C). Complex discharges have also been detected in some 13- to 14-day fetal rat and mouse spinal cord explants after only 2 days in vitro (Figs. IV-2;3) (Crain and Peterson, 1967; Crain et al., 1976; see also Pappas et al., 1975). The appearance of these complex bioelectric activities indicates that polysynaptic networks are beginning to function in the cultured cord tissue (Crain and Peterson, 1963, 1964, 1967). Although intracellularly recorded postsynaptic potentials (PSPs) have not yet been obtained from cultured CNS explants during the first week in vitro (see, however, section D), electrophysiologic analysis of extracellular recordings provides excellent, although less direct, evidence of activities mediated through synaptic pathways. The responses in 3-day and older cultures can often be enhanced with strychnine, picrotoxin, or bicuculline (ca. 10^{-6} M), whereas no significant effects are produced by the application of these drugs during the first 2 days in vitro. Furthermore, all of the complex bioelectric discharges can be rapidly blocked by raising the Mg^{++} concentration of the medium from the usual 1 mM level to 5–10 mM, whereas short-latency spike potentials can still be evoked.[1] This selective interference with complex discharges by increased Mg^{++} levels provides further support for synaptic mediation of these activities (Figs. V-2;8C, VI-8;10) (Chap. VI-E). The marked sensitivity of 13- to 14-day rodent spinal cord explants to strychnine, picrotoxin, and bicuculline by 3 days in vitro suggests, moreover, that inhibitory circuits may already be functioning quite early during CNS synaptogenesis (see sections B–D and Chap. VII-D).

---

[1] On the other hand, introduction of low concentrations of tetrodotoxin (ca. 10^{-8} g/ml), a drug that selectively blocks active Na^+ channels in conductile membranes (Kao, 1966), rapidly abolishes all action potentials in these spinal cord (and other neural) explants, thereby also blocking all of the synaptic network discharges which require conduction through numerous internuncial axon pathways between the synapses.

The complex spike barrage and slow wave responses in cord explants are quite labile, often requiring rest periods of 1–10 sec between stimuli, in contrast to the more rapid recovery of spike potentials which could be reliably evoked at repetition rates of 10–100/sec. The lability of these complex discharges (e.g., Fig. IV-4D) and their relatively long and variable latencies (e.g., Fig. IV-4,5,13) provide strong additional evidence for their mediation by sequential activation through polysynaptic networks (Crain and Peterson, 1963, 1964). The lability and "fatigability" properties are even more pronounced during the first few days after onset of complex network responses, and postdischarge recovery periods may be longer than 1 min (see also similar properties of immature cerebral synaptic network discharges in section D-1).

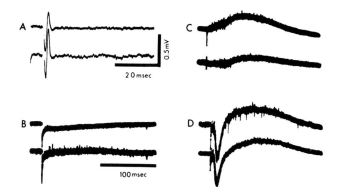

FIG. IV-2. Onset of complex synaptic network functions in fetal mouse spinal cord explants (13–14 days *in utero;* 1–3 days *in vitro*). **A:** Simple early-latency spike potentials evoked in two sites of cord explant (at 1 day *in vitro*) by a single stimulus applied to the third site. No signs of complex discharges were detected following these spikes, either in BSS or after addition of pharmacologic agents (see below). **B:** Long-lasting repetitive spike barrages and small-amplitude slow-wave responses elicited in two sites of cord explant at 2 days *in vitro,* but only after introduction of bicuculline (10^{-5} M) and caffeine (10^{-3} M). See also Figs. IV-1C;31;32. Note the change in time calibration; afterdischarges lasted more than 1–2 sec. **C:** Similar long-lasting repetitive spike barrages, but these are accompanied by much larger-amplitude negative slow-wave responses, evoked in two sites of another cord explant at 2 days *in vitro* (tissue was obtained from a slightly more mature fetus than that in **B**). These complex discharges were observed only after introduction of strychnine (10^{-5} M) and caffeine (10^{-3} M). **D:** Still more elaborate diphasic slow-wave potentials and spike barrages evoked at two sites in a cord explant at 3 days *in vitro* after addition of strychnine (10^{-5} M). Smaller-amplitude slow-wave potentials and shorter spike barrages (as in **C**) could also be elicited in this explant in BSS (prior to strychnine). (From Pappas et al., 1975; Crain et al., 1976.)

During the next few days of culture beyond the critical 2- to 3-day period, the afterdischarges increase in amplitude and complexity; and they can be elicited at lower thresholds with fewer stimuli (Fig. IV-4A–C). These long-lasting "slow-wave" and oscillatory potentials are probably extracellularly recorded field potentials representing summated excitatory and inhibitory postsynaptic potentials (EPSPs and IPSPs respectively) generated in complex sequences during activation of the synaptic networks in these cord explants (see sections B-1b; D-3,4a). Still more elaborate repetitive discharges often occur in older rodent spinal cord explants (Fig. II-1)—e.g., long-lasting rhythmic (7–15/sec) oscillatory afterdischarge sequences (Fig. IV-4E–L; see also section D)—and these patterned repetitive sequences have also been evoked in long-term explants of *human* embryo spinal cord (Fig. IV-5) (Crain and Peterson, 1963; Crain, 1966). The afterdischarges appear in all-or-none fashion at a critical stimulus intensity, and they may also be evoked following facilitation of paired subthreshold stimuli at long test intervals. The oscillatory afterdischarge patterns are often relatively stereotyped, but variations in response to single stimuli of constant strength may occur. The repetitive discharges may continue

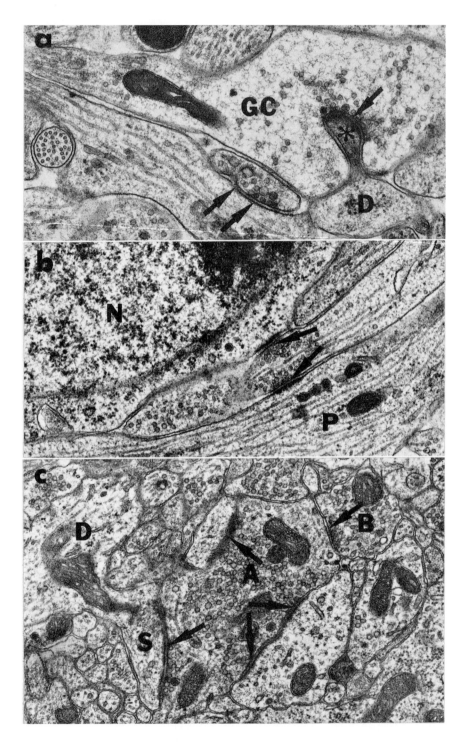

uninterrupted for many seconds after the stimulus. They often occur synchronously over widespread regions of the explant, even after a weak stimulus localized to a few neurites close to a 10-μm stimulating electrode. Nevertheless, the bioelectric responses evoked in 4-day cultures of 14-day fetal rodent spinal cord tissue already include the basic organotypic properties characteristic of mature explants of cord and other CNS tissues (Crain, 1966, 1970b, 1973b, 1974a).

The 2- to 3-day lag in onset of functional interneuronal transmission within these immature spinal cord tissues in culture cannot be attributed simply to depression of activity following surgical trauma at explantation, since complex, long-lasting afterdischarges can already be evoked within 1 day after explantation of 18-day fetal rat cord. It should be noted, moreover, that the 18-day cord tissue appears to undergo more degeneration during the first few days *in vitro* than does the 14-day cord, since a larger fraction of the tissue from the older fetus is composed of longitudinal fiber tracts which are transected during preparation of these 0.5- to 1-mm cord cross sections. The 2- to 3-day lag in onset of complex bioelectric activity in the 14-day fetal cord explants can therefore be considered to be due primarily to the immature state of the neuronal networks developing during the first few days in culture, rather than merely to depression of activity following explantation trauma.

The onset of complex bioelectric activity in 14-day fetal rodent spinal cord explants after 2–3 days *in vitro* correlates closely with the earliest time at which clear-cut synaptic profiles, mainly axodendritic, are regularly seen in electron micrographs of these cultured tissues (Figs. IV-1D$_1$;3a,b) (in rat: Bunge et al., 1967a; Crain et al., 1964b; in mouse: Pappas et al., 1975). Furthermore, formation of functional synaptic networks by 2 days after explantation of 13- to 14-day fetal mouse cord and onset of DRG-evoked cord discharges by 3 days *in vitro* (Crain et al., 1976; see also section B1) correlates well with evidence of spinal reflex activity by 15–16 days in the fetal mouse *in utero* (Vaughn et al., 1975). The marked increase in number of synapses as the cord explants mature in culture [as many as nine synaptic junctions have been found on a single neuron in a thin electron

---

FIG. IV-3. Electron micrographs of 14-day fetal mouse spinal cord explants during early stages of synaptogenesis and after maturation in culture. **a** and **b:** Two days *in vitro* (see bioelectric network discharges in Fig. IV-2B,C). **a:** Portion of a growth cone (GC) which envelops and forms a synaptic junction with a filopodium (*) arising from a presumed dendritic (D) process containing ribosomes. Another immature synaptic contact appears nearby (*double arrow*). Note clusters of presynaptic vesicles at both junctions. **b:** A neuritic shaft forms synaptic contact (*arrows*) with a cell body (nucleus N) and another process (P). **c:** Dorsal horn region of cord with attached DRGs, 6 weeks *in vitro*. A large presynaptic terminal (A) forms junctions with three neuritic elements (*arrows*), including a spine (S) arising from a dendritic shaft (D). This presynaptic terminal also *receives* synaptic input from another neurite (B, at *arrow*). ×26,000. (**a** and **c** provided by E. B. Masurovsky and G. D. Pappas. **b** From Pappas et al., 1975.)

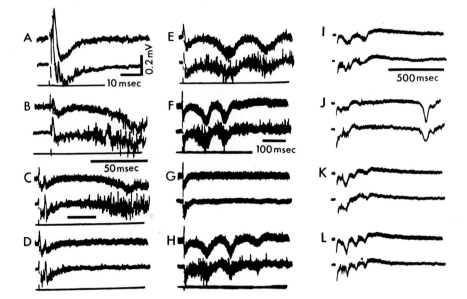

FIG. IV-4. Oscillatory afterdischarges evoked by single, brief, electric stimuli in a long-term culture of rat spinal cord (3 months *in vitro*). **A–C:** Simultaneous recordings of typical repetitive, spike-barrage responses evoked in two regions of the explant (400 μm apart) by a stimulus applied 500 μm from both recording sites. **D:** Short-duration response when stimulus was applied 1 sec after spike barrage in **C. E, F,** and **H:** Long-lasting oscillatory sequences (up to 400 msec) evoked shortly after records **A–D.** Note the regularity of the pattern of these 7–15/sec diphasic potentials and the synchronization of the responses between the two recording sites. **G:** Control record (subthreshold stimulus). **(I–L):** Similar oscillatory afterdischarges at a slower sweep rate. Note the second sequence in **J,** which appears after a silent period of 500 msec. (From Crain and Peterson, 1964; Crain, 1966.)

microscopic section (Bunge et al., 1965)] and the concomitant developments in synaptic membrane density, cleft substances, and presynaptic vesicle accumulation (Figs. IV-1D_2;3C) (Bunge et al., 1965; Pappas et al., 1975; see also Guillery et al., 1968) provide important morphologic parameters which probably underlie the sequential developments in bioelectric activities seen during the first week *in vitro* and thereafter. Although collateral fiber sprouts and neuritic arborizations are also developing in abundance during this period, these are not likely to constitute a critical parameter since similar elaborate neuritic processes develop in explants of DRGs (Figs. I-3, III-1:5) (Levi and Meyer, 1938; Lumsden, 1951; Peterson and Murray, 1955) where no such complex bioelectric activities have been detected (Crain, 1956) in the absence of synaptic junctions [Bunge et al. (1967*b*); see, however, synaptic-like potentials recorded from *some* DRG neurons (Crain, 1971*a*) (Chap. III-A)].

The electrophysiologic studies noted above focused primarily on the

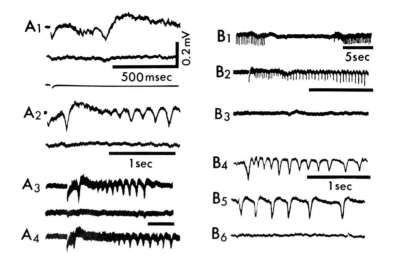

FIG. IV-5. Oscillatory afterdischarges evoked by single stimuli in long-term culture of human spinal cord (6 week embryo; 3–4 months *in vitro*). **A:** Simultaneous recordings from two sites in cord explant (ca. 200 μm apart) during application of cord stimulus 400 μm from both recording sites. Note the regular, 5–10/sec, repetitive sequences (at various sweeps), including an early evoked potential followed by a long delay and then a series of diphasic oscillatory potentials of increasing amplitude. Note also the remarkable similarity to repetitive discharge patterns in Figs. IV-4;37). Responses at other cord site are of extremely small amplitude (lower sweep) but appear to occur synchronously with the larger potentials at the first site. Lowest sweep in **A₁** shows a stimulus signal. **B₁:** Spontaneous (sporadic) sequences of 7–15/sec, diphasic oscillatory potentials recorded from a similar human cord explant. **B₂:** Initial phase of repetitive discharge evoked by a single stimulus to this explant (barrage continued for about a minute). **B₃,₆:** Control records (no stimulus). **B₄:** Spontaneous discharge, at a faster sweep than in **B₁**. **B₅:** Evoked oscillatory sequence similar to those in **A**. (From Crain and Peterson, 1963; Crain, 1966.)

development of internuncial synaptic networks within the interior of relatively thick spinal cord explants. The dense packing of cells in these CNS explants has obscured resolution of contours of the somas and dendrites in the living state (Fig. IV-9B). Although this compromise has interfered with selective microelectrode placements under direct visual control at dendrites and synapses, it has provided an opportunity to demonstrate the degree to which functional organization may develop and be maintained in cultured fragments where the normal cellular interrelationships of CNS tissues are left relatively intact. These bioelectric studies have therefore provided a foundation that has become increasingly fruitful with improvements in culture technique and with greater depth of bioelectric, pharmacologic, and histologic analyses. Correlative electrophysiologic and morphologic studies of specific sensory DRG inputs into fetal spinal cord explants (see section B) and motoneuron outputs to skeletal muscle fibers (see below and Chap. VIII-B) provide significant insights into organotypic *regionally* localized spinal cord functions that can still develop under isolated condi-

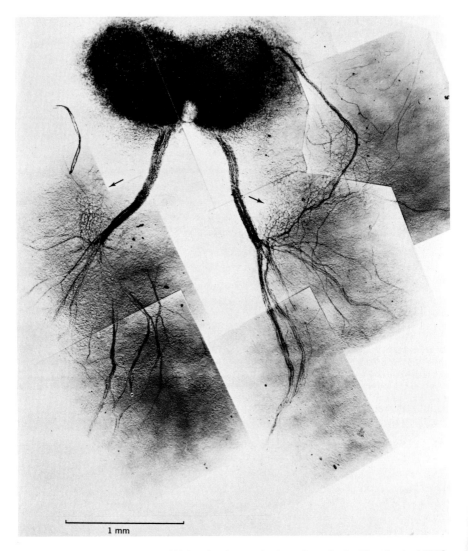

1 mm

FIG. IV-6. Photomicrograph of living fetal rat spinal cord explant with attached DRGs (12-day fetus; 46 days *in vitro*). Only myelinated fibers are seen. Spinal cord segment as well as the ventral and dorsal roots have been preserved on the right (see also Fig. II-1). On the left only the ventral root appears preserved. Actually the left dorsal root is also present but is not seen because the fibers are not myelinated. Further details are revealed after silver impregnation (Fig. IV-7). *Arrows* point to the locations of spinal ganglion cells. Note the spread of myelinated fibers toward the periphery. (From Sobkowicz, Hartmann, Monzain, and Desnoyers, 1973.)

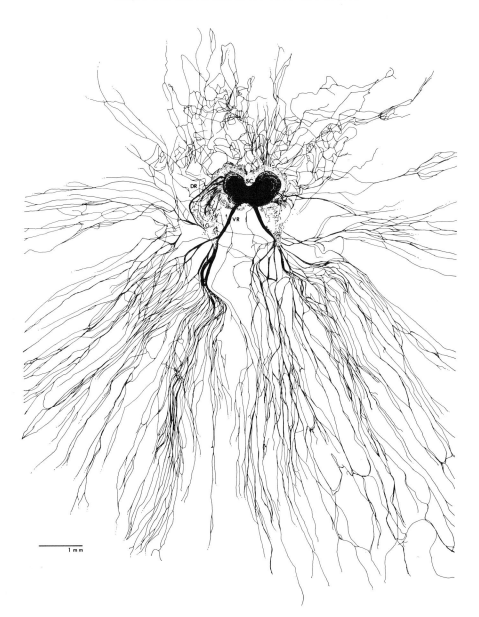

FIG. IV-7. A mirror-image projection drawing of the cord culture shown in Fig. IV-6 after the culture had been fixed and stained with Holmes' silver method. Both myelinated and unmyelinated fibers are present in great numbers, although not all fibers were visualized under low magnification. Note that the fibers which originate in the ventral horn or spinal ganglia tend to grow in braids, taking a fairly straight course. By contrast, fibers that originate in the dorsal horn take a very tortuous course, loop frequently, and tend to return to the explant (cf. Fig. IV-26). (From Sobkowicz, Hartmann, Monzain, and Desnoyers, 1973.)

tions in culture. [See photomicrographs and tracings of mature spinal cord explants and their elaborate, often highly ordered axon tracts, as well as less well-defined neuritic fascicles and arborizations in Figs. II-1, IV-6– 9;14;17;20;22;26 (Peterson et al., 1965; Crain et al., 1968b; Peterson and Crain, 1970, 1972; Guillery et al., 1968; Sobkowicz et al., 1973; Crain and Peterson, 1974a). Studies of the innervation of dissociated sympathetic ganglion cells by neurons in fetal rat spinal cord explants provide valuable data on still another set of neurons in this complex spinal cord model system (Bunge et al., 1974) (Chap. V-A; Figs. V-3;4). These correlative cytologic and bioelectric studies constitute a prototype for similar experi-

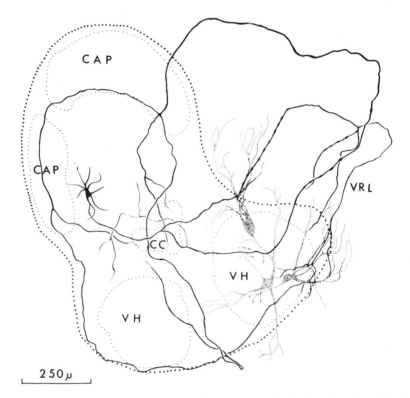

FIG. IV-8. Projection drawing of one-half of a fetal mouse spinal cord explant, 51 days *in vitro,* outlining some of the elaborate neurons and neuritic arborizations that can be resolved in a whole-mount preparation after Holmes' silver impregnation. The heavy dotted line indicates the outline of the explant. Three large ventral horn cells are shown in the stippled area (see also Fig. IV-9); and a single cell of the dorsal horn with its axon is shown in black. Notice the relation between this axon and the dendrites of the ventral horn cells, and the loops that the axon forms in the outgrowth zone; note also that the axon runs from the inner band, deep to the dorsal cap zone, into the outer band. (No DRGs or muscle were present in this culture; cf. Figs. II-1, IV-7.) CAP, dorsal cap zone. CC, central canal. VH, ventral horn. VRL, lateral division of ventral root. (From Guillery, Sobkowicz, and Scott, 1968.)

mental analyses with explants from higher CNS centers—e.g., cerebral neocortex and hippocampus (see section D), cerebellum (see section E), and brainstem (see section C)—where specific input and output circuits have not yet been demonstrated in cultured preparations [except for our recent electrophysiologic studies of selective DRG innervation of dorsal column nuclei in medulla cross-sectional explants; see section C_2) (Crain and Peterson, 1975a).]

Organized synaptic network activities have also been recorded in similar types of spinal cord tissues several weeks after explantation from chick embryos (Crain and Peterson, 1964) and bullfrog tadpoles. The frog spinal cord explants were cultured in the same nutrient media used for mammalian CNS tissues, but diluted 25% with distilled water and maintained at 27°C (see also Grosse and Lindner, 1968). Many of the axons emerging from the cord explants became well myelinated after several weeks in culture [see photomicrographs by Crain (in Murray, 1959)], and complex bioelectric discharges could be evoked in the cord tissue [Crain, *unpublished observations;* see also studies by Corner and Crain (1965) with early frog neurulae explants (section A_3) and by Padjen et al. (1975) with explants of adult bullfrog peripheral ganglia (Chap. II-A1)].

Further insights into cellular mechanisms associated with synaptic functions in spinal cord explants have been obtained through studies of stimulation-dependent uptake of horseradish peroxidase into presynaptic vesicles (Holtzman et al., 1973; Teichberg et al., 1975). When spinal cord synapses are actively releasing neurotransmitters during periods (ca. 30–60 min) of repetitive network discharges elicited by electric stimulation or exposure to 10^{-6} M strychnine (Chaps. VI-A, VII-A), cytochemical analyses at the electron microscope level demonstrate that a substantial fraction of presynaptic vesicles in many of the cord synapses become labeled with endogenous peroxidase (present in the culture medium at a concentration of 10 mg/ml). By contrast, little peroxidase accumulation is seen during incubation of these explants with peroxidase for similar periods in the presence of 10 mM Mg^{++} or 100 μg/ml Xylocaine, both of which appear to depress synaptic network discharges by impeding transmitter release (Chap. VI-E). The experiments were carried out on fetal cord explants primarily during the period of 10–14 days *in vitro,* after abundant synapses had formed, especially in the neuropil covering the surface of the explant (see above), but before extensive growth of a glial and/or connective tissue overlay had formed which might impede penetration of peroxidase to the synaptic junctions in the cord explant (e.g., Guillery et al., 1968).

Up to 30% of the synapses in a cord explant may show at least some peroxidase-labeled vesicles in presynaptic terminals after this period of intense repetitive network activity, and up to 30% of the vesicles in a given synapse may show peroxidase uptake. The wide variability may be related to the presence of many different types of synapses in these cord explants,

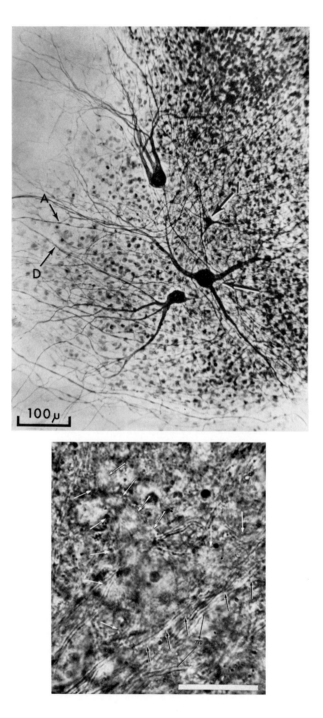

only some of which may have been activated by the mode of stimulation utilized in these experiments. Furthermore, some of the cord synapses may not release transmitter by mechanisms which would lead to peroxidase labeling under these experimental conditions. A similar absence of peroxidase labeling has been observed at the motor nerve terminals in our cord-muscle cultures (e.g., Fig. II-1), even after long periods of repetitive stimulation of motor axons (monitored by visual observation of the neurally evoked repetitive muscle contractions—e.g., Fig. IV-13 and Chap. VIII-B; Crain, Pappas, Masurovsky, Teichberg, and Peterson, *unpublished observations*). Peroxidase was clearly demonstrable in many presynaptic terminals within the cord explant and in the extracellular spaces near the motor endplate, but little or no sign of uptake into presynaptic vesicles at the motor axon terminal was detected, in contrast to the marked uptake which occurs at amphibian and invertebrate neuromuscular junctions (Holtzman et al., 1971; Ceccarelli et al., 1972, 1973; Heuser and Reese, 1973).

In spite of these variables, our experiments confirm, for at least some types of intact mammalian CNS neurons, previous evidence for a close relation between synaptic transmitter release and the retrieval of membrane in the form of small vesicles, as demonstrated at amphibian and invertebrate neuromuscular junctions (Holtzman et al., 1971; Ceccarelli et al., 1972, 1973; Heuser and Reese, 1973). Furthermore, longer-term "chase" experiments with the cord explants in tracer-free medium indicate that vesicles and other structures labeled with peroxidase, in response to stimulation, disappear from the endings through processes that require several hours to produce a marked decrease in the frequency of labeled vesicles. The number of labeled bodies at terminals decreases at an appreciable rate even when cultures are maintained in 10 mM Mg^{++} without tracer. Under these conditions it is unlikely that much loss of tracer occurs through processes such as those associated with transmitter release which account for the initial accumulation of tracer.

The data suggest that much of the depletion of label from terminals during a chase with elevated Mg^{++} reflects retrograde intraneuronal transport of vesicles to the neuron perikarya for further processing. Perikaryal

---

FIG. IV-9. Photomicrographs of ventral horn region of fetal rodent spinal cord explants. **Top:** Ventral horn region of silver-impregnated mouse cord explant drawn in Fig. IV-8. Note the three large ventral horn neurons (stippled areas in Fig. IV-8). A and D indicate an axon and a dendrite from two of these cells. Also note stellate, intermediate neuron (1). **Bottom:** Ventral horn region of living, unstained rat cord explant (36 days *in vitro*). *Arrows* point to the perikaryon and broad dendritic processes of a large neuron (which could be discerned more clearly by systematic focusing at various levels through this complex three-dimensional "figure" embedded in a low-contrast glial "ground"). A band of myelinated axons (m) runs diagonally across the lower right portion of the field. Calibration: 50 μm. (**Top** from Guillery, Sobkowicz, and Scott, 1968; **Bottom** from Peterson, Crain, and Murray, 1965.)

tracer accumulation during chases is much more dramatic when the initial exposure to peroxidase is with strychnine than when the tracer exposure occurs with elevated Mg^{++}. In other words, the amount of tracer that eventually ends up in neuronal perikarya is related to the degree of synaptic activity during the initial loading of presynaptic endings with peroxidase. Such observations carry obvious implications for the use of retrograde transport methods in neuronal mapping. The more rapid (4–8 hr) loss of tracer-containing vesicles which occurs during exposure to strychnine may reflect vesicle membrane reutilization for exocytosis (Teichberg et al., 1975).

This interdisciplinary study of circulation and turnover of synaptic membranes in spinal cord explants provides an excellent example of the potentialities of CNS tissue culture models for correlative analyses of nerve cell functions under conditions which facilitate long-term yet direct experimental manipulations and measurements on intact groups of synaptically connected mammalian neurons. Further experiments involving shorter and more carefully controlled periods of stimulus-regulated peroxidase labeling of presynaptic vesicles may also be fruitful, since our present data do not preclude the alternative possibility that peroxidase uptake may occur concomitantly with transmitter release by a "shutter"-like mechanism; i.e., a membrane-delimited synaptic vesicle may remain only briefly at the presynaptic surface before being retrieved, so that very little alteration may occur in the structure of the vesicle. This is in contrast to the elaborate synaptic vesicle membrane transformations postulated in current hypotheses based on exocytosis coupled with compensating endocytosis. Both modes of release may occur.

The marked stimulus-dependent peroxidase uptake at synapses in CNS explants demonstrates, moreover, the feasibility of studying the direct effects of various enzymes and other macromolecules on CNS functions both extracellularly and after incorporation into synaptic vesicles and other intracellular sites — e.g., acetylcholinesterase (Politoff et al., 1975) — with less serious diffusion barrier problems than in situ.

2. Cord Innervation of Skeletal Muscle In Vitro

Tissue culture models of neuromuscular relationships and related studies of noninnervated or denervated muscle have been the subject of intensive investigations in many laboratories during the past few decades. Since a comprehensive review of these studies would double the size of this volume, only selected aspects of neuromuscular functions in culture are included in this chapter and in Chaps. V-A and VIII-B. A number of extensive reviews are available: Murray, 1965a, 1972; Shimada and Fischman, 1973; Nelson, 1973, 1975; Crain and Peterson, 1974a; Fischbach, 1974, 1976; Fischbach et al., 1974a,b; Harris, 1974a,b.

As noted in Chapter I-B, indirect evidence of the development of functional neuromuscular transmission in cultures of frog embryo spinal cord tissue explanted together with attached myotomes was first reported by Harrison (1907) and then extended by Szepsenwol (1941, 1946,1947) with chick tissues. Direct electrophysiologic recordings from cord-myotome cultures were first begun in 1964 using mouse tissues (Crain, 1964b; see also Crain, 1970a, and morphologic correlates by Bornstein et al., 1968). Cross sections (0.5 mm thick) of the dorsal half of 12- to 13-day mouse embryos were explanted, each fragment containing spinal cord, DRG, paravertebral masses of myoblasts, and various connective tissues, with relatively little disruption of the normal tissue array.

Microscopically visible contractions of large numbers of muscle fibers were generally evoked in these myotome cultures by selective stimulation of spinal cord neurons. Muscle action potentials could be detected with extracellular microelectrodes, and they occurred with latencies ranging from 1 to 15 msec. Cord-evoked muscle responses were generally triggered at a critical stimulus threshold and occurred only with careful positioning of the stimulating microelectrode in the cord tissue. Muscle responses with earliest latencies were evoked with minimal stimulus intensities at critical sites in the ventral cord (or ventral root). Together with observations on *in vitro*-coupled cord-muscle explants (see below), the data suggested that innervation of the muscle fibers in these cultures was provided by motor neurons located in the ventral horn regions of the cord cross sections.

The effects of d-tubocurarine and eserine on the bioelectric activities of cord-myotome explants indicated that neuromuscular transmission was mediated by cholinergic synaptic mechanisms as *in situ*. Introduction of d-tubocurarine (0.3–10 μg/ml) produced a characteristic rapid block of cord-evoked muscle responses, while cord afterdischarges were unaffected (as in Fig. IV-13). Presynaptic neural spikes could still be elicited and the muscle fibers could still be activated by *direct* electric stimuli. The anti-cholinesterase agent eserine, on the other hand, produced characteristic excitatory effects on myotome explants at low concentrations (0.1–0.5 μg/ml). Single cord stimuli, which evoked single muscle responses in control media, now began to elicit repetitive muscle twitches even though the cord discharges showed no enhancement (Crain, 1970a). Strychnine also produced "convulsive" muscle contractions in the myotome cultures, but in this case the effects were mediated by action on the *cord* tissue (e.g., Fig. VII-1; see also Chap. VII-A). Long series of repetitive muscle spikes (and contractions) were now associated with long-lasting cord afterdischarges evoked by single stimuli or occurring spontaneously.

These studies provided the first direct demonstration that immature neurons of mammalian spinal cord retain the capacity *in vitro* to form *functional* neuromuscular junctions with skeletal muscle fibers. The organotypic bioelectric properties of cord-myotome explants are in good agreement with histologic evidence of characteristic cholinesterase-loaded neuromuscular synapses on cross-striated muscle fibers (Bornstein et al., 1968). It should

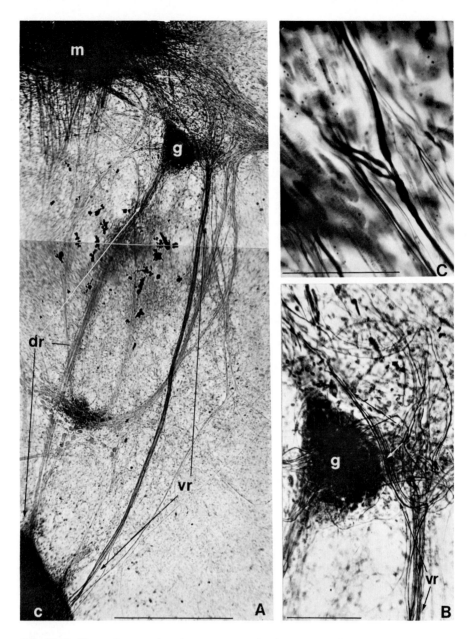

FIG. IV-10. Photomicrographs of motor axons that have grown from fetal rodent spinal cord explants and formed neuromuscular junctions in separate explants of skeletal muscle (5–9 weeks in culture; Holmes' silver impregnation). **A:** Low-power view shows the organized neuritic bundles that have grown *in vitro* across the gap between fetal rat cord and muscle explants. Dorsal root fibers (dr) can be traced from the spinal cord (c) into the DRG (g). A portion of these fibers passes into the muscle (m). Deeply impregnated ventral root fibers emerge from the cord (lower left), pass close to but *around,* the ganglion, and enter the muscle region. Scale 500 μm. **B:** Higher-power view shows more clearly the ventral root (vr) coursing around the ganglion (g). Scale: 50 μm. **C:** Detail of a ventral root fiber (*white arrow* in **A**) which branches as it enters the muscle tissue. Scale:

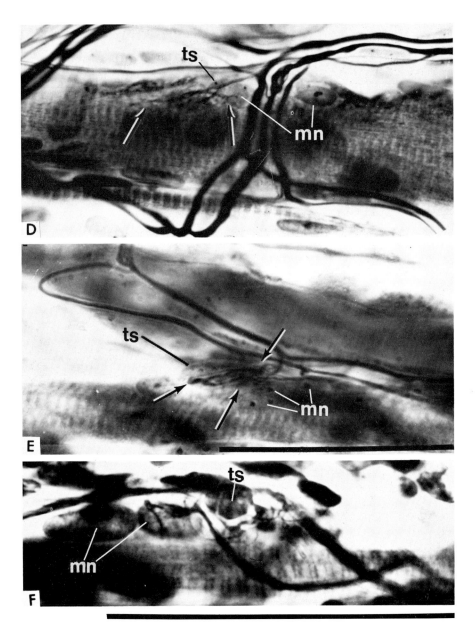

50 μm. **D–F:** Terminals of motor axons from fetal mouse cord to explant of regenerating *adult* muscle fibers (see low- and high-power views of living culture in Figs. II-1 and VIII-5, and electron micrograph of typical motor endplate in Fig. IV-11). **D:** Fine terminal arborization (*arrows*) of a delicate branch of a study axon on mature muscle fiber. Note the terminal Schwann cell (ts) and the subneural specialization of sole plate myonuclei (mn). **E:** Terminal branch with delicate arborization and bouton structures (*arrows*) on a well-differentiated muscle fiber. Note the terminal Schwann cell (ts) and sole plate myonuclei (mn). **F:** Complex arborization of a nerve terminal in a well-differentiated endplate structure. Note myonuclei (mn) and terminal Schwann cell (ts). Scale: 50 μm. **A–C** from Peterson and Crain, 1970. **D–F** from Peterson and Crain, 1972.)

be emphasized that neuromuscular junctions have probably not yet formed in the immature 12- to 13-day mouse embryo tissue explanted for these experiments. Clear-cut junctions in the rat fetus have not been detected by electron microscopy until 17–18 days *in utero* (Teräväinen, 1968; Kelly and Zacks, 1969), in agreement with physiologic studies (Windle et al., 1935; Diamond and Miledi, 1962). Critical developmental processes associated with formation of neuromuscular junctions must therefore have occurred after explantation of 12- to 13-day cord-myotomes.

Techniques were then developed to permit innervation *in vitro* of isolated skeletal muscle explants positioned within 1 mm of the ventral edge of previously explanted fetal rodent spinal cord (Fig. II-1) (Peterson and Crain, 1970, 1972). Electrophysiologic studies demonstrated that characteristic neuromuscular transmission developed not only after innervation *in vitro* of fetal rodent muscle (Fig. IV-10A) (Crain, 1968, 1970*a*) but also after innervation of muscle fibers regenerating in *adult* rodent (Figs. IV-10C–E;11;12) and even *human* (Fig. IV-14) muscle explants (Crain et al., 1970). After coupling periods of 2–7 weeks *in vitro*, selective stimulation of ventral horn regions of the spinal cord explants (or ventral root loci) evoked widespread coordinated contractions in all of these types of muscle fibers (Figs. IV-13;15;16). Simultaneous microelectrode recordings of ventral cord and muscle responses to local cord stimuli show that muscle action potentials (and contractions) generally occurred with latencies of several milliseconds after onset of the cord discharges. The cord potentials appear to be due to activation of motoneurons, which then propagate impulses toward the muscle fibers (Figs. IV-14;15) (Crain, 1970*a*). Similar temporal relations were often seen during spontaneous rhythmic discharges of the coupled cord and muscle tissues. Long series of repetitive discharges at 2- to 5-sec intervals may occur synchronously between these cord and muscle explants in response to single cord (or DRG) stimuli, and they may also appear spontaneously (Chap. VII-A). As in the cord-myotome cultures, *d*-tubocurarine (1–10 μg/ml) selectively and reversibly blocked neuromuscular transmission (Figs. IV-13B,E;16A) and eserine accelerated recovery of normal function (Fig. IV-16B). Repetitive cord and muscle discharges were greatly augmented after introduction of strychnine. Complex rhythmic oscillatory (ca. 10/sec) afterdischarges generated in strychninized cord explants led to similarly patterned muscle discharges (and contractions), which may also occur in normal medium (Fig. IV-13A).

The organotypic bioelectric properties of these cultured neuromuscular tissues correlate well with histologic evidence of silver-impregnated axons arborizing among cross-striated muscle fibers (Fig. IV-10) and terminating at characteristic neuromuscular junctions with marked cholinesterase localizations (Fig. VIII-5B) (Peterson and Crain, 1970, 1972) and typical motor endplate ultrastructure (Figs. IV-11,12) (Pappas et al., 1971*a,b*). Some of these cord-innervated muscle cultures have remained in healthy

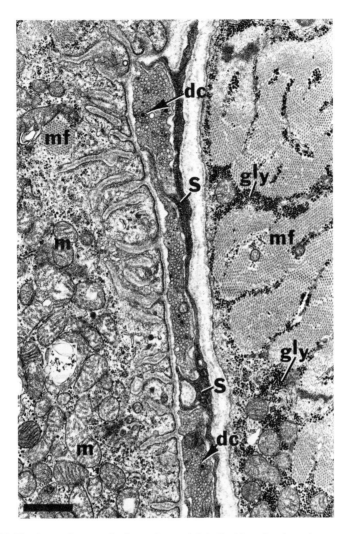

FIG. IV-11. Electron micrograph of a motor endplate that has developed on a regenerated adult mouse skeletal muscle fiber after innervation by a motoneuron in a fetal mouse spinal cord-ganglion explant, 3 months in culture. (Low-power views are shown in Figs. II-1 and IV-10D-F). The axon terminals are filled with presynaptic vesicles, some of which are of the dense-core variety (dc). The postsynaptic infoldings of the sarcolemma, characteristic of mature neuromuscular junctions, extend along the entire region of synaptic contact. The axon terminals are ensheathed by Schwann cell processes (S) (Fig. IV-10), except at the synaptic contact surface. The myofilament lattices (mf) are seen here in cross section; in longitudinal section they appear similar to those in Fig. IV-12; note also the mitochondria (m), glycogen particles (gly), and ribosomes. Scale: 1 μm. (From Pappas, Peterson, Masurovsky, and Crain, 1971a.)

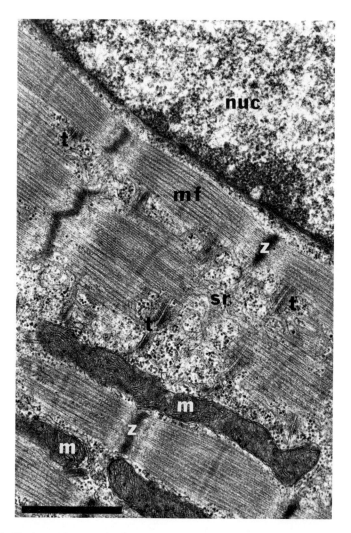

FIG. IV-12. Electron micrograph of a regenerated, spinal cord-innervated muscle fiber in a culture similar to that in Fig. IV-11 (5 weeks *in vitro*). The cytoplasm is filled with highly ordered myofilament lattices (mf) aligned in register across the girth of the fiber (see living muscle fiber in Fig. VIII-5), and part of a subsarcolemmal nucleus (nuc) is visible (see lower-power view in Fig. IV-10). Note the network of sarcoplasmic reticulum (sr) cisternae associated with the Z-line region (z) and insinuated elsewhere among the lattices. Triad configurations (t) appear in the A-1 junction area; and typical mitochondria (m), glycogen granules, and ribosomes are present. Scale: 1 μm. (From Crain and Peterson, 1974a; electron micrograph provided by E. B. Masurovsky and G. D. Pappas.)

condition for more than 1 year, suggesting that neurotrophic effects may play an important role in maintaining the structural and functional integrity of the muscle fibers (Crain and Peterson, 1974a) (Chap. VIII-B). This view is supported by our demonstration of serious muscle atrophy within 2–4 weeks

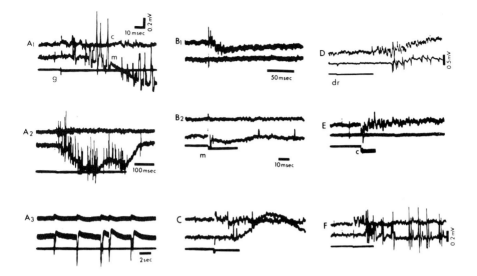

FIG. IV-13. Neuromuscular transmission between separate explants of fetal mouse spinal cord and *adult* mouse skeletal muscle in 6- and 8-week cultures; the muscle tissue was "presented" to the isolated cord explant at 4 days *in vitro*. $A_{1,2}$: Simultaneous recordings from cord and muscle explants (8-week culture) show a brief burst of spike potentials in cord (first sweep, c), evoked by a single stimulus to attached DRG (third sweep, g), and a much longer-lasting barrage of spikes superimposed on a large slow wave in muscle (second sweep, m). The muscle discharge in A_2 actually included approximately 10 additional spikes of large amplitude (up to 1 mV) — similar to the first four extending above the first sweep. They occurred in groups of two or three, every 20–40 msec, as in A_1, but were barely visible at the slower sweep rate in A_2 (only the first few were retouched, to avoid undue complexity). Synchronous contractions of large numbers of muscle fibers occurred concomitantly with the slow wave (see text). A_3: Cord-muscle discharge sequence (and contractions) occurs repetitively at 2- to 5-sec intervals following the initial responses evoked by a single ganglion stimulus. B_1: Neurally evoked muscle discharge (and contraction) is blocked under *d*-tubocurarine (10 µg/ml) while the spike burst is still elicited in cord explant by ganglion (or cord) stimuli. B_2: Muscle spike potential (and contraction) can still be evoked by *direct* electric stimulus to muscle tissue (third sweep, m). **C:** After return to normal medium, characteristic muscle discharges (and contractions) can again be elicited with cord (or ganglion) stimuli. **D:** Cord and muscle discharges evoked by dorsal root stimulus in another culture (6 weeks *in vitro*) showing much longer latencies — in this case approximately 30 msec for the onset of cord barrage and an additional delay of 20 msec before the appearance of the muscle response. *d*-Tubocurarine produces a selective block of cord-evoked muscle discharge **(E),** and characteristic responses can again be elicited after a return to normal medium (cf. **F** and A_1). (From Crain, Alfei, and Peterson, 1970.)

after surgical denervation of these *in vitro*-matured muscle fibers (Fig. VIII-6). Furthermore, muscle denervation atrophy after cord extirpation is markedly postponed if sympathetic (but not dorsal root) ganglia were previously explanted close to the muscle fibers (Fig. VIII-7). Although these neurotrophic effects were observed in the apparent absence of direct synaptic connections between sympathetic ganglion and muscle cells, some of the muscle fibers in these cultures appeared to have become innervated by the

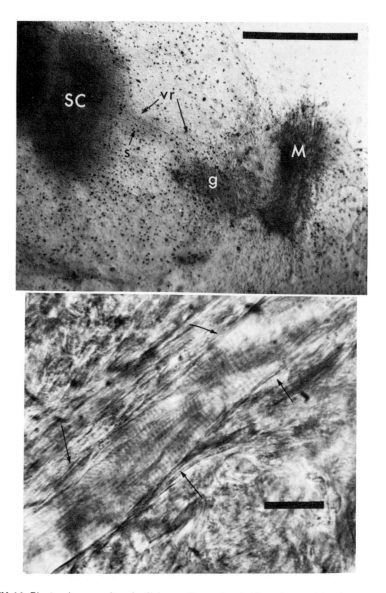

FIG. IV-14. Photomicrographs of a living culture of paired explants of *fetal mouse* spinal cord and *adult human* muscle (quadriceps). **Top:** Low-power view of cord (SC) and muscle (M) explants (2 weeks *in vitro*). DRG (g) attached to cord had migrated *in vitro* to a position near the muscle explant. Ventral root neurites (vr) that have grown across the gap between cord and muscle explants could be seen more clearly at higher magnification (electric stimuli were applied at site "s"—see Figs. IV-15;16). Scale: 500 μm. **Bottom:** High-power view of one of the human striated muscle fibers that matured in culture under neurotrophic influence of mouse cord neurites (4 weeks *in vitro*), as occurs with rodent muscle (Figs. II-1; IV-10–12). Scale: 20 μm. (From Crain, Alfei, and Peterson, 1970.)

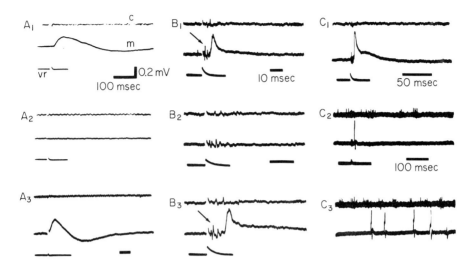

FIG. IV-15. Neuromuscular transmission between explants of *fetal mouse* spinal cord and *adult human* muscle (4-week culture; see Fig. IV-14). **A₁**: Simultaneous recordings from cord and muscle explants show small, brief spike potentials in cord (c) evoked by a single stimulus to ventral root neurites (vr) near the edge of the cord (see "s" in Fig. IV-14), and a large negative potential in muscle (m) after a latency of 15 msec and lasting more than 150 msec (concomitant with coordinated muscle twitch). **A₂**: After slight withdrawal of the stimulating electrode from the root, the entire cord and muscle responses disappear. **A₃**: Muscle potential (and contraction) can again be evoked after returning the stimulating electrode to the root (note the slower sweep rate). **B₁,₃**: Muscle action potential is recorded from a nearby site in the same explant following a ventral root stimulus. Note the small, brief neural spike potentials arising prior to generation of the muscle potential. The muscle spike lasts several milliseconds and is followed by a negative afterpotential of long duration. **B₂**: After a slight decrease in stimulus intensity, the muscle response and largest neural spike (*arrows* in **B₁,₃**) disappear, but some components of the neural spike burst are still evoked. **C₁**: Maintenance of neuromuscular transmission for a short period after introduction of *d*-tubocurarine (1 μg/ml), and transient appearance of spontaneous repetitive spike barrages in cord (**C₂,₃**). Repetitive muscle action potentials (and contractions) may also occur in relation to some of these cord discharges (**C₃**), similar to the evoked potential in **C₂**. (From Crain, Alfei, and Peterson, 1970.)

sympathetic neurites which arborized over the muscle tissue (Chaps. III-B, VIII-B). Similarly unexpected formation of connections in culture between dissociated sympathetic ganglion cells and skeletal myotubes were recently demonstrated by Nurse and O'Lague (1975) (Chap. V-A).

3. Frog Neurulae with Presumptive Muscle

A far more extreme test of the capacity of isolated neuromuscular tissue to self-differentiate *in vitro* has been carried out with explants of frog neurulae (Corner and Crain, 1965). The prospective spinal cord was excised together with underlying presumptive axial muscle and cultured in a relatively simple amphibian balanced salt solution. Since each of these amphibian

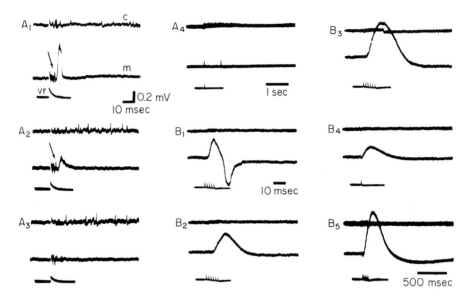

FIG. IV-16. Block of neuromuscular transmission in curarized mouse-innervated human muscle explant and recovery after eserine. **A₁**: Simultaneous cord and muscle recordings, as in Fig. IV-15, showing neuromuscular transmission several minutes after exposure to *d*-tubocurarine (1 μg/ml). **A₂**: Shortly afterward, the muscle action potential (and contraction) fails to develop following cord-evoked, early-latency neural spikes (*arrows* in **A₁,₂**); small-amplitude negativity resembling a muscle endplate potential occurs instead, with the same latency. **A₃**: After a slight reduction in stimulus intensity, this "endplate potential" and the presynaptic neural spike both disappear. **A₄**: Neuromuscular transmission is still blocked several minutes after a return to normal medium. Note the long-lasting spike barrage evoked in the cord explant by the vr stimulus. **B:** After introduction of eserine (10 μg/ml), vr stimuli evoke coordinated muscle contractions concomitantly with recordings of slow waves (as in Fig. IV-15A). Tetanic stimuli (40–50/sec) are required during the early stage of recovery (**B₁₋₃**), but single stimuli soon become effective (**B₄**), and repetitive stimuli then produce summation effects (**B₅**). (From Crain, Alfei, and Peterson, 1970.)

embryonic cells contains a substantial quantity of yolk vesicles, the neural and muscle cells can continue to grow and differentiate (for at least 1–2 weeks) without dependence on special nutrients in the extracellular culture environment. Spontaneous muscle twitches began to occur in many of these explants during the first week *in vitro* [as observed by Harrison (1907) in his pioneering experiments with older frog cord myotome cultures (Fig. I-1)]. The twitching often occurred regularly in bursts, at a rate of 5–8/sec, each burst lasting 0.5–5 sec and appearing at intervals of 1–20 sec. Electrophysiologic studies after 1–2 weeks *in vitro* demonstrated that long-lasting spike barrages could be evoked in the neural regions of these explants by brief electric stimuli. The response patterns were indeed remarkably similar to those characteristic of more mature cultures of mammalian spinal cord and indicate that synaptic networks may develop even from this primordial neurula tissue within 1–2 weeks *in vitro*. Preliminary electrophysiologic data suggested, moreover, that regular, rhythmic endogenous bursts of muscle contractions may be triggered by periodic bursts of neural activity. These results are consistent with microscopic observations during ontogenetic development of amphibian neuromuscular systems *in situ* (Corner, 1964*a,b*) as well as with analysis of cultured mouse cord-myotomes (see above).

B. SPINAL CORD INNERVATION BY DORSAL ROOT GANGLIA

1. DRGs Attached to Cord

A. Cytologic Aspects

Initial electrophysiologic studies of 13- to 14-day fetal rat cord cross sections with attached pairs of DRGs demonstrated that synaptically mediated cord responses could be evoked by DRG stimuli by 6 days after explantation of the "presynaptic" tissues (Crain and Peterson, 1967). More recent extension of this work to 13- to 14-day fetal mouse cord-DRG cultures indicates, however, that DRG stimuli may be effective in eliciting complex cord discharges as early as 2–3 days after explantation when tested in the presence of appropriate pharmacologic agents, e.g., strychnine and bicuculline (e.g., Fig. IV-2; see also section D) (Crain et al., 1976). Onset of sensory-evoked cord network responses in 13- to 14-day fetal cord DRG explants at 2–3 days *in vitro* correlates quite closely with evidence of spinal reflex activity as early as 15–16 days in the mouse fetus *in situ* (Vaughn et al. 1975), as in the rat fetus (Windle and Baxter, 1935–1936; Narayanan et al., 1971; see also May and Biscoe, 1975).

Although DRG-evoked cord network responses could be obtained in some explants even after months in culture, we were concerned that a substantial fraction (up to 90%) of the DRG neurons in these embryonic rodent cord-ganglion explants atrophied or degenerated during the first few days in our control culture medium (Fig. IV-17A,B). In earlier studies with 15- to 18-day fetal rat cord-DRG explants, on the other hand, a much larger fraction of the ganglion cells generally survived and matured in control cultures (Peterson et al., 1965; Bunge et al., 1967*b*) (Figs. I-3, IV-20) possibly due to decreased dependence of more mature DRG neurons on exogenous nerve growth factor (NGF) (Levi-Montalcini and Booker, 1960) or other trophic factors. Introduction of NGF at explantation, in concentrations ranging from 10^{-8} to 10^{-5} g/ml (i.e., 1–1,000 biologic units (BU)/ml), led to a higher survival rate of DRG neurons (Crain and Peterson, 1974*b*) in addition to the characteristic dose-dependent enhancement of neuritic outgrowth (Levi-Montalcini, 1958; Levi-Montalcini and Angeletti, 1968*a,b*). Vastly increased neuronal survival occurred in higher concentrations of

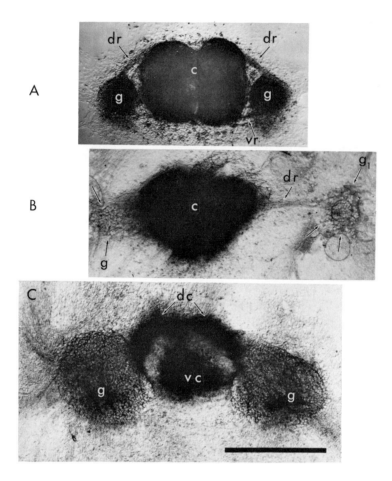

FIG. IV-17. Photomicrographs of 14-day fetal mouse spinal cord explants (cross sections) with attached DRGs; these are living, unstained cultures. Scale: 1 mm. **A:** Shortly after explantation (1 day *in vitro*). Note size of DRGs (g) relative to cord tissue (c); also dorsal (dr) and ventral (vr) roots. **B:** One month in normal culture medium. Many of the ganglion cells degenerated during the first few days *in vitro*, leaving a small thinly spread array of DRG neurons (g), which have matured and retained characteristic (myelinated) dorsal root (dr) connections to the cord (see also Figs. II-1; IV-6;10). Note that the DRGs are of similar size, although only one (g₁) shows the characteristic "migration" away from the cord. Most of the other control cultures showed even lower survival of DRG neurons (see text). **C:** Another cord-DRG explant after 1 month in the same culture medium, but NGF was added to explantation (1,000 BU/ml). Note remarkable enlargement of DRGs (g) relative to their initial size at explantation **(A)** and in contrast to the control culture **(B)**. Many hundreds of ganglion cells form densely packed clusters close to the cord. (The major DRG volume increase was reached by the second week *in vitro*). Relatively dense appearance of dorsal cord (dc) is due to large numbers of myelinated axons which represent central branches of DRG neurons (see text). Dense region in ventromedial cord (vc) is due primarily to a "necrotic core" which generally develops in both treated and control explants. (From Crain and Peterson, 1974b.)

NGF (100–1,000 units/ml) concomitant with more abundant neuritic out-growths from the DRG cells, as in cultures of NGF-"hypertrophied" mouse sympathetic ganglia (Crain et al., 1964*a;* Chap. III-B). These *in vitro* effects resemble the remarkable selective hypertrophy of sensory DRGs and sym-pathetic ganglia in 7- to 10-day chick embryos *in ovo* within 3–4 days after daily injection of microgram quantities of NGF (Fig. IV-18) (Levi-Montal-cini, 1958; Levi-Montalcini and Cohen, 1960). At the higher NGF levels, massive DRGs containing many hundreds of neuron perikarya developed during the first week *in vitro* and often remained densely packed in close proximity to the spinal cord tissue (Fig. IV-17C). This is in sharp contrast to the sparse, irregular array of several dozen DRG neuron perikarya (rarely more than 100) in control cultures (Fig. IV-17B; see also Figs. II-1; IV-6;7;20), which generally "migrate" approximately 0.5–1 mm away from the cord (Peterson et al., 1965; Sobkowicz et al., 1973), retaining characteristic dorsal root connections (Peterson and Crain, 1972; Crain and Peterson, 1974*b*). The NGF-stimulated DRG neurons continued to mature during the following weeks in culture even though no additional NGF was introduced beyond that included in the medium at explantation. Some of the DRGs ac-tually became comparable in volume to their associated spinal cord segment (cf. Fig. IV-17C and IV-17A). Examination of the living cultures at high magnification indicates that the enlarged DRGs were composed of many layers of healthy neuron perikarya; and normal neuronal and supporting cell morphology has been observed in preliminary histologic analyses at the light- and electron-microscopic level (Peterson et al., 1974; *in preparation*).

These experiments are consonant with the earlier demonstrations that NGF is necessary for the survival and development of dissociated sensory ganglion cells in culture (Levi-Montalcini and Angeletti, 1963; Varon et al., 1973). Moreover, our present data show that NGF may play an essential role, at least at a critical developmental stage, in determining the survival of fetal rodent sensory ganglion cells, even when they remain within an or-ganized ganglion in close association with the normal array of supporting cells. Most of the NGF-stimulated DRG cells can then mature and be main-tained for months in culture. Further controls will be required to clarify the degree to which the NGF-enlarged DRGs represent a real hypertrophy *in vitro* or simply a closer approximation to their *in situ* counterparts. In addi-tion to NGF-induced DRG "hypertrophy," the dorsal regions of the asso-ciated spinal cord segment appear to develop unusual enlargements which become increasingly prominent in long-term culture. Preliminary observa-tions indicate that these dorsal cord regions contain far more abundant ar-rays of densely packed axons, which as they become myelinated during the second and third weeks *in vitro* can be traced to, and appear in continuity with, the entering dorsal roots of the ganglion (Fig. IV-17C) (Peterson et al., *in preparation*).

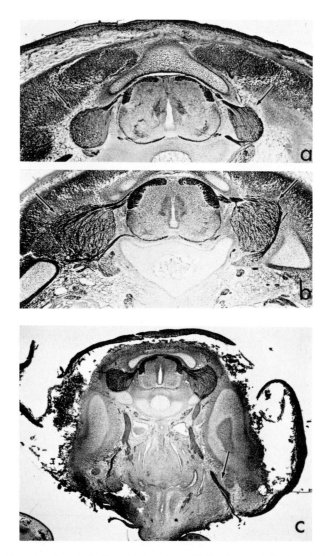

FIG. IV-18. Hypertrophy of 10-day chick embryo DRGs *in ovo* following 3 days of injections with purified salivary gland NGF extract. **a,b:** Transverse sections through the thoracic level of embryos. *Arrows* point to ganglia. **a:** Control. **b:** Injected with NGF. Note the increase in size of the spinal ganglia. **c:** Transverse section through sacral level of the same NGF-treated embryo as in **b.** *Arrow* points to the sensory nerve, which has increased in length; the nerve perforates the skin and appears at the free surface of the body. (Note: sacral DRGs in control embryo were much smaller than those in **c;** see Levi-Montalcini and Cohen, 1960.) All sections were silver-impregnated. (Modified from Levi-Montalcini and Cohen, 1960.)

B. Electrophysiologic Aspects

Correlative electrophysiologic experiments have been carried out on these fetal mouse cord-DRG explants to determine whether the NGF-stimulated growth and development of DRG neurons leads to enhancement of organized synaptic relationships with spinal cord neurons or if the additional neuritic bundles and arborizations are merely unregulated growth processes leading to "deadends" or to aberrant functional connections – as occurs in some types of NGF-stimulated sympathetic ganglion cells *in situ* (e.g., Olson, 1967).

Extracellular recordings were made with Ag-AgCl electrodes via micropipettes (3- to 5-μm tips) filled with isotonic saline. In control cultures application of a focal stimulus close to the DRG or dorsal root (via a 10-μm electrode) often evokes a small negative slow-wave potential in the dorsal regions of the spinal cord, with a rapid rising phase and a slower falling phase (Fig. IV-19A,B). The amplitude and duration of this potential are quite variable, ranging up to approximately 0.5 mV and 100 msec, depending on the stimulus intensity, geometry of the cellular array, and proximity of the stimulating and recording electrodes to the excitable neuronal elements. This negative slow-wave response appears after a latency of 2–3 msec when the stimulus is applied to the DRG perikarya or the dorsal root (Fig. IV-19A,B_3). [No clear-cut evidence of these dorsal cord potentials was obtained in our earlier studies of 14-day fetal rat cord-DRG explants during development in normal media (Crain and Peterson, 1967).] Simultaneous recordings in the ventral regions of the spinal cord segment generally show longer-latency (>5–10 msec) responses, often including a positive slow-wave potential (ca. 100 msec) and a spike barrage of variable complexity (Fig. IV-19A,B).

Application of similar stimuli to NGF-hypertrophied DRGs evoked comparable negative slow-wave responses in the dorsal cord with similar latency and a sharp rising phase, but the amplitude and duration were now remarkably larger (Fig. IV-19C) (Crain and Peterson, 1974*b*, 1975*a;* see also Crain, 1976). The cord potentials often reached 2 mV in response to a single large DRG stimulus, and a prominent negative slow wave could be evoked even after a 10-fold reduction in stimulus strength to these low-threshold neurons (Fig. IV-19C_3,E_2). Furthermore, the duration of the DRG-triggered dorsal cord responses was often more than 500 msec (Fig. IV-19C) – far longer-lasting than generally observed in control cultures. Single stimuli applied to peripheral branches of NGF-stimulated DRG cells, as much as 2–3 mm beyond the explant zone (e.g., Figs. IV-6;7;20), were also effective and elicited responses comparable to those in Fig. IV-19C_3,E_2 but with longer latencies (ca. 5–10 msec).

The temporal patterns of the dorsal cord potentials evoked by stimulation of NGF-hypertrophied DRGs *in vitro* contain components that are remark-

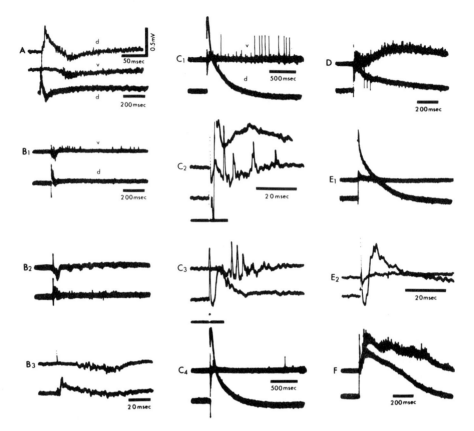

FIG. IV-19. Enhanced responses evoked in dorsal regions of fetal mouse spinal cord explants by stimuli applied to NGF-hypertrophied DRG. **A:** Control culture, 4 weeks *in vitro* (Fig. IV-17B). Early-latency negative slow-wave potential (resembling PAD — see text) is evoked in dorsal cord (d) by single DRG stimulus (via focal 10-μm tip electrode), and is followed by a positive slow-wave concomitant with a high-frequency spike barrage (dorsal cord response is shown at slower sweep rate on lowest record). Ventral cord response (v) begins after longer latency and involves primarily a positive slow-wave and spike barrage. **B$_1$:** Smaller PAD elicited in dorsal cord (d) of another control explant (2 weeks *in vitro*); ventral cord response (v) again consists of a primary positive slow-wave and a repetitive spike barrage. **B$_{2,3}$:** After introduction of strychnine (10^{-6} M), the ventral cord discharge becomes larger and more complex, but PAD is relatively unchanged although it is now followed by a long spike barrage. Fast sweep (**B$_3$**) shows that PAD begins shortly after DRG stimulus, whereas ventral cord response occurs at longer latency (as **A**). **C$_1$:** Similar explant, 2 weeks *in vitro*, but NGF was added at explantation (1,000 BU/ml). A PAD-like potential evoked in the dorsal cord (d) by a single stimulus to NGF-hypertrophied DRG (Fig. IV-17C) is much larger in amplitude and longer in duration (cf. **A** and **B$_1$**), whereas the ventral cord response (v) is similar to the control pattern. **C$_2$:** An early-latency, sharp rising phase and the complexity of the PAD response are seen at a faster sweep rate. **C$_3$:** Tenfold reduction of DRG stimulus intensity evoked smaller but still prominent PAD, and the ventral cord discharge now begins after a longer latency, during the falling phase of PAD (as in **A** and **B$_3$**). **C$_4$:** Larger DRG stimulus (as in **C$_1$**) again elicits characteristic large PAD just before drug application. **D:** Introduction of bicuculline (10^{-5} M) leads to a marked decrease in amplitude of PAD concomitant with the onset of a convulsive negative slow-wave and repetitive-spike discharge in the ventral cord (v). **E$_1$:** After transfer to 10^{-3} M GABA, the large PAD response is restored (cf. **C$_4$**) in contrast to almost complete block of the ventral cord discharge. **E$_2$:** Tenfold reduction of DRG stimulus intensity still evokes relatively large PAD (cf. **C$_3$**, in BSS). **F:** Return to bicuculline (10^{-5} M) leads to partial depression of PAD and appearance of the secondary longer-lasting negative slow wave in the dorsal cord, concomitant with the onset of a huge negative slow-wave and oscillatory discharge in the ventral cord (cf. Figs. VI-2;3) (From Crain and Peterson, 1974*b*.)

ably similar to those characteristic of the primary afferent depolarization (PAD) response in mammalian spinal cord *in situ* (Eccles, 1964). The PAD-like component recorded with extracellular microelectrodes in the cord explants appears to be a field potential produced by summated excitatory postsynaptic potentials (EPSPs) generated following DRG activation of dorsal cord circuits (see below). The weak PAD-like response generally observed with focal DRG stimulation in control cultures may be due partly to the lower density of excitable DRG neurons developing in the absence of added NGF, as well as to less extensive (or less effective) synaptic connections of each DRG cell with cord neurons. In contrast to the dramatic enhancement of the "PAD" potentials in the dorsal cord of NGF-treated explants, no substantial alterations in the response patterns of *ventral* cord regions have been observed (cf. Fig. IV-19A,C).

Marked temporal facilitation of PAD responses in explants occurs following brief application of 100/sec DRG volleys at low stimulus strength — resembling characteristic facilitation of PADs evoked by repetitive afferent stimuli *in situ* (Eccles, 1964). Furthermore, whereas strychnine showed relatively little effect on PAD potentials in dorsal cord [even at concentrations (ca. 10^{-5} M) which greatly enhanced complex long-latency spike-barrage and slow-wave discharges in both dorsal and ventral cord (cf. Fig. IV-19B$_2$ and IV-19B$_1$)], bicuculline and picrotoxin (10^{-5} M) produced marked attenuation of the PADs concomitantly with the onset of the convulsive discharges, especially in the ventral cord regions (Fig. IV-19D,F). On the other hand, after introduction of 10^{-3} M γ-aminobutyric acid (GABA) into the culture bath the PAD responses in dorsal cord were generally maintained or even *augmented* (Fig. IV-19E), in contrast to the rapid and sustained depression of almost all detectable synaptically mediated discharges in ventral cord regions as well as long-latency discharges in dorsal cord (Fig. IV-19E; upper sweep). GABA enhancement of PADs occurred in control as well as in NGF-treated cord explants and was especially marked during brief 100/sec DRG volleys. Generation of the PADs by Ca^{++}-dependent synaptic transmitter release is suggested by the rapid and complete block of PAD potentials after increasing the Mg^{++} concentration from 1 to 10mM, whereas spikes could still be directly evoked (Crain, 1974*b,c*) (see also Figs. VI-8;10; Chap. VI-E).

Although the PADs recorded in our explants probably include field potentials due to summated EPSPs in the dorsal cord interneurons triggered by DRG collaterals, the marked selective attenuation of these responses in bicuculline and picrotoxin suggests that a major component is generated by GABA-mediated EPSPs, possible at DRG terminals as *in situ* (Davidoff, 1972*a,b;* Barker and Nicoll, 1973; Benoist et al., 1974). (Attempts are being made to obtain more direct evidence for this interpretation by selective recordings from dorsal root fibers during generation of these PAD potentials in dorsal cord regions of the explants.) Depolarization of DRG terminals (by these GABA interneurons triggered by DRG collaterals) presumably decreases both the amplitude of the presynaptic action potential and quantity of transmitter released, and this presynaptic inhibition provides a potent regulatory mechanism that depresses the central excitatory actions of many primary afferent fibers in the mammalian CNS (Eccles, 1964; Wall, 1964; cf. Curtis et al., 1971b). Analyses of dorsal and ventral cord responses to selective single and paired stimuli applied to various neural elements in these cord-DRG explants provide additional evidence that the observed PADS are associated with inhibitory mechanisms (Crain, in preparation). The longer-latency negative slow-wave and oscillatory potentials elicited by DRG stimuli in bicuculline probably represent summated postsynaptic potentials synchronously and sequentially activated after interference with GABA-mediated inhibitory postsynaptic potentials (IPSPs) of cord neurons involved in these complex network responses (Crain, 1974b, 1975c, 1975d; Crain and Bornstein, 1974; see also Zipser et al., 1973). Introduction of 10^{-3} M GABA, on the other hand, may block convulsive network discharges by enhancing GABA-mediated IPSPs of cord neurons as well as GABA-mediated EPSPs (or other depolarization) of DRG terminals.

Sensory-evoked circuits leading to GABA depolarization of DRG terminals may not necessarily require mediation by axoaxonic synapses between GABA-inhibitory interneurons and DRG axons[2] (Curtis, 1975). Since GABA appears to depolarize all regions of DRG neurons (DeGroat, 1972; DeGroat et al., 1972; Obata, 1974) (Chap. V-A), perhaps simple diffusion of GABA from neighboring axosomatic synapses may increase the local extracellular concentration of GABA sufficiently to depolarize the terminal regions of DRG axons. If the relatively large surface area of DRG terminals contains abundant GABA receptor sites within reasonable distance of the presynaptic transmitter zone, effective depolarization of DRG terminals may well be produced by such a nonsynaptic mode of "presynaptic inhibition." This "diffuse" type of DRG-triggered GABA depolarization of DRG terminals may in turn be regulated or limited by the particular mode of glial envelopment of DRG axons in the terminal region. The glial investment

---

[2] The serial synaptic array in the electron micrograph of the dorsal horn region of a mature spinal cord explant with attached DRGs (Fig. IV-3c) is compatible with such an axoaxonic synapse, but the junction cannot be characterized in the absence of selective labeling of the DRG terminals. Recent electron microscopic-immunocytochemical techniques developed by McLaughlin et al. (1975) have allowed the demonstration of clear-cut labeling with the GABA-synthesizing enzyme glutamate decarboxylase (GAD) of terminals presynaptic to other axonal terminals (which in turn are presynaptic to other dendrites). These GAD-positive terminals are concentrated in the dorsolateral region of the dorsal horn precisely where GABA-ergic interneurons involved in presynaptic inhibition have been located by correlative biochemical and electrophysiologic data (Miyata and Otsuka, 1972; Otsuka and Konishi, 1975). The data are "consistent with the growing evidence that GABA may . . . be the transmitter mediating presynaptic inhibition of primary afferent terminals," but further studies of the distribution of GAD-positive terminals after dorsal rhizotomies are needed to determine if the labeled terminals are indeed presynaptic to degenerating DRG terminals (McLaughlin et al., 1975).

might not only provide a diffusion barrier to restrict and demarcate the surface area of DRG terminals exposed to interneuron-released GABA, it
may also permit active glial uptake of extracellular GABA so as to regulate
the local GABA concentration in CNS interstitial fluid—as appears to occur in satellite and Schwann cells in DRG and sympathetic perikaryal regions (Iversen et al., 1973, 1975).[3]

Enhancement of PADs in cord explants by exposure to 10^{-3} M GABA
may be due primarily to depolarization of DRG neurons to a level that
produces decreased threshold for excitation by applied stimulating current
or by impulses invading terminal DRG branches in the spinal cord. [Still
higher GABA concentrations may actually lead to sustained block of conduction, as shown by Sabelli et al. (1974) in frog dorsal (but not ventral) root
fibers exposed to 5×10^{-3} M GABA.] Alternatively, introduction of exogenous GABA may lead to greater GABA uptake into inhibitory interneurons, followed by increased GABA transmitter release. Although these
facilitating effects of exogenous GABA on PAD potentials may merely be
related to special conditions occurring in cord-DRG explants in culture,
they may nevertheless provide clues to regulatory mechanisms *in situ*.

This study demonstrates for the first time that at least some of the abundant additional neurites which develop after exposure of fetal DRG cells
to NGF can proceed to make characteristic long-term synaptic relationships with *specific* types of spinal cord neurons. The data also indicate that
responses resembling PADs can be generated in organized spinal cord-
DRG explants with remarkable mimicry of these specialized synaptic network functions *in situ*. Moreover, if further analyses of the greatly enhanced
PADS generated in spinal cord explants in response to the unusually large
input from NGF-hypertrophied DRGs do indeed demonstrate their relationship to presynaptic inhibitory functions, this may be evidence of an
intrinsic CNS regulatory system, involving development of compensatory
(homeostatic) inhibitory circuits proportional to the magnitude of the excitatory synaptic input (Crain, 1974a).

2. Innervation of Cord by Isolated DRGs

It has been noted in previous tissue culture studies that fetal rat DRGs
detached from spinal cord and explanted in close proximity to deafferented
spinal cord explants did not invade the CNS tissue (Peterson et al., 1965;
Bunge and Wood, 1973). Attempts have been recently made to clarify the
mechanisms underlying these complex cellular "barriers" by more systematic alterations of the experimental conditions under which DRG and

---

[3] This dramatic uptake and selective localization of GABA in DRG supporting cells may indeed represent a peripheral extension of the blood-brain barrier to prevent excessive sustained
depolarization of DRG neurons by fortuitous increases in circulating GABA levels following
ingestion of foods with high GABA concentrations, during metabolic disorders, etc.

cord neurons, and their associated supporting cells, may interact in culture. When a series of individual fetal mouse DRGs are positioned at various sites around a cross section of deafferented fetal mouse spinal cord, the NGF-stimulated neuritic growth pattern in relation to the cord explant is essentially similar to that observed without NGF. Although the DRG neuritic outgrowth is greatly enhanced, it still appears to bend away from the CNS tissue. (Meningeal covering of CNS tissues, which would present a formidable block to DRG invasion, was totally stripped prior to explantation.)

In order to provide experimental conditions more favorable to NGF-stimulated DRG invasion of CNS tissues, regions of the CNS rich in sensory target neurons, e.g., strips of *dorsal* cord instead of whole cross sections, were placed in close proximity (ca. 0.5 mm) to clusters of three to six DRGs (Peterson and Crain, 1975). Under these conditions neurites from at least some DRGs of a cluster readily invaded the target CNS explants and formed characteristic functional connections (Crain and Peterson, 1975c). Focal stimuli to initially isolated DRGs evoked prominent negative slow-wave potentials in dorsal cord explants, as in dorsal cord with attached DRGs (Fig. IV-19C) arising abruptly after latencies of a few milliseconds, with amplitudes up to 2 mV and often lasting more than 500 msec, resembling PAD responses *in situ*. In contrast to the successful DRG innervation of CNS target tissues, when strips of *ventral* cord were presented to similar DRG clusters most of the DRG neuritic outgrowth appeared to be deflected from the CNS explant. PADs were not elicited by stimuli to DRGs paired with ventral cord explants, although longer-latency, positive slow-wave or spike barrages were occasionally evoked. All of the DRG-evoked ventral cord responses were rapidly blocked in 10^{-3} M GABA, whereas the DRG-evoked PADs in dorsal cord were unaffected or enhanced at this GABA concentration (as in Fig. IV-19E). The DRG-evoked PADs were, however, depressed in 10^{-5} M bicuculline and blocked in 10^{-2} M Mg^{++}, as in cord with attached DRGs.

In cases where longitudinal slabs of *whole* spinal cord were used, neurites from isolated DRGs formed prominent fascicles which appeared to be preferentially directed toward dorsal cord target zones (thereby reconstituting "dorsal roots" *in vitro*: Crain and Peterson, *in preparation;* see also section C_2), whereas no evidence of functional DRG neurites could be detected by systematic focal stimulation in the adjacent growth zone associated with ventral cord regions. Furthermore, focal stimuli within nearby ventral cord regions (100–200 μm away) evoked only early-latency spike potentials in dorsal cord, whereas large PADs could be readily elicited with stimuli to distant DRGs (>2 mm away).

Besides the greatly increased density of outgrowing DRG neurites in high NGF, the rate of neurite elongation is also markedly enhanced. Migration of Schwann cells and meningeal tissue (the latter explanted with the DRGs) lags far behind the neuritic outgrowth. Under these conditions the

DRG neurites are essentially naked for at least the first 3 days, and they are therefore unencumbered by cellular elements which might interfere with successful DRG invasion of CNS explants. When the slowly migrating Schwann cells finally arrive at the zone of glial outgrowth from the CNS tissue, they stop abruptly.

Under the equivalent geometric conditions provided by these explant arrays, the apparently selective growth of DRG neurites toward specific regions of CNS tissue rich in sensory target neurons provides further support for the theory of "chemoaffinity in the orderly growth of nerve fiber patterns and connections" (Sperry, 1963), which may now be accessible to more direct analysis under rigidly controlled physicochemical conditions in CNS tissue cultures. Correlative histologic studies after selective labeling of the DRG cells innervating cord cross-sectional explants may clarify whether the central DRG neurites arborize *diffusely* throughout the cord tissue (as they often do when growing on homogeneous collagen gel substrates, e.g., Figs. IV-7;26) — making initial transitory contacts with all types of neurons including the final target cells — or whether they do indeed tend to be restricted to the dorsal horn regions as suggested by the microelectrode mapping experiments described above. Furthermore, if the DRG fibers are in fact concentrated primarily in the dorsal cord, is this due to "repulsion" by ventral cord tissue (see above) or to "tropic" (or trophic) effects exerted by target cells in the dorsal cord?

C. BRAINSTEM: SPECIFIC AND NONSPECIFIC NETWORKS

After showing that DRG neurons could establish characteristic functional synaptic networks in dorsal regions of spinal cord explants, we proceeded to prepare model systems suitable for analyzing further development of central DRG neurites up the neuraxis. Our earlier electrophysiologic studies showed that complex synaptic interactions could develop between neurons in explants of fetal rodent spinal cord and brainstem tissues after growth of neurites across gaps of 0.5–1 mm, but no signs of selective synaptic connections between specific types of neurons were detected (Crain and Peterson, 1966; Crain et al., 1968*b*). The neurites and glial cells often spread diffusely between the explants, requiring careful study under high magnification to detect the existence of neurites which had bridged the gap (Fig. IV-20). In some cases, on the other hand, a densely packed neuritic-glial bridge formed between the explant (Fig. IV-22).

1. Nonspecific Cord-Brainstem Connections

Simultaneous microelectrode recordings from paired spinal cord-brainstem explants demonstrated that spontaneous discharges arising in one explant may be regularly followed, after a latency ranging from several to

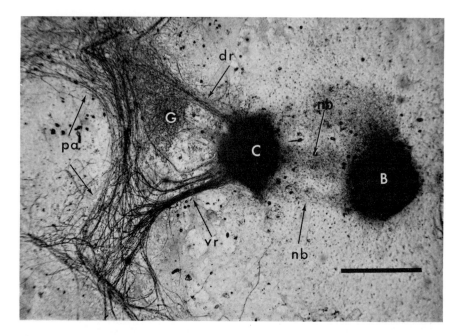

FIG. IV-20. Explant of rat spinal cord (C) with an attached DRG (G) located approximately 1 mm from an explant of rat brainstem (B); from 16-day fetal rat, 6 weeks *in vitro;* living, unstained culture. Note the long dorsal (dr) and ventral (vr) roots connected to the cord and the peripheral arborizations (pa) of these neurites. Note also the dense bands composed of neurites (and supporting cells) that have formed a "bridge" (nb) across the gap between the cord and brainstem explants (cf. Figs. IV-24;26). (Neurites in the bridge could be clearly seen at higher magnification.) A relatively large population of DRG neurons survives and matures in the absence of exogenous NGF when the DRGs are explanted from 16-day or older fetal rodents (as in Fig. 1-3; cf. 14-day fetal mouse DRGs in Fig. IV-17B). Scale: 1 mm. (From Crain, Peterson and Bornstein, 1968*b*.)

several hundred milliseconds, by long-lasting discharges in the other explant (Figs. IV-21;23). The synchrony between the onset of activity in each explant did not generally apply to the temporal pattern or duration of the discharges in the two tissues. Selective stimulation of DRGs attached to the cord explant (Fig. IV-21B) was utilized to ensure synaptic excitation of cord neurons without direct application of a stimulating electrode to the vicinity of the cord explant (see section B). This procedure precludes fortuitous antidromic excitation of brainstem neurites which had bridged the gap and may then have arborized within the cord explant. Under these conditions a brief DRG stimulus evoked an early discharge in the cord explant, which was sometimes followed by a longer-lasting discharge (ca. 1 sec) in the brainstem explant (Figs. IV-21B;23A$_3$). The latency between the onset of evoked activity in the two explants varied widely, as was also observed during spontaneous discharges, and is probably due to gradual activation of brainstem neurons through polysynaptic pathways from cord neurons (or vice

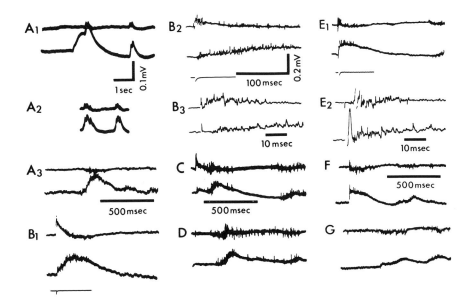

FIG. IV-21. Functional interneuronal connections between separate explants of fetal rat brainstem and spinal cord ganglia after maturation in culture. Simultaneous recordings from spinal cord (upper sweep) and brainstem explants, connected only by a *de novo* neuritic bridge across a 1-mm gap (Fig. IV-20). **A$_{1-3}$**: Spontaneous slow-wave potentials occurring synchronously in both explants. Activity appears to arise earlier in the brainstem explant (**A$_3$**). **B$_{1,2}$**: Long-lasting spike barrage and slow-wave potentials evoked in both explants by stimulus to the DRG attached to the spinal cord explant (located 1 mm away from the cord, in a direction opposite to the brainstem). Note the similarity between the response evoked in brainstem via the DRG-cord pathway and the spontaneous discharge (**B$_1$** and **A$_3$**, lower sweeps). Note also the 5-msec latency in onset of the brainstem barrage compared to the early appearance of cord activity (**B$_3$**). **C**: Stimulus to ventral root (500 μm from edge of cord) evokes a similar (but smaller) cord response as with DRG stimulation, and the latency of the major brainstem discharge is now greater than 100 msec. Note the resurgence of activity in both explants after a 400-msec silent period **(C)** and the spontaneous appearance shortly afterward of a discharge **(D)** similar to those evoked by cord stimulation. **E$_{1,2}$**: Stimulus to a small group of brainstem neurites (in growth zone, approximately 50 μm from the edge of the explant) also evokes long barrages in both explants, but now the cord response shows a minimum latency of several milliseconds (cf. **E$_2$** to **B$_2$**). **F**: Similar cord and brainstem responses are elicited by a stimulus applied within the brainstem explant (remote from the neuritic bridge). **G**: Spontaneous discharges again occur synchronously between the explants. (From Crain, Peterson, and Bornstein, 1968*b*.)

versa when the brainstem explant triggered the cord; e.g., Figs. IV-21A,E;23B). Spontaneous discharges occurred more commonly in the brainstem than cord explants in normal culture medium (Figs. IV-21A;23B), although the cord tended to become the pacemaker during exposure to strychnine (Fig. IV-23A$_{1,2}$). Functional connections between cord and brainstem explants were often difficult to detect prior to introduction of strychnine or bicuculline (10^{-6} M), even though complex activities could be generated within each explant. This suggests that inhibitory pathways may

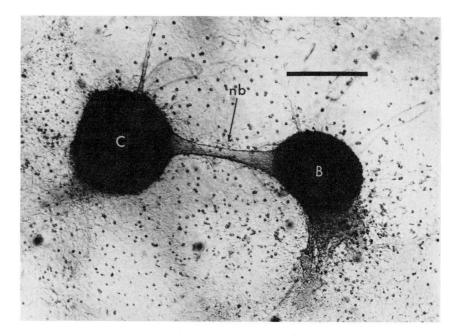

FIG. IV-22. Explant of rat spinal cord (C) located approximately 1 mm from an explant of rat brainstem (B), similar to the culture in Fig. IV-20 (16-day fetal rat; 1 month *in vitro;* living, unstained culture). Note the prominent neuritic bridge (nb) that has formed between the explants, in contrast to the diffuse bridge in Fig. IV-20. The DRG is out of the field, located approximately 1 mm from the cord, in a direction opposite to the medulla. Scale: 1 mm. (From Crain, Peterson, and Bornstein, 1968*b*.)

be involved in the circuits connecting the explants (Figs. VII-4;5; Chap. VII-B), although inhibitory circuits within each explant could also account for the effects of these pharmacologic agents. GABA (10^{-3} M), on the other hand, generally blocked transmission between these explants (see section B and below).

The essential role of the neuritic pathways in mediating the interactions between these nearby CNS explants is demonstrated by the complete abolition of transmission from one explant to another after microsurgical transection of the neuritic bridge across the gap (Figs. IV-22;23C). Additional controls have been made in a number of cultures to clarify the possible role of non-neural spread of current. In the first place, these bioelectric interactions between CNS explants are not seen in cases where neurites have not grown across the gap—even when the tissues are located less than 100 μm apart—although widespread complex activity may be evoked within each explant. Moreover, after acute midline transection of an explant, electric stimuli applied to the neural tissue on one side of the slit produced the usual bioelectric responses within the confines of the surgical boundary, but no activity was detected in the tissue beyond the incision (even when the gap was less than 10 μm wide). Controls demonstrating the absence of significant spread of applied stimulating currents have also been made systematically (e.g., Fig. IV-15A) (Crain et al., 1968*b*).

2. Specific Sensory Inputs to Medulla

In our more recent experiments aimed at facilitating *direct* DRG innervation of medulla target neurons, a midline section of the spinal cord cross section was made from the central canal through the dorsal cord and menin-

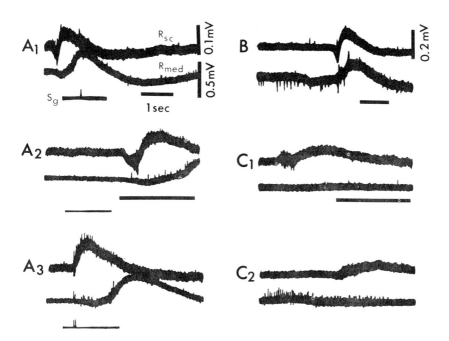

FIG. IV-23. Effect of surgical transection of the neuritic bridge between functionally coupled spinal cord and brainstem explants, similar to the array in Fig. IV-22 (14-day mouse fetus; 12 days *in vitro*). $A_{1,2}$: Simultaneous recordings of spontaneous activity of the spinal cord (R_{sc}, upper sweep) and medulla (R_{med}) explants connected by a neuritic bridge across a 300-μm gap (after application of strychnine at 10 μg/ml). A stimulus (S_g) was applied after the onset of spontaneous discharges and was ineffective (cf. A_3). Note synchronization of the slow waves generated by these explants and the long but regular latency of the medulla wave after the onset of cord activity. A_3: Application of a stimulus to the DRG, located approximately 400 μm from the edge of the cord (in a direction opposite to the medulla), evokes a similar cord-medulla discharge sequence as observed spontaneously (but the initial negative phase of the spontaneous cord slow wave does not occur). **B:** Synchronized spontaneous activity is still present after strychnine has been replaced by the control medium. Note that the *medulla* discharge now arises first (cf. $A_{1,2}$). C_1: Shortly after microsurgical transection of the neuritic bridge between the cord and medulla explants. Spontaneous (as well as electrically evoked) discharge in the cord no longer triggers the medulla, and the discharge in the latter can occur independently of cord activity (C_2). (From Crain, Peterson, and Bornstein, 1968*b*.)

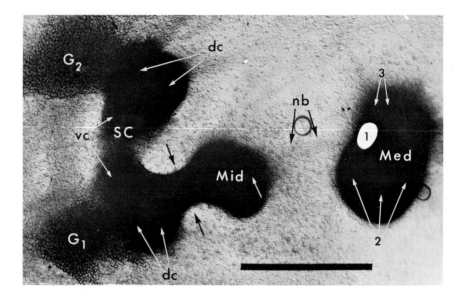

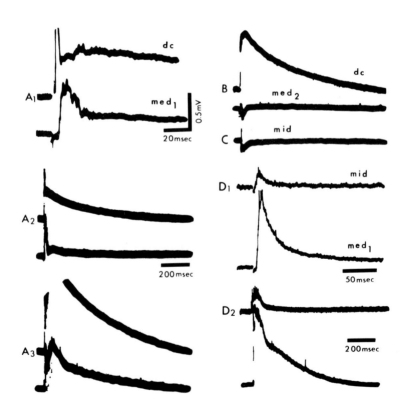

ges prior to explantation of fetal cord-DRG explants (Fig. IV-17). In the younger fetuses only the meninges required cutting since dorsal closure of the cord was not yet completed. This ensured outgrowth of CNS neurites and glial cells, including DRG fibers that have passed through the cord, comparable to dorsal column axons. Previous studies showed that "peripheral-type" neurites (invested by Schwann cells) did not invade separate CNS explants [Peterson et al., 1965; Bunge and Wood, 1973; however, see recent procedures which facilitate direct innervation of CNS tissues by isolated DRGs (section B2 and below)]. Fetal mouse brainstem explants were therefore carefully positioned near the dorsal edge of the cord cross sections so as to be in the path of the outgrowing "dorsal column" (Figs. IV-24;26) (Crain and Peterson, 1975a). Tissues from various regions of the medulla and midbrain were presented to the cord-DRG explant, including complete cross sections through the medulla at the level of the cuneate and gracilis nuclei (Figs. IV-25;26).

PADs similar to those evoked in dorsal cord explants have now been detected in small regions of medulla explants connected to cord with NGF-hypertrophied DRGs. The medulla PADs evoked by single DRG stimuli ranged up to 1 mV and arose after longer (ca. 3–10 msec) latencies (Figs. IV-24;25). The large amplitude of these PADs indicates that relatively large numbers of DRG terminals probably make synaptic connections with target neurons in the medulla explants. In cord-DRG cultures without added NGF, where only a few dozen DRG neurons may survive (Fig. IV-17B), dorsal cord PADs are often much smaller than these medulla PADs in spite of the abundant dorsal cord neurons available for establishing sensory synap-

---

FIG. IV-24. Negative slow-wave potentials resembling PADs evoked in spinal cord and brainstem explants by DRG stimuli (14-day fetal mouse tissues; 14 days in culture). **Top:** Photomicrograph shows spinal cord cross section (SC) with attached DRG ($G_{1,2}$). The dorsal edge of one-half of the cord is "fused" to the midbrain (Mid) explant (*black arrows*); a thinly spread array of neurites and glial cells have formed a bridge (nb) to the medulla (Med) explant (barely visible at this low magnification). Midline section of dorsal cord (see text) resulted in lateral displacment of the dorsal horns and DRGs at either end of the ventral cord (vc). Scale: 1 mm. **Bottom:** Simultaneous recordings of PADs in dorsal cord (dc, *lower left arrow* in photomicrograph) and medulla (Med, site 1) in response to a single DRG stimulus (G_1). Note abrupt onset and long duration of these potentials; also longer latency of medulla response. A_2: Same, but at slower sweep rate. A_3: Brief 100/sec DRG volley (at smaller, near-threshold stimulus strength) elicits much larger and longer-lasting PADs in both cord and medulla. **B:** Large DRG_1 stimulus evoked only small, positive slow-wave responses in other regions of medulla explant (Med_2); the dorsal cord PAD is still large. Microelectrode mapping showed no signs of medulla PADs in response to DRG stimuli, except in the zone indicated in white around site 1, and none in the entire midbrain (Mid) explant (e.g., at *white arrow;* record **C**). D_1: After adding 10^{-3} M GABA, PAD in medulla (Med_1) shows marked increase in amplitude and duration (as in Fig. IV-25B), and it can now also be evoked in adjacent region 3; the polarity of the midbrain response (Mid) has now become negative, although still relatively small. D_2: Brief 100/sec DRG volley elicits still larger and longer-lasting PAD in the medulla "target zone" (Med_1). (From Crain and Peterson, 1975a.)

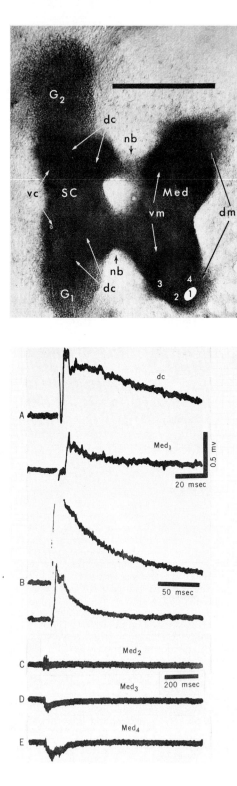

FIG. IV-25. PAD responses evoked in dorsal region of spinal cord (SC) and medulla (Med) explants (complete cross sections) by DRG stimuli (14-day fetal mouse tissues; 14 days in culture). **Top:** Medulla cross section is at the level of the cuneate and gracilis nuclei; dorsal closure has not yet occurred at this fetal stage so that the dorsal medulla tissues (dm) are laterally displaced. Note the bridges (neurites and glia) which have formed between the dorsal edge of the cord (dc) and the ventral edge of the medulla (vm) explants in two regions (nb); DRGs ($G_{1,2}$) are located more laterally in this explant (cf. Fig. IV-24), further away from the ventral cord (vc). Scale: 1 mm. **Bottom: A:** Simultaneous recordings of PADs in dorsal cord (dc, *lower left arrow* in photomicrograph) and dorsal medulla (Med, site 1) in response to a single DRG_1 stimulus. **B:** After adding 10^{-3} M GABA, PADs at this site in medulla (Med_1) and in dorsal cord are augmented (as in Fig. IV-24D). **C:** A large DRG_1 stimulus evokes only a spike burst at site 2 in the medulla (Med_2) and small positive slow-wave responses at $Med_{3,4}$ **(D,E).** Systematic mapping of entire medulla explant showed no signs of PADs in response to DRG stimuli except in a small zone indicated in white around Med_1 (ca. 0.1×0.2 mm), even during GABA exposure. (Mapping was not attempted in this culture with stimuli to DRG_2.) (From Crain and Peterson, 1975a.)

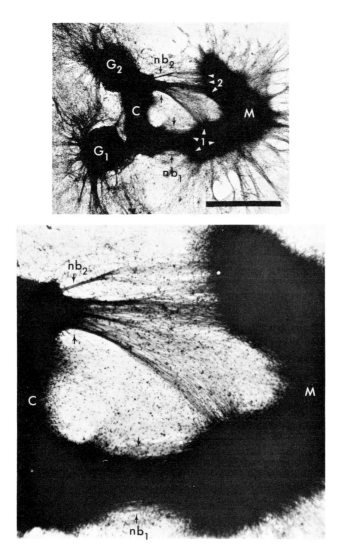

FIG. IV-26. Photomicrographs of a pair of spinal cord-DRG and medulla explants (as in Fig. IV-25 but separated by a larger gap), showing details of the neuritic bridges that formed between the two explants (14-day fetal mouse tissues). **Top:** Medulla explant (M) consists of à cross section at the level of the cuneate and gracilis nuclei, and is positioned so that the dorsal edge faces the dorsal edge of the cord explant (C) (cf. Fig. IV-25 where the ventral edge of the medulla faces the dorsal cord). The cord-DRG explant was added to a 1-week-old medulla culture, and the paired array was then maintained for two additional weeks *in vitro*. Note the broad neuritic bridge (nb_1) which formed between the dorsolateral regions of the lower parts of the cord and medulla explants (including the "dorsal column" fibers; see text). Note also the prominent array of neurites (nb_2), which appears to have emerged from the dorsolateral edge of the upper part of the cord explant and then to have fanned out so that a major component reached the "contralateral" dorsal medulla region (near area 1); there is also a direct bridge to the "ipsilateral" medulla (near area 2). **Bottom:** Higher-power view of these complex neuritic bridges. Large PAD responses were evoked in area 1 in the lower part of the medulla explant by stimuli to lower DRG (G_1; as in Fig. IV-25A), but no PADs could be detected in the contralateral (upper) side of the medulla explant. On the other hand, stimuli to upper DRG (G_2) elicited smaller but clear-cut PADs in "target" areas in *both* sides of medulla, in areas 1 and 2. All of these DRG-evoked PAD responses were maintained or enhanced during exposure to 10^{-3} M GABA (as in Figs. IV-24;25). Furthermore, no PADs could be detected in the entire medial region of the medulla explant (between areas 1 and 2) even with maximal stimuli to G_1 or G_2. (From Crain and Peterson, *in preparation*.)

tic networks with ingrowing DRG neurites (e.g., Fig. IV-19A,B) (Crain and Peterson, 1974b, 1975b). Introduction of 10^{-3} M GABA generally augmented the brainstem and dorsal cord PADs (Figs. IV-24D;25B), whereas various cord-evoked brainstem network discharges were seriously depressed, as were ventral cord responses. Moreover, in cases where a midbrain explant was positioned between the cord and medulla, prominent DRG-evoked PADs were detected only in the latter explant, even when it was located more than 1 mm distal to the interposed midbrain tissue (cf. Fig. IV-24A and IV-24C). Weak PADs, however, could be detected in some midbrain regions, especially when medulla target neurons were relatively distant (Fig. IV-24D) or absent. Using this pharmacologic marker technique, we have been able to map more than 20 DRG-cord-brainstem cultures, and in most cases PADs were sharply localized to one or two small zones (ca. 100–300 μm) in each medulla explant. In 10 cultures where cross sections of the entire medulla at the level of the cuneate and gracilis nuclei were presented to the DRG-cord explant with controlled orientation, prominent PADs were evoked only in the *dorsal* medulla regions (Fig. IV-25), precisely where dorsal column sensory fibers normally terminate and lead to PADs *in situ* (Andersen et al., 1964; Eccles, 1964; Wall, 1964; Davidson and Southwick, 1971). Similar results were obtained in cultures where the medulla cross section was rotated 90° or 180° (Fig. IV-26) with respect to its orientation to the cord explant in Fig. IV-25 (note the interesting divergence of part of the neuritic bridge, containing "dorsal column" fibers, to the "contralateral" medulla).

These *in vitro* experiments demonstrate that DRG neurites, after passing through spinal cord tissue, can grow across a homogeneous collagen-film substrate and, in mimicry of dorsal column fibers *in situ*, establish characteristic functional synaptic networks with programmed target neurons in brainstem explants, even in the presence of a variety of alternative CNS neurons with abundant synaptogenic receptor sites (see also Olson and Bunge, 1973). Furthermore, although the initial neuritic and glial spinal cord outgrowth in relation to these nearby medulla explants was comparable to that extending toward nontarget CNS tissues, preliminary analyses in suitably arrayed cultures suggest that prominent fascicles of "dorsal column fibers" may become organized toward the target neuron zones in the medulla (Fig. IV-26) (Crain and Peterson, *in preparation*). In more recent studies with *isolated* DRGs positioned near medulla explants (see section B2), we have also demonstrated that DRG neurites can, under favorable NGF stimulation, grow directly into medulla cross sections. Focal stimulation of DRG neurites located 1–2 mm from the medulla explant could evoke characteristic PADs in dorsolateral medulla target zones, whereas similar stimuli applied within nearby ventral or medial regions of the medulla explant (100–200 μm away) were often ineffective. The remarkable degree of characteristic pharmacologic sensitivity and regional specificity of these sensory-evoked spinal cord and brainstem networks provides the basis for a powerful new model system to analyze mechanisms underlying formation and development of specific synaptic connections in the mammalian CNS (Sperry, 1963, 1965) under isolated conditions in culture (see also Weiss, 1955, 1966; Jacobson, 1970).

3. Monoaminergic Brainstem Systems

Although no systematic electrophysiologic studies have yet been reported on brainstem monoaminergic neurons *in vitro,* a number of preliminary biochemical and histofluorescence analyses of brainstem cultures demonstrate the feasibility of maintaining functional noradrenergic, serotonergic, and dopaminergic systems in culture. Biochemical analyses of explants from newborn rat brainstem raphe nuclei, after 1–3 weeks *in vitro,* indicate maintenance of characteristic serotonin turnover properties (Halgren and Varon, 1972). Furthermore, explants from newborn rat substantia nigra, after 3–6 days *in vitro,* show increasing ability to take up ^{3}H-dopamine as well as characteristic histofluorescence patterns (Coyle et al., 1973). Brief reports by Shoemaker et al. (1974) and Schlumpf and Shoemaker (1975) noted that explants of locus ceruleus and substantia nigra from 17- to 19-day fetal rats show a characteristic capacity to synthesize norepinephrine and dopamine, respectively, during assays of both culture media and cells after 2–3 weeks *in vitro.* The neurons in these brainstem explants appeared to be "healthy . . . as judged by morphological appearance, process formation, the ability to produce spontaneous and induced action potentials [as well as] synthesis of catecholamine neurotransmitters" (Shoemaker et al., 1974).[4] Although no evidence of synaptic network activities was noted in these brainstem explant studies, similar types of explants have indeed been shown to generate complex synaptically mediated discharges (e.g., Figs. IV-20;22; VII-4-6). In the latter studies, however, no attempt was made to determine if any of the bioelectric activities were associated with monoaminergic neurons.

An exciting brainstem tissue culture model was also developed by Levitt et al. (1975) involving histofluorescence analyses during the reaggregation *in vitro* of dissociated cell suspensions derived from 13- to 18-day embryonic mouse midbrain regions and allowed to differentiate in rotating-shaker cultures for 1–7 days (Chap. II-A2). Dopaminergic (DA) neurons retained histofluorescence immediately after dissociation and could be followed

---

[4] Recent studies of the uptake of ^{3}H-noradrenaline and ^{3}H-serotonin in explants of 18-day fetal rat medulla and pons after 10–28 days in culture showed a strong selective accumulation in a small proportion of the neurons within the explants and in the outgrowing neurites (Hösli et al., 1975b). In contrast, previous studies of uptake of amino acid transmitters into spinal cord and brainstem explants demonstrated that glycine, GABA, and glutamate were not only taken up by neurons but to a great extent also by glial cells (Hösli et al., 1973, 1975a).

throughout their development in culture. Randomly dispersed DA neurons in suspension were observed to associate selectively, first grouping into several small clusters within each aggregate by 48 hr and then forming a single thick, elongated band across one side of the aggregate by 4–5 days in culture. This reorganization within an aggregate of a structure closely resembling the morphology of the substantia nigra during its migratory phase *in situ* was accompanied by increasing levels of dopamine, as determined by radioisotopic assay.

These preliminary studies of brainstem explants in culture provide encouraging evidence that monoaminergic neurons may develop and maintain localized concentrations of characteristic neurotransmitters after isolation *in vitro*. It will be of great interest to extend these experiments with correlative electrophysiologic, pharmacologic, and histofluorescence analyses of locus ceruleus, raphe, and substantia nigra explants, suitably paired with various CNS target explants, e.g. cerebellum and hippocampus. Deplants (1 mm³) (Chap. I-A) of these types of fetal rat monoaminergic brainstem tissues were recently studied during development in the rat anterior eye chamber (Olson and Seiger, 1972, 1973, 1974). Fluorescence histochemical analyses demonstrated that noradrenergic (NA), DA, and serotonergic (5-HT) neurons sprouted neurites in the eye chamber, and all were able to form characteristic plexuses within denervated host iris to which the brainstem deplants became attached and from which they became vascularized. The neuritic arborizations produced in iris musculature by brainstem monoaminergic neurons deplanted into the eye chamber appear to be comparable to those observed by Silberstein et al. (1971) in cultures of sympathetic ganglia where neurites formed patterned plexuses in nearby iris explants (Chap. III-B). In both cases the pattern of iris reinnervation may be determined by the Schwann cell plexus remaining in the iris after sympathetic denervation, and the ingrowing fibers seem to adapt to this pattern without the fibers losing their transmitter identities (Olson and Seiger, 1972, 1974). Olson and Seiger (1975) demonstrated, moreover, that NA neurons in deplants of locus ceruleus and 5-HT neurons in raphe deplants also grew neurites which arborized within the muscle layers of separate deplants of vas deferens positioned near the brainstem tissues in the rat eye chamber. The transmitter mechanisms of grafted central NA, DA, and 5-HT fibers innervating sympathetically denervated iris were also studied recently. It was shown that all three types of monoamine neurons are able to accumulate labeled transmitters *in vitro* and to release them on electric field stimulation in the same way as their normal CNS counterparts (Seiger et al., 1976).

These elegant deplant experiments provide a valuable new model system for analyses of brainstem monoaminergic systems, and they will undoubtedly encourage extension of the studies from *in oculo* to *in vitro* chambers [just as our earlier analyses of the development of organotypic activities in cultures of fetal mouse cerebral explants (Crain and Bornstein, 1964; Crain,

1966) (see section D) probably stimulated recent developmental studies of cerebral *deplants* in the rat eye chamber (Chap. I) (Seiger and Olson, 1975; see also Hoffer et al., 1975*b*, 1976; Olson et al., 1976)]. As Olson and Seiger (1974) remarked, "intraocular brain tissue transplantations [provide] a most useful experimental model for a number of different purposes to complement other available methods of experimental neurosurgery and tissue culture. Defined areas of the developing CNS can be isolated from normal input and output connections and its further development studied. Rapid vascularization permits a good taking and growth of the transplants. No adverse immunological reactions have been observed using inbred rats." Correlative studies of deplants and explants of neural tissues will undoubtedly lead to many fruitful insights as the same isolated tissues are analyzed during development in different physicochemical environments. Neural deplants growing in isolation from all other parts of the nervous system, but in relatively normal contact with the host's circulatory system, should provide valuable guides and baselines for a variety of experimental manipulations and simplifications which can be more easily introduced into the culture environment of similar neural explants growing *in vitro* (Chap. I-A).

An interesting difference between development of brain explants in culture and similar-sized (ca. 1 mm³) deplants in the rat eye chamber is the remarkable increase in volume which occurs as the deplant matures intraocularly — to as large as 10–30 mm³ (Olson and Seiger, 1974; Olson et al., 1976). This is in contrast to the relatively small change in volume of CNS explants even after months of maturation of the neuronal networks. Comparison of the functions of similar CNS tissues after this marked divergence in structure during maturation *in vitro* and *in oculo* may provide valuable information regarding the role of the additional cellular elements that develop in the deplants.

One aspect of the studies with brainstem deplants that is important to analyze more critically in culture relates to Olson and Seiger's (1974) conclusion that "there seems to be a *general lack of specificity* between different monoamine neurons towards various receptor areas, since any type of central or peripheral monamine neurons can reinnervate a sympathetically denervated iris. Regardless of the neuronal input, the innervation pattern is determined by the receptor organ. . . . Many CNS monoamine neurons thus seem to have a general programming to fill up receptor areas, which may explain the readiness by which the iris becomes reinnervated. In this respect, the monoamine neurons seem to be the absolute opposite to the highly specified neurons of the retinotectal projection with an almost cell to cell specificity." Furthermore, the possible role of NGF in regulating growth of embryonic CNS monoaminergic neurons and the demonstrated NGF enhancement of sprouting of injured adult brainstem catecholaminergic neurons (Bjerre et al., 1973; Stenevi et al., 1974) should be amenable to more direct analyses in brainstem cultures (see also Crain, 1973*c*).

D. CEREBRAL NEOCORTEX, HIPPOCAMPUS, AND LIMBIC REGIONS

1. Early Functions

Explants of late fetal or newborn mouse cerebral neocortex (frontal region) (Fig. IV-27) show a sequence of developmental changes in bioelectric properties similar to those in 13- to 14-day fetal rodent spinal cord cultures during the first week after explantation (Crain, 1964a; Crain and Bornstein, 1964, 1974; morphologic correlates in Bornstein, 1964; Kim, 1972a; Seil et al., 1974). Serial microscopic examinations of the cultures grown in Maximow slide chambers provide cytologic evidence of the growth and differentiation of the cerebral tissue *in vitro* (Bornstein, 1964) and facilitate selection of suitable cultures for bioelectric experiments. During the first few days, many neuritic processes grow out from the explanted fragment (e.g., Fig. IV-27B). They are particularly numerous in the region near the original cortical surface (Fig. IV-27A) and eventually surround the fragment with a dense felt-like layer. Neuroglia cells migrate from the edges of the fragment and mingle with the fine neurites in the outgrowth zone (Fig. IV-27B). Neurites are also observed within the explant itself where numerous cell bodies nestle into the dense, intertwining neuropil. Within 4–5 days neuron somas become distinguishable within the explant. In the region near the original cortical edge of the explant, they are small (ca. 20 μm in diameter) but extremely numerous and closely packed. In other areas of the fragment, particularly those derived from the deeper layers of the cerebral cortex, neurons appear somewhat larger and more widely separated by neuroglia and neuritic processes. Laminar arrays of neurons can be observed in living cerebral explants after months in culture (Fig. IV-28B), and they have also been demonstrated with selective histologic stains (Fig. IV-28A,C) (Seil et al., 1974; see below). In the deepest zone of the explant containing subcortical tissue (near SCE in Fig. IV-27), some of the axons may become myelinated after 2–3 weeks *in vitro* (Bornstein, 1964).

Only simple spike potentials could be evoked during the first 2 days after explantation of newborn mouse cerebral neocortex (Fig. IV-29A). Up to this stage, there have been no clear-cut signs of long-lasting excitatory phenomena or other complexities indicative of synaptic interactions. Analogous with cerebral recordings *in situ*, regions near the original surface of the cortex (e.g., zone 1 in Fig. IV-27) are referred to as superficial in contrast to those at greater "cortical depths" (e.g., zones 2 or 3). Diphasic action potentials, recorded simultaneously from two cortical areas of these immature explants in response to a brief stimulus applied to a deeper region of the tissue (Fig. IV-29A), indicate propagation of impulses toward the cortical surface. One group arrives at a deep recording locus after a latency of approximately 1 msec, and another at the more superficial locus after 1.8 msec. The duration of the negative phase of these

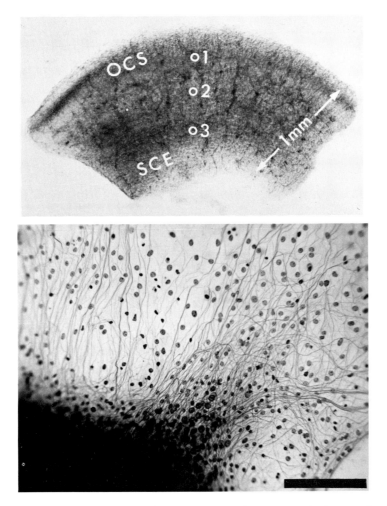

FIG. IV-27. Photomicrographs of explants of neonatal mouse cerebral neocortex. **Top:** Low-power view shortly after explantation (ca. 0.5 mm thick). OCS, original cortical surface. SCE, subcortical edge. The tissue has assumed the characteristic crescent shape it generally maintains for months *in vitro.* Focal recording electrodes were often positioned in contact with the tissue, at 1 and 2; and a cathodal stimulating lead is placed at 3. Indifferent electrodes were located near each active electrode, in fluid just below tissue. The distance of the locus from the original cortical surface is referred to as "cortical depth" (see text). **Bottom:** Higher-power view of the edge of the explant (lower left) after 3 weeks *in vitro,* showing numerous neurites which grew out from cerebral tissue during the first week after explantation along with many neuroglia cells. Bodian silver impregnation. Calibration bar: 100 μm. (From Crain and Bornstein, 1964.)

spikes is approximately 2–3 msec, and their amplitudes may reach 600 μV. Only crude estimates of conduction velocity along these neurites can be made at present because of difficulty in determining the actual pathways traversed. The values appear to be of the order of 0.4 meters/sec, which

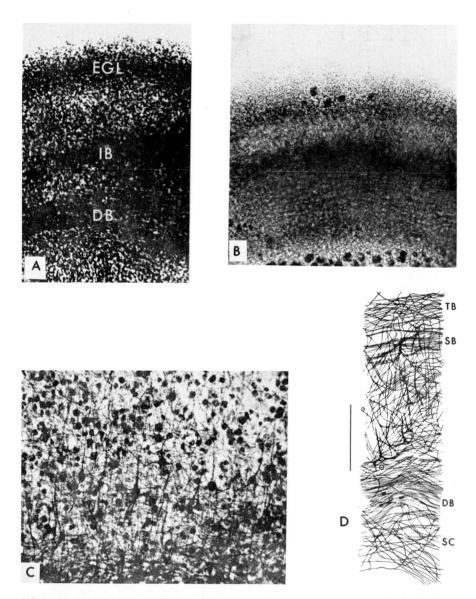

FIG. IV-28. Laminar organization of neonatal mouse cerebral neocortex explants. **A:** Horizontal laminar organization is demonstrated, after 3 weeks *in vitro,* with Holmes' silver impregnation. An external granular layer of neurons (EGL) can be clearly distinguished (lying between the tangential and submarginal bands), as can an intermediate band (IB) and a deep band (DB) of fibers. Subcortical tissue is seen ventral to the deep band. ×64. **B:** Laminar organization is still clearly evident in living unstained cerebral explant after 3 months *in vitro* (slightly lower magnification than in **A**). **C:** Pyramidal cell neurons in a cerebral neocortex explant similar to that in **A** (3 weeks *in vitro*) are distinguished by their vertically oriented apical dendrites and appear prominently in the lower two-thirds of the explant, ventral to the submarginal band. Holmes' silver impregnation. ×240. **D:** Drawing based on a camera lucida tracing of a Holmes-stained cerebral neocortical culture (3 weeks *in vitro*) (lower magnification than in **C**). Shown are the tangential band (TB), submarginal band (SB), and deep band (DB) of fibers, as well as subcortical neurites (SC). Also shown are some impregnated neurons. (This explant has no organized intermediate band.) Vertical bar: 200 μm. (**A, C, D** from Seil, Kelly, and Leiman, 1974. **B:** Photomicrograph provided by M. B. Bornstein; see also related figures in Bornstein, 1964.)

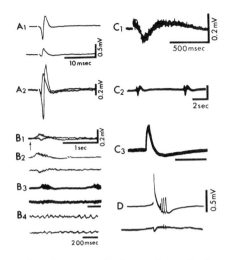

FIG. IV-29. Onset of complex slow-wave discharges in cerebral neocortex tissue cultures by 3 days after explanation from newborn mice. A_1: Simultaneous recordings of brief early-latency spike potentials evoked at "cortical depths" of 200 μm (upper sweep) and 400 μm by a single stimulus applied near the subcortical edge of the explant (ca. 800 μm from OCS; see Figs. IV-27;28). A_2: Superimposition of responses as in A_1, at a higher gain. Note the longer latency of the negative phase of the superficial as compared to the deep action potential. B_1: At slow sweep rate, the long-duration negative slow-wave potential rises, with a long latency (ca. 100 msec) following the early spike at a superficial site (shown alone in upper sweep of record B_2); also note the long-duration positivity (shown alone in the lower sweep of B_2) which develops with a still longer latency after the early deep spike. *Arrow* indicates onset of the stimulus in record B_1. Small-amplitude repetitive potentials (ca. 10–20/sec) occur during the falling phase of the slow waves. B_2: Similar responses evoked by a pair of stimuli spaced 50 msec apart, resulting in decreased latency as compared to B_1. Note that the second pair of stimuli in B_2, applied 1 sec after the first pair, is ineffective. B_3: Spontaneous bursts of 10–20/sec potentials lasting approximately 1 sec. B_4: Single spontaneous repetitive burst at a faster sweep. C_1: Long-duration triphasic response, including barrages of spikes, evoked in another 3-day explant by a single stimulus located in another region of the explant, approximately 0.5 mm away. C_2: Spontaneous bursts similar to the evoked response in C_1, but at a lower gain and slower sweep rate. C_3: Large, spontaneous, negative "sharp wave" after introduction of strychnine (10^{-5} M), lasting more than 600 msec and followed by a 2-sec positivity (cf. Figs. IV-30A_4 *in situ* and Fig. IV-32A,B in a younger explant). **D:** In 6-day cerebral explant, strychnine "sharp wave" is larger in amplitude and shorter in duration (cf. Fig. IV-30B_4). Lower sweep shows a simultaneous recording in another region of the explant. (From Crain, 1964a.)

agree with those obtained by Purpura et al. (1960) and Grafstein (1963) for conductile elements in neonatal cerebral cortex *in situ*. Attempts to evoke responses in these regions of the explant (zones 1 and 2) by application of stimuli near the original cortical surface were ineffective at this early stage *in vitro*. Application of dual stimuli shows that these action potentials arise in conductile neural elements which display characteristic refractoriness following electric excitation (as in immature spinal cord explants; Fig. IV-1A). The potentials are due to the summation of spikes from small groups of synchronously active neurons, as shown by the graded increase in response amplitude with increasing stimulus strength (Crain, 1964*a*) (see also Fig. IV-1A). At times the action potentials occur spontaneously and resemble repetitive unit-spike activity as seen in cultured cerebellum (Hild and Tasaki, 1962) (see section E), in contrast to the larger-amplitude compound action potentials evoked by electric stimuli.

Within 3 days after explantation from newborn mice, much more complex response patterns may be evoked in cerebral cultures under the same stimulus and recording conditions as described above. A long-duration negativity may arise, for example, with a latency of approximately 100 msec after the early superficial spike (Fig. IV-29B) and a long-duration positivity, with a still greater latency after the early deep spike. The long-lasting responses (ca. 400 msec) may be only 50–100 μV in amplitude, whereas the early spikes often reach 600 μV (Fig. IV-29A$_2$). In these cultures, as in explants maintained for longer periods *in vitro* (Fig. IV-37B,C), the slow waves recorded from superficial loci are generally negative while those from deep loci are positive (even when the stimulus is applied to more superficial regions). The slow waves and superimposed rhythmic, repetitive discharges may appear spontaneously (Fig. IV-29B) in bursts (ca. 1 sec) occurring sporadically several times per minute. The amplitude and duration of these complex discharges were greatly enhanced by strychnine (Fig. IV-29C), resembling the onset of strychnine sensitivity in electro-corticographic recordings of 4-day-old rat cerebral neocortex *in situ* (Fig. IV-30) (Crain, 1952, 1970*b*, 1975*a*). Most other electrophysiologic studies of neonatal rodent cerebral cortex have also failed to detect synaptically mediated activities until 3–4 days after birth (Kobayashi et al., 1963; Deza and Eidelberg, 1967; see reviews by Ellingson and Rose, 1970; Myslivecek, 1970). Armstrong-James and Williams (1963, 1964), on the other hand, obtained complex evoked potentials by direct electric stimuli in 1-day-old rat cerebral cortex *in situ* (section 2). Because of the drugs that have generally been used to immobilize these neonatal animals for physiologic studies, as well as technical problems involved in bioelectric recording from fragile CNS tissues *in situ,* data on the onset and early development of cerebral synaptic network activities are still quite fragmentary and ambiguous, especially with regard to the possible role of inhibitory systems at the earliest stage of synaptogenesis.

Explants of *fetal* mouse cerebral tissues have therefore been used in more recent studies as a model system to facilitate direct microelectrode recordings and pharmacologic manipulations during the critical developmental period just before birth (Crain and Bornstein, 1974; Crain et al., 1975*b*). Only simple early-latency spike potentials could be elicited by large single, or repetitive, electric stimuli in 18-day fetal hippocampus and neocortex explants after 1–2 days *in vitro* (Fig. IV-31A; see also Fig. IV-29A). This restricted activity was all that could be detected, even after altering the chemical environment in various ways that greatly enhance

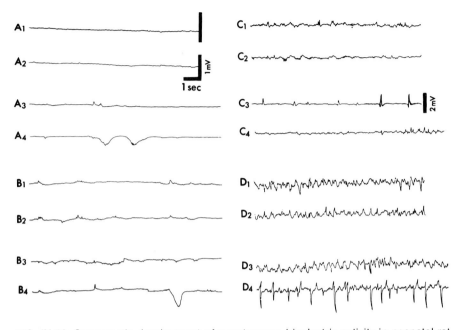

FIG. IV-30. Ontogenetic development of spontaneous bioelectric activity in neonatal rat cerebral cortex *in situ* and effects of strychnine. **A:** Four days after birth. **A₁:** Spontaneous activity recorded from the left frontal-parietal skull. **A₂:** Simultaneous recording from the right frontal-parietal cortex. (**A₃,₄**): Same as **A₁,₂** after application of strychnine crystals near the electrode on the right parietal cortex. Note the two large waves in **A₄**, each approximately 1 sec in duration (cf. Fig. IV-29C₃). **B:** Seven days after birth. **B₁:** Spontaneous activity recorded from left frontal-parietal cortex. **B₂:** Simultaneous recording from left parietal-occipital cortex. Note the development of sporadic burst activity as compared to **A₁,₂**. **B₃,₄:** Same as **B₁,₂** after application of strychnine to left occipital cortex. Note that the "sharp wave" in **B₄** is shorter in duration and larger in amplitude than in **A₄** (cf. Fig. IV-29D; see also Fig. IV-32A,B). **C:** Ten days after birth. **C₁:** Spontaneous activity recorded from left frontal-parietal cortex. **C₂:** Simultaneous recording from right frontal-parietal skull. Note the more regular, rhythmic activity compared to that in **B₁,₂**. **C₃,₄:** Same as **C₁,₂** after application of strychnine to the left parietal cortex. Note the much shorter duration and larger amplitude of sharp waves in **C₃** (gain was reduced threefold). **D:** Fourteen days after birth. **D₁:** Spontaneous activity recorded from right frontal-parietal skull. **D₂:** Simultaneous recording from left frontal-parietal cortex. Note the larger amplitude and still greater regularity of these EEG patterns compared to those in **C₁,₂**. **D₃,₄:** Same as **D₁,₂** after application of strychnine to left frontal cortex. Note the greater frequency of occurrence of sharp waves in **D₄**. [*Note:* Bipolar recordings were made with chloridized silver-core wick electrodes and were fed through a differential input, DC amplifier into an oscillograph. Rats were paralyzed with *d*-tubocurarine (0.2–1 mg/kg), artificially respired, and maintained at approximately 37°C.] (From Crain, 1952, 1970*b*.)

generation of complex discharges in older cultures (e.g., strychnine, picrotoxin, bicuculline, chloride-free medium; Chap. VI). The early spike responses were often of large amplitude and indicated propagation of impulses through many of the neurites in the explant, but no spike barrages or slow-wave potentials could be elicited at these stages.

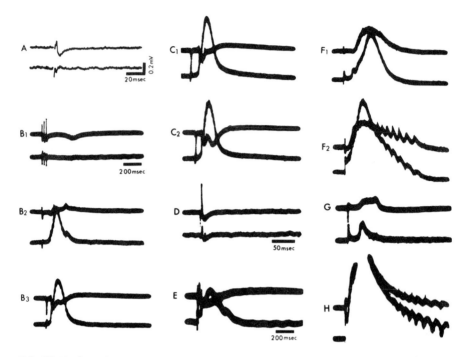

FIG. IV-31. Complex bioelectric discharges evoked in explants of 18-day fetal mouse hippocampus after 3–5 days in culture. **A:** Only simple, early-latency spike potentials could be elicited in this 3-day explant in response to single or repetitive stimuli in normal medium (BSS). (All recordings were made with electrodes at two sites approximately 0.5 mm apart in response to a stimulus applied to a third region of the explant about 0.5 mm away.) **B$_1$:** Shortly after introduction of strychnine (ca. 10^{-5} M), positive slow-wave potentials with small amplitude and long latency could now be evoked at one site (upper sweep) with repetitive stimuli (three or four at 50/sec). **B$_2$:** Several minutes later the negative slow-wave potentials with larger amplitudes and shorter latencies could be elicited at both sites, even with single stimuli (cf. Fig. IV-29C). These responses were quite labile, and rest periods of approximately a minute were generally required even with large stimuli. **B$_3$:** Similar but larger-amplitude responses were evoked occasionally after a return to BSS (lower sweep). **C$_1$:** Within 1 min after replacing regular BSS with a chloride-free BSS (propionate substituted for all chloride ions), the amplitude of the negative slow-wave response at one recording site (lower sweep) increased by nearly 50%. **C$_2$:** Shortly afterward, the response at other recording site (upper sweep) became more complex, involving an additional positive phase followed by an enhanced, longer-lasting negative phase. **D:** In another hippocampal explant from the same batch, only simple spike potentials could be evoked in BSS even after 5 days *in vitro*. **E:** Introduction of strychnine (ca. 10^{-5} M) led to the appearance of prominent slow-wave responses as in the 3-day explant (cf. **B$_{2,3}$**). **F:** Removal of chloride ions by introducing propionate-BSS dramatically enhanced the evoked responses, i.e., doubling of the amplitude of the negative slow-wave potential (lower sweep), inversion of the positive slow-wave potential at the other recording site (upper sweep), and onset of long-lasting repetitive oscillatory (ca. 10/sec) potentials at both sites (**F$_2$**). **G:** Responses became much smaller again after returning to the regular BSS. **H:** Huge primary negative slow-wave potentials and secondary oscillatory discharges can be evoked again after removal of the chloride ions, as in **F**. (From Crain and Bornstein, 1974.)

On the other hand, by 3 days *in vitro,* although most 18-day fetal explants still showed only simple spike responses to electric stimuli when bathed in normal medium (Fig. IV-31A), much more complex discharges could be evoked after introducing relatively low concentrations of strychnine (Figs. IV-31B;32), picrotoxin, or bicuculline (ca. 10^{-5} M), or by transfer to a chloride-free medium (Fig. IV-31C). Negative slow-wave potentials reached large amplitudes, especially in a chloride-free medium (Chap. VI-D). These trends were still more evident in 5-day-old explants (cf. Fig. IV-31F_2,H and IV-31C). The complex responses in 3-day cultures were extremely labile and generally required rest periods of approximately a minute even with large stimuli. The thresholds were often high, and stimulus intensities approximately 10 times larger than usual were necessary to evoke slow-wave discharges at this early stage. The response latencies were also generally much longer than in older cultures, ranging up to 100 msec (Figs. IV-31;32). Adding caffeine (10^{-3} M) to the above drugs was often quite effective in reducing the threshold and decreasing the postdischarge depression period, and frequently led to the onset of spontaneous discharges. This effect may be related to the potency of caffeine and other phosphodiesterase inhibitors, as well as exogenous cyclic AMP, in facilitating synaptic transmission in CNS explants during depression produced by calcium-ion deficits (Chap. VI-E) (Crain and Pollack, 1973; Crain, 1974*a,b*). Generation of the drug-induced slow-wave discharges by Ca^{++}-dependent synaptic transmitter release is indicated by the rapid and complete block of these complex potentials after increasing the Mg^{++} concentration from 1 to 5–10 mM, whereas spikes could still be directly evoked (Chap. VI-E) (Crain, 1974*a,b*). The complex network discharges often occurred synchronously over widespread regions of the explant (Fig. IV-32C_2), even at these early stages of synaptogenesis. The onset and early development of complex synaptically mediated network discharges occurred similarly in 18-day fetal mouse neocortex explants after 3 days *in vitro,* in contrast to the relatively precocious activity of hippocampus (compared to neocortex) in the neonatal kitten *in situ* (Purpura et al., 1968). The threshold for activating these discharges was often much lower, however, in 3-day explants of hippocampus compared to neocortex.

Even in the 5-day-old cultures (from 18-day fetuses)—which might be equivalent in maturity to 1- to 2-day postnatal mouse tissue *in situ* (assuming a gestation period of 21 days)—evoked responses in normal BSS were relatively simple and brief (Fig. IV-31D). Furthermore, recordings in chloride-free medium after 5 days *in vitro* revealed that these relatively primitive synaptic networks had already developed the capacity to generate characteristic rhythmic (ca. 10/sec) oscillatory afterdischarges lasting more than a second (Fig. IV-31F_2,H). After several more days of maturation in culture, similar organotypic primary slow-wave and secondary repetitive-

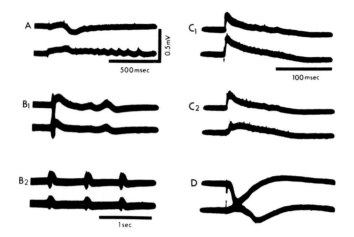

FIG. IV-32. Complex synaptic network discharges evoked in explants of 18-day fetal mouse cerebral neocortex and hippocampus after 3 days in culture. **A:** Single stimulus to cerebral neocortex explant evoked diphasic slow-wave response (lasting several hundred milliseconds) at one recording site and a much longer-duration negative potential together with an oscillatory (ca. 10/sec) afterdischarge at another site (electrodes ca. 0.5 mm apart; in 10^{-5} M strychnine). Short-duration spike potentials occur with brief latency after the stimulus (not distinguishable from shock artifacts at this slow sweep rate). See electron micrographs of this explant in Fig. IV-33. B_1: Complex slow-wave discharges evoked at two sites in a similar cerebral neocortex explant by a single stimulus at a third site (in 10^{-5} M strychnine plus 10^{-3} M caffeine). Responses began after a shorter latency and showed greater degree of synchrony between the recording sites; they also occurred spontaneously (B_2). C_1: Prominent negative slow-wave responses evoked at two sites in another 3-day neocortex explant. C_2: Generation of these complex discharges over widespread regions of the explant is demonstrated by recording of a substantial negative slow-wave potential and a repetitive spike barrage even after moving one recording electrode (lower sweep) to the opposite end of the explant (> 1 mm from stimulating and other recording electrode). **D:** Large slow-wave discharges evoked at two sites in a hippocampus explant cultured on the same coverglass as the neocortex explant in record **A** (in 10^{-5} M strychnine). See electron micrographs of this explant in Fig. IV-34 and comparable discharges in a similar explant in Fig. IV-31. (From Crain, Raine, and Bornstein, 1975b.)

discharge sequences (Crain, 1966) could often be elicited in normal BSS, and they may then also occur spontaneously (Fig. IV-29B) (section 4).

Although cultures of 15-day fetal mouse hippocampus have not developed as uniformly as 18-day explants, in at least two cases complex slow-wave discharges could be evoked at 5 days *in vitro* (again only after the stated pharmacologic maneuvers), whereas 3- to 4-day cultures showed only simple spike responses. On the other hand, within 1 day after explantation of 20-day fetal mouse hippocampus, characteristic negative slow-wave responses could be evoked (after adding bicuculline), although they were much smaller in amplitude than in 18-day fetal explants after 3 days *in vitro*. In previous studies of newborn mouse cerebral neocortex explants, complex activity was not observed until 3 days *in vitro* (Crain and Bornstein, 1964) (see also Fig. IV-29). The capacity for generating slow-wave discharges during the first 2 days in culture may have remained undetected in those experiments because of inadequate pharmacologic manipulation of the medium (only strychnine was used), or perhaps the newborn cerebral explants required a longer recovery period following surgical isolation *in vitro.*

2. Morphologic Correlates of Early Network Discharges

Electron microscope studies indicate that neocortex (Caley and Maxwell, 1971; Model et al., 1971), as well as hippocampus (Fig. IV-35) (LaVail and Wolf, 1973), are indeed quite immature in the newborn rodent. Characteristic synaptic junctions are rarely seen in these cerebral tissues at birth, although poorly defined cellular contacts and clusters of vesicles in axon terminals suggest that immature synapses may have already developed. Nevertheless, Johnson and Armstrong-James (1970) were able to detect in 1-day rat cerebral neocortex a "small number of . . . unequivocal synapses which in many respects resembled those in the adult," and they estimated that the numbers of synapses per unit volume were only a few percent of adult levels. Although these electron microscopic data correlate well with the complex slow-wave discharges recorded in 1-day rat neocortex by Armstrong-James and Williams (1963, 1964), these workers concluded, on the contrary, that "the neurons [in 1-day rat cortex] were electrically excitable, but no synaptically produced propagation was found" (Johnson and Armstrong-James, 1970). The absence of "propagation" of the cerebral-evoked potentials in the 1-day rat does not, however, preclude generation of these "directly evoked" slow-wave discharges by complex cortical synaptic networks (e.g., Purpura, 1959).

No typical synapses were detected in fresh fragments of 18-day fetal mouse cerebral neocortex or hippocampus, or in explants sampled after 1–2 days *in vitro,* in agreement with the absence of complex slow-wave discharges at these stages. Membrane thickenings suggestive of synaptic junctions were indeed seen often, but *not* in association with clusters of vesicles. In other cases vesicle arrays were seen in the absence of characteristic membrane thickenings. On the other hand, in the same 18-day fetal cerebral neocortex and hippocampus explants which showed synaptic network discharges at 3 days *in vitro* (Fig. IV-32A,D), ultrastructural analyses showed that at least some characteristic, although immature, synaptic complexes could be detected in each thin section (Crain et al., 1975*b*). Both axosomatic and axodendritic synapses were observed (Figs. IV-33;34). Similar types of synapses were also noted in explants of 18-day fetal rat hippocampus after 3 days in culture (Wenzel et al., 1973). The synaptic junctions showed morphologic features comparable to those observed during early stages of synaptogenesis in other CNS tissues *in situ*

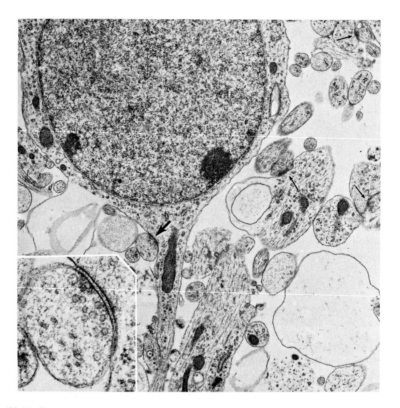

FIG. IV-33. Electron micrograph of synapses in an explant of 18-day fetal mouse cerebral neocortex after 3 days in culture (synaptic network discharges generated by this explant are shown in Fig. IV-32A). A small cortical neuron shows a large process, probably a dendrite, at the base of which is a prominent axosomatic synapse (*large arrow*). Several axodendritic synapses are present nearby (*small arrows*). (The abnormal extracellular space and debris are primarily due to preparative artifacts, e.g., fixation and residual explantation trauma.) ×8,800. **Inset:** Detail of the axosomatic synapse depicted above. Note the membrane specialization and the characteristic but low number of synaptic vesicles. ×35,200. (From Crain, Raine, and Bornstein, 1975*b*.)

and *in vitro* (Bunge et al., 1967*a;* Johnson and Armstrong-James, 1970; Model et al., 1971; LaVail and Wolf, 1973) (Fig. IV-35). Only small numbers of vesicles were clustered near the electron-dense thickening of the presynaptic membrane, and mature synapses were quite sparse in these 18-day fetal cerebral explants after 3 days in culture. A similar paucity of definitive synapses were observed in freshly isolated fetal cerebral tissues at 20 days *in utero*. After only 1 day in culture, however, cerebral explants from 20-day fetal mice showed synaptic densities comparable to 18-day fetal explants after 3 days *in vitro,* concomitant with the onset of complex synaptic network discharges (Crain and Bornstein, 1974).

The presence of axosomatic synapses at this early stage (Figs. IV-

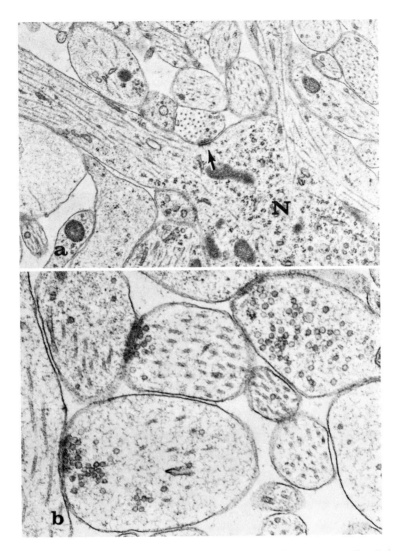

FIG. IV-34. Synapses in an explant of 18-day fetal mouse hippocampus after 3 days in culture (synaptic network discharges of this explant are shown in Fig. IV-32D). **a:** Portion of a neuronal perikaryon (N) shows two dendrites emerging, between which is a primitive axosomatic synapse (*arrow*). ×11,200. **b:** Several immature axodendritic synapses are present in another area of the same explant. ×38,400. (From Crain, Raine, and Bornstein, 1975*b*.)

33;34) was particularly striking, and agrees with observations in 1-day rat cerebral neocortex (Johnson and Armstrong-James, 1970), 18-day fetal rat hippocampus explants after 3 days *in vitro* (Wenzel et al., 1973), and *Xenopus* embryo spinal cord (Hayes and Roberts, 1973). On the other hand, delayed appearance of axosomatic synapses has been noted in cat

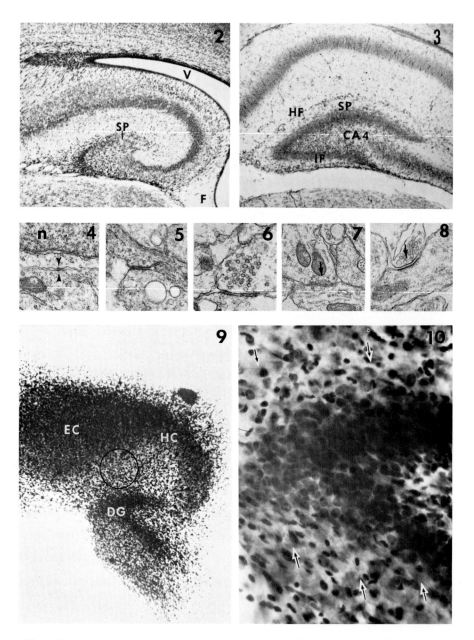

FIG. IV-35. Neonatal mouse hippocampus *in situ* and *in vitro*. **2:** Frontal section of hippo-campal formation of a newborn mouse. The suprapyramidal limb of the dentate gyrus has already assumed a linear form, but the infrapyramidal limb is as yet only suggested. F, fornix. SP, suprapyramidal limb. V, ventricle. Toluidine blue preparation. ×61. **3:** Hippo-campal formation of a 5-day-old mouse. Same orientation as in **2.** The suprapyramidal (SP) and infrapyramidal (IP) limbs are well defined and much larger at this age. HF, hippocampal fissure. Toluidine blue preparation. ×61. **4:** Example of membrane speciali-

cerebral neocortex (Voeller et al., 1963), cat hippocampus (Schwartz et al., 1968), monkey and chick spinal cord (Bodian et al., 1968; Foelix and Oppenheim, 1973; Vaughn and Grieshaber, 1973), and cultured rat spinal cord (Bunge et al., 1967*a*).

The data therefore indicate that, in spite of the sparse distribution of synapses in these immature cerebral explants, prominent, organotypic slow-wave discharges can be recorded with extracellular microelectrodes. They further suggest that some types of complex synaptic networks may already be functioning during late fetal or newborn stages in mouse cerebral neocortex and hippocampus — assuming a gestation period of 21 days (Crain and Bornstein, 1974; Crain, 1975*a*). Since birth may occur in mice after 19–20 days of gestation, the stage of cerebral maturation of newborn mice may vary. This ambiguity must be considered in comparisons between different studies on "newborn" mice, as well as between fetal cerebral explants and their *in situ* counterparts. Regional differences in rates of synaptogenesis and species differences (e.g., between mice and rats; see above) must also be considered. These factors may account for the recent electron microscope demonstration that characteristic synapses are already present in fetal rat temporal cortex by 16–17 days *in utero* (König et al., 1975). Comparative developmental studies of frontal and temporal cortex in culture as well as *in situ* should clarify the significance of these surprisingly precocious synapses in fetal rat temporal cortex.

3. Early Onset of Inhibition

The primitive cerebral synaptic networks appear, moreover, to be under tonic inhibition at these early stages of synaptogenesis *in vitro,* since the pharmacologic procedures which revealed or greatly augmented the complex discharges in immature explants have been shown to produce selective interference with CNS inhibitory mechanisms *in situ,* e.g., picrotoxin, bicuculline, strychnine, or chloride-free medium (Figs. IV-31;32) (Crain and Bornstein, 1974; see also Chaps. VI and VII-D). Simple cell assemblies connected by excitatory synaptic connections probably develop first during

---

zation (*arrowheads*) between granule cell somas in the suprapyramidal limb of the dentate gyrus of a newborn mouse. The nucleus (n) of a granule cell is at the top of the figure. *In situ.* ×12,750. **5-6:** Examples of immature contacts found rarely in the molecular layer of the suprapyramidal limb of the newborn mouse. *In situ.* **5,** ×13,175. **6,** ×22,950. **7-8:** Examples of synaptic contacts (*arrows*) found in the molecular layer of the suprapyramidal limb in a 5-day-old mouse. *In situ,* **7,** ×13,600. **8,** ×22,950. **9:** Whole mount of a hippocampal culture that was explanted from a newborn mouse and maintained for 12 days *in vitro.* The infrapyramidal limb appears distinct. The apex of the dentate gyrus is illustrated in **10.** EC, entorhinal cortex. DG, dentate gyrus. HC, hippocampus, proper. Holmes' silver impregnation. ×78. **10:** Enlargement of the apex of the dentate gyrus in **9.** Delicately impregnated fibers course in the presumptive molecular layer and pass into the granule cell layer (*arrows*) of the explant. ×315. (From LaVail and Wolf, 1973.)

CNS synaptogenesis (Purpura, 1972; Crain, 1974a), but tonic inhibitory mechanisms may appear shortly thereafter which maintain a restraining influence on these primitive networks until they reach critical stages of development in forward reference to their ultimate functions (Crain, 1971b,c, 1974a; Pollack and Crain, 1972).

Correlative extra- and intracellular recordings in older hippocampal explants (Fig. IV-42) (Zipser et al., 1973) provide strong additional evidence that the large negative slow waves evoked in these explants after 3–5 days *in vitro* represent, or at least include, summated EPSPs (Crain, 1966, 1975b,c). Furthermore, the large "primary" positive slow-wave components may represent summated IPSPs. Demonstration of abundant synapses with characteristic ultrastructure during maturation of fetal rodent hippocampal explants in culture (LaVail and Wolf, 1973) (e.g., Fig. IV-36) provides valuable morphologic correlates for these organotypic functional networks (see section 4b). The enhancing effects produced by

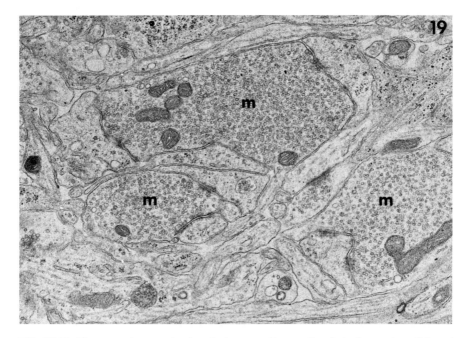

FIG. IV-36. Electron micrograph of typical mossy fiber ending (m) of granule cell found near the large, modified pyramidal neurons of the CA4 region in a mature hippocampus explant (several weeks *in vitro*). These endings are identified by their unusually large size (up to 5 μm in some profiles), multiple synaptic contacts, and numerous vesicles. ×15,725. (See lower-power views of similar explant in Fig. IV-35, parts 9 and 10.) (From LaVail and Wolf, 1973.)

agents which interfere with CNS inhibitory mechanisms *in situ* may not, however, be necessarily confined to inhibitory postsynaptic sites in cerebral explants *in vitro*. This may be particularly relevant during embryonic development (or denervation) in relation to the widespread acetylcholine sensitivity of vertebrate skeletal muscle fiber membranes prior to formation of neuromuscular junctions (Diamond and Miledi, 1962) and after denervation. Perhaps embryonic or denervated CNS neurons have similarly widespread sensitivities to *inhibitory* as well as excitatory transmitters, which only gradually become restricted to receptor sites at postsynaptic junctions (Crain, 1975c), as occurs, for example, after denervation and reinnervation of excitatory cholinergic synapses on parasympathetic ganglion cells in the frog (Kuffler et al., 1971). The early tonic inhibition that appears to occur in these CNS explants could be produced, therefore, not only by sustained inhibitory interneuronal impulse activity at synaptic junctions but also by spontaneous leakage of inhibitory transmitter from nerve terminals to neighboring extrajunctional receptor sites.

This view is strengthened by recent studies with selective inhibitors of glutamate decarboxylase (GAD) in adult brain suggesting that GABA transmitter release may be primarily regulated by the rate of its synthesis in inhibitory neurons rather than by the absolute GABA levels (Tapia, 1974). Furthermore, since a wide variety of agents that depress GAD activity lead to increased cerebral excitability and convulsive activity (Tapia, 1974), widespread tonic inhibition may be maintained in the CNS by this continuous synthesis-dependent GABA transmitter release (Chaps. VI-B, VII-D). Substantial levels of GAD activity are indeed already present in newborn rat brain (Van den Berg et al., 1965). Preliminary analyses indicate that the level of GAD activity in our cerebral explants increases sharply during the first few days *in vitro* and correlates well with the electrophysiologic evidence of early onset of GABA-mediated tonic inhibition (Lehrer, Bornstein and Crain, *in preparation;* see also Lehrer et al., 1970; Seeds, 1971, 1973) (Chap. V-C).

Llinás (1975) emphasized the increasing electrophysiologic data "which demonstrate that inhibition can also occur at the dendritic level and that it may have a rather decisive role in neuronal integration. The apparent conclusions are that dendritic inhibition may have a rather tonic action on the neuronal system by hyperpolarizing the neuron without significantly changing the resistive properties of the soma or initial dendrites. In this manner, a tonic depression in some ways similar to the 'central inhibitory state' can be obtained without a grave shunting of the synaptic inputs terminating in the somatic and proximal dendritic region." The abundant axodendritic synapses which form and predominate in early CNS networks may well provide the morphologic substrate for this tonic dendritic inhibition (Chaps. VI-B, VII-D).

4. Organotypic Synaptic Networks in Older Cerebral Explants

A. Neocortex

In older cerebral cultures complex evoked responses may be of much larger amplitude and briefer duration than those seen at 3–4 days (Crain and Bornstein, 1964), as occurs *in situ* (e.g., Bishop, 1950; Purpura et al., 1960; Himwich, 1962). Large negative superficial responses and positive deep responses can be evoked by a deep stimulus in a 10-day culture (Figs. IV-37C;38A), but the initial slow wave (after the early-latency spikes) lasts generally less than 100 msec, compared to 400 msec in younger cultures (cf. Fig. IV-29B; see also *in situ* records in Fig. IV-30A$_4$,B$_4$,C$_3$). Here too the deep positive evoked response occurs after a longer latency than that of the superficial negative response (Figs. IV-37C;38A). Many of the response patterns described in this as well as in subsequent sections have also been seen in cerebral explants maintained for more than 2 months *in vitro* (e.g., Figs. IV-39, VI-9). Careful probing at various cortical depths in some of the cerebral explants indicates that the polarity of the evoked responses reverses at a critical depth, ranging from 200 to 400 μm in different cultures (Figs. IV-37B,C;38). At times this polarity reversal occurs after the recording microelectrode is displaced by less than 10 μm away from the critical cortical depth noted above. These bioelectric properties— analogous to phase-reversal patterns characteristic of depth recordings in cerebral cortex *in situ* (Li et al., 1956)—indicate maintenance in culture of at least some laminar organization of neural elements parallel to the original cortical surface (Figs. IV-27;28).[5] Analysis of extracellular recordings from multiple sites in the cerebral explants suggest that the superficial-negative and deep-positive slow waves represent summated PSPs (section A$_1$) that are predominantly excitatory (depolarizing) and inhibitory (hyperpolarizing), respectively (Crain, 1964a; Crain and Bornstein, 1964). This interpretation draws an analyses of mechanisms that appear to underlie cortical evoked responses *in situ* (Purpura, 1959; Eccles, 1964). It is also in agreement with intracellular recordings by Purpura et al. (1965) in neonatal cat cerebral cortex *in situ,* which demonstrate IPSPs of "extraordinary duration," i.e., 200–600 msec (Fig. IV-37B, lower sweep) (Crain, 1969, 1972a, 1974a; Purpura, 1969, 1972). The prominent PSP-like activity recorded in older cerebral explants is consonant, moreover, with the development of abundant axosomatic and axodendritic synapses during the first week *in vitro* (Pappas, 1966; Model et al., 1971; Crain et al., 1975b), as in older hippocampal explants (e.g., Fig. IV-36) (LaVail and Wolf, 1973).

---

[5] Similar polarity reversal of evoked slow-wave field potentials was observed in fetal rat hippocampal deplants *in oculo* as the recording microelectrode was advanced 200–300 μm below the superficial region, past the pyramidal cell layer (Olson et al., 1976; see Chap. I-A).

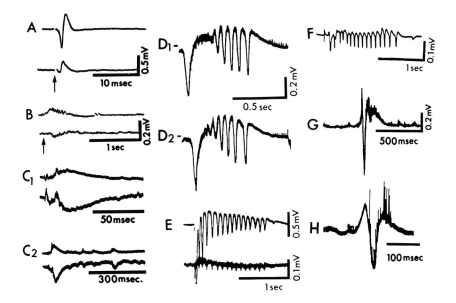

FIG. IV-37. Transition from simple to complex evoked responses and oscillatory after-discharges in cultured cerebral neocortex tissue, during the first 2 weeks after explantation from a newborn mouse. **A:** Three days *in vitro*. Simultaneous records showing simple spikes evoked, at "cortical depths" (Fig. IV-27) of 200 μm (upper sweep) and 400 μm, by stimulus applied near the subcortical edge of the explant (same records as in Fig. IV-29A$_1$). **B:** Early signs of complex response patterns recorded, at a much slower sweep rate, in the same culture and at the same electrode loci as in **A**. Long-duration slow waves are evoked after long latencies and small-amplitude repetitive potentials (ca. 10–20/sec) occur during the falling phase of the slow waves (same records as in Fig. IV-29B$_2$). **C$_1$:** Ten days *in vitro*. Simultaneous records of characteristic evoked potentials at "cortical depths" of 250 μm (upper sweep) and 650 μm following a single stimulus applied at a depth of 700 μm (but 300 μm from the deep recording site). Note the 60-msec negative evoked response in the superficial region and the positive response in the deep zone, which is similar but of longer duration and greater latency. **C$_2$:** Same as **C$_1$**, but at a slower sweep rate. Note that the small-amplitude repetitive potentials at 10–20/sec follow primary responses at both sites and are also of opposite polarities (see also Fig. IV-38). **D** and **E:** Two to six weeks *in vitro*. Repetitive oscillatory afterdischarges evoked in two mouse cerebral explants by a single stimulus applied several hundred micrometers from the recording site. Lower record in **E** shows a simultaneous recording from another region of the explant (800 μm away). Note the variation in latency of onset of the repetitive discharge following the initial, positive evoked potential (**D$_{1,2}$**). **F:** Characteristic repetitive afterdischarge evoked in cerebral cortical slab in a 5-day-old kitten, 3 days after neuronal isolation, *in situ*. Note similarity between this response pattern and those obtained from cerebral explants. **G:** Spontaneous discharge recorded in a mouse cerebral explant (2 weeks *in vitro*). **H:** Characteristic paroxysmal abnormal wave recorded in the epileptic cortex of an adult monkey, *in situ*. Note the similarity of the triphasic, initially negative complexes in **G** and **H**, with superimposed bursts of unit spikes. (**A–E** and **G** from Crain, 1964a; **F** from Purpura and Housepian, 1961; **H** from Schmidt, Thomas, and Ward, 1959.)

Systematic studies of the effects of various pharmacologic and metabolic agents on the bioelectric activities of these cerebral explants (e.g., bicuculline, strychnine, d-tubocurarine, xylocaine) have helped to clarify some of the synaptic network components which mediate the complex evoked potentials recorded in these cerebral explants (Chaps. VI and VII-D). Analyses of the alterations in the complex evoked potentials recorded from superficial and deep regions of cerebral neocortex explants during exposure to d-tubocurarine (Fig. IV-38), for example, reveal significant clues regarding mechanisms underlying generation of these regionally distinct responses. Of particular interest in Fig. IV-38B$_3$ is the sudden, large increase in amplitude of *one* of the positive repetitive potentials in the deep response. Concomitantly there occurred a reversal of the polarity of the corresponding potential in the superficial record, suggesting increased synchronization of the activity in these two regions (400 μm apart). Within 1 min the amplitude of all of the positive repetitive potentials increased greatly, from less than

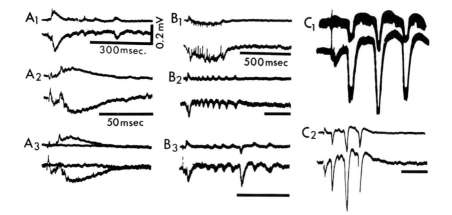

FIG. IV-38. Paroxysmal, repetitive discharges in a newborn mouse cerebral neocortex explant following d-tubocurarine (10 days *in vitro*). **A$_1$**: Simultaneous records at "cortical depths" of 250 μm (upper) and 650 μm (see Fig. IV-27) showing complex responses following a single stimulus applied at a depth of 700 μm (but 300 μm from the deep recording site). Note the 60-msec negative evoked response in the superficial region and a similar positive response in the deep zone (same record as in Fig. IV-37C$_2$). **A$_2$**: Response similar to that in **A$_1$** but at a faster sweep rate (same record as in Fig. IV-37C$_1$). **A$_3$**: Same as **A$_2$**, with superimposed baselines. **B$_1$**: After d-tubocurarine (10 μg/ml) evoked responses are more complex, with spikes of increased amplitude. **B$_2$**: d-Tubocurarine was increased to 100 μg/ml. Note the greater regularity of the repetitive discharge pattern. **B$_3$**: Sudden increase in amplitude of *one* of the positive potentials in deep response (lower) and a reversal of polarity of the corresponding potential in the superficial response. **C$_1$**: Large increase in amplitude of *all* positive potentials in deep response (within 1 min after record **B$_3$**) and reversal of polarity of *all* corresponding potentials in superficial response (as well as an increase in their amplitude). Note the marked decrease in frequency of the repetitive discharge. **C$_2$**: Decrease in amplitude of the large paroxysmal waves (shortly after record **C$_1$**: still larger-amplitude paroxysmal discharges which developed after longer exposure to d-tubocurarine are shown in Fig. VI-5. (From Crain, 1964a.)

100 μV to as much as 800 μV (Fig. IV-38C$_1$, lower record). Simultaneously, all of the corresponding superficial potentials reversed to positive polarity, also with relatively large amplitudes (Fig. IV-38C$_1$, upper record). The selective inversion of only *one* of the negative potentials in the repetitive sequence recorded at the superficial critical site (Fig. IV-38B$_3$) supports the view that these potentials represent summated PSPs generated *locally* and that the inversion to large positive waves may result from selective depression by *d*-tubocurarine of cholinergic excitatory synapses, thereby unmasking powerful repetitive IPSPs (Crain, 1969). Correlative intracellular recordings are required, however, to verify these interpretations (see further discussion in Chap. VI-C).

The analogy between the distance from the original cortical surface of a cerebral explant with actual depth below the cortical surface *in situ* may be complicated by the growth of neurites (and neuroglia) so as to form a neuropil layer over the entire cut surface of the fragment (Bunge et al., 1965; Guillery et al., 1968). An electrode may therefore have to penetrate this neuropil to contact the neuron somas in the main part of the explant. The polarity reversals described above suggest that development of such an overlying neuropil need not seriously interfere with maintenance of laminar organization parallel to the original cortical surface (OCS) edge of the explant. The presence of this neuropil may account, however, for the large shifts in response latency which under certain conditions are produced by small displacement of the stimulating electrode. An unusually long 100-msec response latency was obtained, for example, simply by withdrawing the stimulating (cathodal) electrode approximately 5–10 μm away from direct contact with the neuron soma layer, thereby producing local excitation of the overlying neuropil (cf. Fig. VI-5C and VI-5B). Furthermore, the same striking increase in response latency could be produced by applying a local electric stimulus to neurites which had grown out from the OCS edge of this explant (Fig. IV-27A) for more than 100 μm into the growth zone of the culture (as in Fig. IV-27B). This suggests that impulses generated in the neuropil overlying the "deep" region of the explant (zone 3 in Fig. IV-27A) may not pass directly to the neural elements generally excited by a stimulating electrode which penetrates the tissue in this region. The impuses may instead have to spread through more circuitous pathways, similar to those activated by impulses arriving at the OCS edge of the explant from neurites far out in the growth zone. These pathways may also be involved in cases where stimuli are applied to subcortical regions of the explant as far as 1 mm from the cortical recording sites (cf. Fig. VI-9B$_2$ and VI-9B$_1$). Propagated impulses reach the latter region within less than 5 msec (Fig. VI-9C$_3$), but spike barrages and slow waves do not appear until at least 35 msec later (Fig. VI-9D$_3$,B$_2$).

In recent studies of bioelectric activity in explants of 2- to 3-day-old mouse cerebral neocortex, Leiman et al. (1975) confirmed some of our earlier data on development of complex evoked slow-wave responses *in vitro*. However, the transition from simple spike potentials to complex slow waves occurred much later, after 5–8 days (versus 3 days in our cultures prepared from newborn mice). In addition, they rarely observed phase reversals in the slow-wave potentials during microelectrode mapping at various "cortical depths," and "complex large amplitude responses provoked by surface stimulation were never elicited by deep fiber stimulation." These and other deficits in functional capacity (e.g., extremely slow recovery after each slow-wave response and unusually large stimulating currents required to elicit both spike and slow-wave responses) may be related to their use of cerebral explants from 2- to 3-day-old mice which may not adapt to the tissue culture environment as well as our explants from newborn mice. This view is further supported by the even more rapid onset of prominent complex slow-wave discharges when the cerebral explants were prepared from late fetal instead of newborn mice (Crain and Bornstein, 1974). Leiman et al. (1975) interpreted the functional deficits in their cerebral explants — which also included an absence of "any regular, progressive modifications such as increments in complexity of waveforms or prominence of oscillatory activity" — as indicative of "the constraints on maximal functional development imposed by the isolation of a portion of an emerging nervous system."

It is obvious that a tiny fragment of CNS tissue isolated from its normal complex interrelationships in the CNS will show significant deficits and alterations during development in culture (Crain and Bornstein, 1964). "Customary input pathways" undoubtedly provide "triggers . . . for more elaborate sequential and progressive modifications with aging" (Leiman et al., 1975). Our studies of deficient PAD circuits in dorsal regions of spinal cord explants in the absence of adequate sensory DRG innervation (Crain and Peterson, 1974*b;* see also section B) provide, in fact, a clear-cut illustration of this principle. However, in view of our demonstration of characteristic regionally patterned slow-wave activities in at least some types of cerebral explants (Figs. IV-29;31;37;38, VI-2;5;9) and similar data by Calvet (1974) (Fig. IV-40), the negative findings by Leiman et al. do not provide compelling evidence regarding the *limits* to which significant components of the intrinsic cerebral circuitry may develop under optimal conditions of isolation *in vitro* (see also Chap. VII-B and Fig. VII-7). Similarly, the absence of bioelectric signs of synaptic activity in *some* types of cerebellar cultures (Hild and Tasaki, 1962) certainly did not warrant their generalization regarding the inability of CNS neurons to form functional synapses when isolated in culture (as discussed in Chap. I and below in section E). The deficiencies observed by Leiman et al. may in fact have been related to suboptimal conditions of culture (e.g., in relation to details of culture medium, explant size, age, etc.), and this relatively trivial alternative interpretation is not excluded or even acknowledged by the authors. The elegant morphologic studies of these same cerebral explants demonstrating a "remarkable degree of neuronal and architectural maturation after several weeks *in vitro*" (Seil et al., 1974) (Fig. IV-28) do not preclude functional deficits of the types under discussion. Furthermore, their use of <1 μm recording electrodes may have impeded adequate sampling of *population* responses related to increased synchronization of neuronal groups in these cultures (and which may underly the complex slow wave discharges which develop in our explants). On the other hand, some of the apparent deficits in functional maturation in the cerebral explants studied by Leiman et al. may be due to increased development of inhibitory circuits which prevented overt expression of the intrinsic circuitry by the modes of electric stimulation used in this study. Systematic pharmacologic studies with selective inhibitory antagonists may clarify this ambiguity.

Burns' (1968) comments on the discharge patterns generated by our fetal cerebral neocortex explants are of special interest in view of his extensive studies with acutely isolated cerebral slabs in the adult cat (Burns, 1958): "Indeed, the responses to single stimuli [recorded by Crain and Bornstein (1964) in cerebral cortex explants] come to resemble in many ways the burst responses of cortex that has been neurologically isolated in the adult cat. The prolonged, irregular afterdischarge that follows a single stimulus suggests that a network of self-reexciting neurones has been formed."

The other major type of complex bioelectric activity that appears during maturation of fetal or newborn mouse cerebral tissue *in vitro* consists of oscillatory afterdischarges similar to those described above in long-term spinal cord cultures (see section A). These afterdischarges are often well developed by 1–2 weeks in culture (Fig. IV-37D,E) and occur more regularly than in cord explants. The cerebral repetitive afterdischarge generally consists of three to six large diphasic potentials each lasting 25–50 msec and occurring at a rate of 5–15/sec (Figs. IV-37D,E;38;39) (Crain, 1966). As in the cord cultures (Fig. IV-4), simultaneous recordings from regions of cerebral explants located more than 1 mm apart indicate that both spontaneous and evoked repetitive slow-wave discharges may involve activity synchronized over large areas of the explant (cf. Figs. IV-37–40) (Crain, 1964*a;* Calvet, 1974). A large, early evoked potential is often followed by a long delay prior to the appearance of a repetitive sequence of potentials of gradually increasing amplitude (Figs. IV-37D;5A; cf. Fig. IV-37E). The response patterns are remarkably similar to those found by Purpura and Housepian (1961) to be characteristic of slabs of neonatal cat cerebral cortex *in situ* several days after neuronal isolation (Fig. IV-37F), and also to "spindle-like activity" (Chap. VII-B) recorded from adult cat neocortex after acute surgical isolation of a cortical area (Kristiansen and Courtois, 1949; see also Andersen and Andersson, 1968). Similar oscillatory afterdischarges with lower amplitudes have been detected in cerebral explants as early as 4 days *in vitro,* superimposed on prolonged (ca. 400 msec) primary

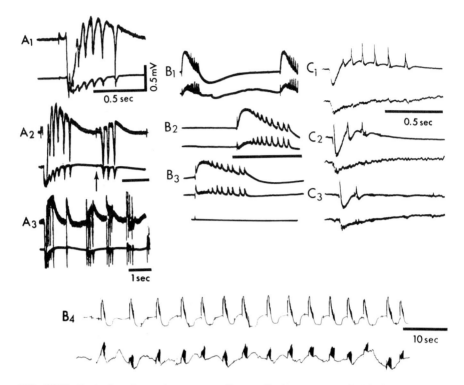

FIG. IV-39. Evoked and spontaneous oscillatory discharges recorded in long-term cultures of mouse cerebral neocortex (1–2 months *in vitro*). **A**$_{1,2}$: Repetitive afterdischarge evoked in two regions of the explant by a single stimulus applied several hundred micrometers away from both recording sites. Note the decreased amplitude and increased latency of the primary evoked response following stimulus applied (at arrow) 1 sec after onset of first afterdischarge (**A**$_2$). **A**$_3$: Similar to **A**$_2$ at a slower sweep rate. Note the marked variations in response pattern to successive stimuli at 1/sec. **B**$_{1,2,4}$: Simultaneous recordings of spontaneous negative slow-wave and oscillatory (ca. 5–10/sec) discharge sequences in another cerebral explant, at two sites 150 μm apart. Note rhythmic network discharges arising at 5–10 sec intervals (recorded at slower sweep rate) in **B**$_4$. **B**$_3$: Similar discharges evoked, at the same recording sites, by a single stimulus (cf. **B**$_2$). **C**$_1$: Repetitive discharge evoked in another region of the same cerebral explant. Note the graded decrease in total duration of the response sequence as the temperature is lowered from 34° to 29°C (**C**$_2$) and then to 27°C (**C**$_3$). (From Crain, 1964a, 1966.)

evoked potentials (Fig. IV-37B). Although these complex repetitive discharges in cerebral slabs *in vitro* show marked hyperexcitability properties as *in situ* (Crain, 1969; Purpura, 1969), the most significant point is the mimicry displayed by the cultured tissues of intricate bioelectric patterns characteristic of organized cerebral cortex *in situ*. Analyses of similar rhythmic bioelectric activities in various regions of the CNS *in situ* suggest that they may be produced by complex circuits involving sequential generation of inhibitory as well as excitatory PSPs (Andersen and Eccles, 1962; Andersen and Andersson, 1968). Development of these complex, yet

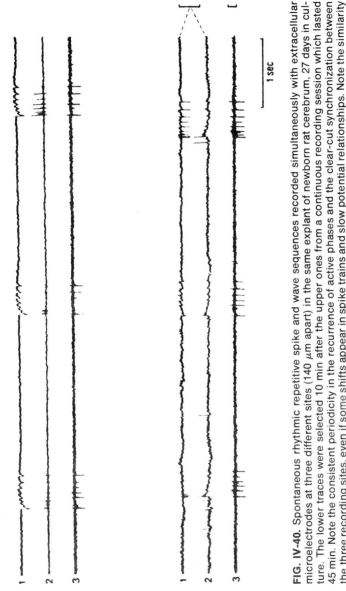

1 sec

FIG. IV-40. Spontaneous rhythmic repetitive spike and wave sequences recorded simultaneously with extracellular microelectrodes at three different sites (140 μm apart) in the same explant of newborn rat cerebrum, 27 days in culture. The lower traces were selected 10 min after the upper ones from a continuous recording session which lasted 45 min. Note the consistent periodicity in the recurrence of active phases and the clear-cut synchronization between the three recording sites, even if some shifts appear in spike trains and slow potential relationships. Note the similarity to characteristic repetitive discharge sequences in mouse cerebral explants (e.g., Figs. IV-37;39 and VII-5;6). Calibration: 1 mV. Negativity is downward in these records (and in Fig. IV-44), whereas negativity is upward in all other extracellular recordings in this monograph (see note in Fig. IV-1). (From Calvet, 1974.)

stereotyped, repetitive discharges that can be triggered by single brief electric stimuli in such diverse CNS tissues, neuronally isolated under widely
different environmental conditions *in situ* and *in vitro* (cf. Figs. IV-4;5;37;
42), suggests that a basic type of neural internuncial CNS network underlies
generation of this common pattern of bioelectric activity (Crain, 1966)
(see also Chap. VII-B; Fig. VII-7). Analysis of this network may be of
significance for clarifying mechanisms leading to generation of complex
rhythmic activities of the CNS, not only under pathologic conditions of
isolation but also in the normal state. Development of these stereotyped
repetitive slow-wave discharge patterns in CNS explants of diverse origin
does not of course preclude concomitant organization of highly specialized
functions generated by *specific* neuronal networks in each type of cultured
tissue, depending on its intrinsic circuitry as well as the particular cellular
inputs incorporated into the *in vitro* assembly.

B. Hippocampus

During the second week in culture, complex slow-wave and oscillatory
(ca. 10/sec) afterdischarges become still more prominent in hippocampus
(Fig. IV-42A) as in neocortex explants (Fig. IV-37). Correlative intracellular microelectrode recordings in these organotypic hippocampal explants
demonstrate that characteristic graded, long-lasting EPSPs are generated
in response to presynaptic impulses initiated by single electric stimuli to
other neurons in the explant (Zipser et al., 1973) (Fig. IV-41A,B; cf. Figs.
V-9–11). Spike potentials occur following orthodromic (Fig. IV-41C,D,G)
or antidromic (Fig. IV-41E) stimuli.

Depolarizing potentials with amplitudes and durations far greater than
those of typical EPSPs have been elicited in cultured hippocampal neurons
after two procedures that are known to reduce postsynaptic inhibition in
the CNS. First, bicuculline and strychnine block the long-lasting IPSPs and
evoke seizure-type activity (Fig. IV-41F) at low concentrations (ca. 10^{-6} M)
comparable to the dosage which produces selective reduction of synaptic
inhibition in the CNS of the adult cat (Curtis et al., 1971*a,b*) (Chap. VI-
A,B). Second, repetitive stimulation of hippocampal explants in some cases
appears to reduce inhibitory and increase excitatory synaptic mechanisms
(Fig. IV-42C_{2-6}), as occurs *in situ* (Purpura, 1969) and in freshly isolated
hippocampal slices (Deadwyler et al., 1975) (see also Chap. VIII-A).

The large depolarizing potentials may reach amplitudes of up to 40 mV
and may last for more than 3 sec (Fig. IV-42C_6,D). They may appear
sporadically, in response to stimuli which generally evoke normal EPSPs
and spikes (Fig. IV-41F), as well as spontaneously. Complex bursts of
spikes may occur at high frequency (up to 50/sec) during the long-lasting
depolarization shifts (Fig. IV-42$C_{4,6}$; see also Figs. V-9–11). Smaller
potentials, several millivolts in amplitude and 25–100 msec in duration,
occur sporadically during the long-lasting depolarizations (Fig. IV-42C_{2-5}).

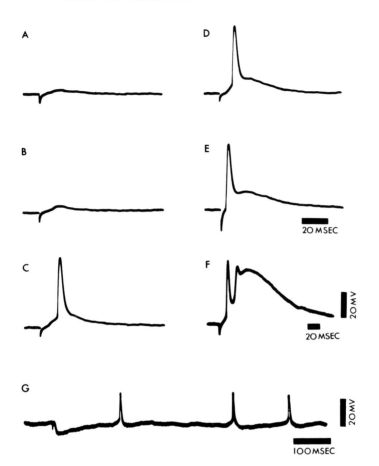

FIG. IV-41. Excitatory and inhibitory PSPs generated by neurons in explants of 18-day fetal mouse hippocampus in response to presynaptic impulses initiated by single electric stimuli to other neurons in the explant (24 days *in vitro*). **A:** Intracellular recording of EPSP of small amplitude evoked by a weak stimulus (after introduction of strychnine at 3×10^{-6} M). As the stimulus strength is progressively increased, EPSP becomes larger **(B)**; the spike potential appears during the rising phase of EPSP **(C)**, with a decreasing latency after the larger stimulus **(D)**. **E:** A still stronger stimulus evokes an antidromic spike potential which occludes the synaptically evoked spike, but large EPSP continues after the end of the spike. **F:** A depolarizing ("paroxysmal") potential (PDS: see text) with a much larger amplitude (ca. 40 mV) and longer duration (>100 msec) than the usual EPSPs is sometimes evoked by a stimulus of intermediate strength. **G:** IPSP evoked in a neuron in another hippocampal explant (15 days *in vitro*), lasting approximately 100 msec and followed by repetitive spikes. [*Note:* In this figure, time and amplitude calibrations apply to all *preceding* records, unless otherwise noted.] (From Zipser, Crain, and Bornstein, 1973.)

They may be due to simple EPSPs (or in some cases possibly IPSPs), and remarkably prolonged rhythmic (5–10/sec) sequences of these potentials (lasting up to 4 sec) have been seen in several neurons that did not generate spikes (Fig. IV-42D). Some components of the prominent long-lasting negative slow-wave potentials which occur synchronously over large regions

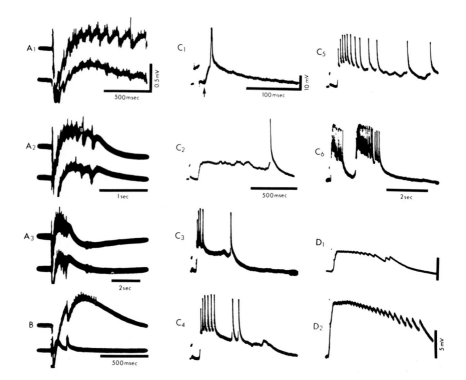

FIG. IV-42. Complex rhythmic oscillatory afterdischarge responses in fetal mouse hippocampus explants recorded with extra- and intracellular microelectrodes. **A:** Simultaneous
extracellular recordings of the network discharge evoked at two sites (1 mm apart) in a
hippocampal explant (2 weeks *in vitro*) by a stimulus to a third site (in 10^{-5} M strychnine).
An early positive slow wave is followed by a much longer-lasting negativity (1–2/sec),
and a rhythmic oscillatory (ca. 10/sec) sequence occurs concomitantly with the latter.
Note the stereotyped features of this complex response pattern in successive records at
various sweep rates ($A_{1,2,3}$; cf. Figs. IV-31F,H and IV-37D,E) and the synchrony between
activity at the two recording sites. **B:** After another 10 min of strychnine exposure, the
amplitude of the negative slow-wave response became larger and rhythmic oscillatory
potentials disappeared. C_1: Intracellular recording from a neuron in a similar hippocampal
explant (10 days *in vitro*). Note EPSP and subsequent spike potential which occur in response to a single stimulus (*arrow*) applied to another region of the explant (initial square
pulse in this and subsequent sweeps is only for calibrations: 10 mV in amplitude and 10
msec in duration). Following a period of repetitive activity, responses drastically increase
in duration. Note the large paroxysmal depolarizing shifts (PDS) in membrane potentials,
5–10 mV in amplitude and 1–2 sec in duration (C_{2-6}), even in the absence of early spike
generation (C_2). Complex bursts of spikes may occur at high frequency (up to 50/sec)
during these long-lasting depolarization potentials (C_{3-6}), each sequence in response to a
single stimulus. Also note the smaller potentials, 25–100 msec in duration and several
millivolts in amplitude, which occur sporadically during the long-lasting responses of this
cell (C_{2-5}) and more rhythmically (ca. 5–10/sec) during impalement of another neuron
($D_{1,2}$) in a similar hippocampal explant (3 weeks *in vitro*). The depolarizing shift lasts more
than 4 sec in D_2 and may have been due to introduction of bicuculline (cf. Fig. VI-2;3).
Note the resemblance of the repetitive oscillatory discharges and long-lasting negative
slow waves recorded extracellularly (with a 5-μm electrode) from small groups of neurons
and the temporal patterns of the potentials recorded intracellularly (with a 0.1-μm electrode) from individual neurons in these explants; also note the additional complex positive slow-wave components which occur at early as well as later stages of the "population"
discharges **(A,B).** Negativity is *upward* in records **A,B** and downward as usual in all of the
intracellular recordings **(C,D** and Fig. IV-41). (From Zipser, Crain, and Bornstein, 1973;
Crain, 1975*c*.)

of the explant in multiple extracellular recordings (Fig. IV-42,A,B) may be due to similar depolarizations (Crain, 1969, 1975a) (Chap. VI). Characteristic IPSPs, approximately 100 msec in duration, have been evoked in other neurons in these hippocampal explants, occurring alone or in more complex EPSP-IPSP sequences (Fig. IV-41G). Early-latency IPSPs may be the basis for the large "primary" positive slow-wave potentials which are often recorded extracellularly in these and other CNS explants in normal culture media (e.g., Figs. VI-2A,9A; VII-4A) and which can be antagonized by various pharmacologic agents that produce selective block of inhibitory synapses *in situ* (Chap. VI-B). The complex synaptic potentials and spike bursts recorded intracellularly from these neurons during generation of organotypic patterned discharges in hipppcampal explants show striking resemblances to some of the complex patterns obtained during intracellular recordings of hippocampal neurons in adult cats *in situ,* especially during seizures (Spencer and Kandel, 1969). The long-duration depolarizing potentials in these hippocampal explants show particularly remarkable mimicry of the large, long-lasting membrane depolarization which occurs in pyramidal neurons coincident with an interictal cortical paroxysm, and which has been named the "paroxysmal depolarizing shift" (PDS) by Matsumoto and Ajmone Marsan (1964). The PDS has been hypothesized to be a "giant recurrent EPSP" (Ayala et al., 1973) generated by multisynaptic and/or repetitive inputs on the impaled neuron (see also Spencer and Kandel, 1969).

Since the PDS in these hippocampal explants appears to be normally suppressed by tonic inhibition and can be readily released by specific drugs or repetitive stimuli, as *in situ,* factors regulating this important type of cerebral hyperexcitability may now become accessible to more direct study *in vitro.* Similar PDS responses have also been recorded intracellularly in freshly isolated slices (0.3 mm thick) of adult guinea pig hippocampus in chloride-deficient medium or after addition of strychnine (Yamamoto, 1972; see also Schwartzkroin, 1975). Their presence in long-term explants, however, permits more flexible environmental manipulations and rigorous control of the tissue during extended excitability studies. These experiments with cultures may help to clarify mechanisms underlying generation of epileptic interictal spikes (Ayala et al., 1973). The PSP studies of neurons in hippocampal explants may also provide valuable correlative data to supplement intracellular recordings from immature hippocampus and neocortex in neonatal kittens *in situ* (Purpura et al., 1968; Purpura, 1969; Prince and Gutnick, 1972). Although many significant deficits undoubtedly exist in the hippocampal explant preparations relative to their *in situ* counterparts, the degree of mimicry of synaptic and spike-generating systems is certainly adequate to warrant serious application of this model system for further analyses of complex mammalian synaptic networks. Furthermore, morphologic studies demonstrate maturation of characteristic neurons, glial cells, and synapses in long-term cultures (LaVail and Wolf, 1973; see also Crain et al., 1975*b*) comparable to the cytologic features of cerebral neocortex explants. Mature hippocampal pyramidal and granule cells with characteristic axodendritic and axosomatic synapses have also been observed in electron microscopic studies of similar Maximow slide cultures of newborn mouse hippocampal explants (Fig. IV-36) (LaVail and Wolf, 1973; Wenzel et al., 1973). In addition to the value of these intracellular recordings for analysis of mechanisms underlying generation of patterned CNS network discharges, they also provide important validation and "calibration" of extracellular microelectrode recordings which can be carried out more routinely and systematically in a wide variety of biologic studies during and after development of synaptic networks *in vitro*.

Chronic recordings from hippocampal explants using extracellular microelectrodes (3- to 5-μm tips) in our sterile closed micrurgical culture chambers (Chap. II-B1) recently demonstrated that these isolated tissues can generate remarkably regular, rhythmic spike-burst and slow-wave network discharges (1 per 2–10 sec) for periods of hours or even days while metabolizing in normal culture medium (Crain et al., *in preparation*). Mechanisms regulating generation of sustained repetitive discharges of these explants and intermittent shifts in their excitability properties are now under systematic study. These studies confirm and extend earlier chronic recordings by Cunningham (1962) of spontaneous discharges in chick embryo cerebral explants, which demonstrated characteristic rhythmic slow-wave activities generated for periods up to 2 weeks in culture (Chap. VII-B) [in spite of technical limitations imposed by the use of large metal recording electrodes embedded in the tissue at explanation (see also Shtark et al., 1974)].

Quantitative analyses of spike firing patterns have also been carried out on neurons in neonatal rat hippocampal explants (Shtark et al., 1972, 1976) (see also similar analyses in cerebellar cultures in section E). Microelectrode recordings of long sequences of complex spontaneous spike discharges from the explants (after 1–4 weeks *in vitro*) and from similar regions of the dorsal hippocampus *in situ* were subjected to elaborate computer analyses. The spike firing patterns recorded from hippocampal neurons *in vitro* showed significant similarities to their *in situ* counterparts,[6] and the data

---

[6] On the other hand, no spontaneous spike discharges were recorded from pyramidal neurons in deplants of fetal rat hippocampus *in oculo* (Olson et al., 1976). In similar deplants of cerebellar tissue *in oculo,* however, Purkinje cells showed characteristic spontaneous spike firing rates *in situ* (Hoffer et al., 1974). Although the data from deplants *in oculo* suggested that spontaneous spike activity of hippocampal pyramidal neurons is "critically dependent on some external input" (Olson et al., 1976), the recordings by Shtark et al. (1976) and our own long-term studies in sealed micrurgical chambers (see above) indicate that, at least under some conditions of culture, fetal rodent hippocampal neurons (presumably pyramidal) can also generate characteristic spontaneous spike activity by endogenous mechanisms as in cerebellar deplants and explants (see also section E).

provide a foundation for further analyses of the complex networks in these hippocampal explants after various experimental manipulations *in vitro* (Shtark et al., 1976).

5. Limbic Regions

A. Hypothalamus

Analyses of spontaneous spike firing patterns of neurons in explants of neonatal rat tuberal hypothalamus show significant similarities to their *in situ* counterparts (Geller, 1975). Recordings of electrical activity in hypothalamic neuroendocrine regions *in situ* have shown characteristic phasic discharge patterns which are thought to correlate with periods of hormone release (Wakerly and Lincoln, 1971; Dreifuss and Kelly, 1972). The observation of spike bursts or cyclic irregular discharges with a cycle period of 1–2 min in these isolated explants suggests that bioelectric mechanisms associated with hormone release may be accessible to direct analyses *in vitro*. It has been suggested, for example, that a peak of cyclic firing in the hypothalamus may facilitate coordinated release of peptide hormones. The mean rate of spontaneous spike firing in the hypothalamic cultures was 2.37/sec, which is close to the mean rate of 2.95/sec found in hypothalamus *in situ* (Feldman and Dafny, 1970). These values, however, are significantly lower than the mean rate of 9.23/sec observed in similar analyses of cerebellar explants (Geller and Woodward, 1974) (see section E). The remarkably small differences in mean firing rate between intact and isolated hypothalamic neurons suggests that this parameter may be modulated only to a small degree by activity in afferent pathways. The relatively low mean rates of spontaneous firing of hypothalamic neurons *in situ* and *in vitro* implies that tonic activity in the afferent pathways to this region is very low and that hormone levels may be the primary modulators of mean neuronal activity. Excitatory and inhibitory synaptic networks occur in neuroendocrine regions of the hypothalamus *in situ,* and complex arrays of synaptic junctions form in explants of fetal and newborn mouse hypothalamus during the first weeks in culture (Masurovsky et al., 1972). Multiple synaptic junction complexes containing a variety of characteristic granular vesicles were observed more frequently as these organized explants matured during the next 2 months *in vitro*. [Elegant histologic analyses have also been made by Sobkowicz et al. (1974*a,b*) in explants of neonatal mouse hypothalamic mammillary tissues, up to 7 weeks *in vitro,* where remarkable organotypic arrays of fiber tracts ramify in complex, highly ordered patterns in the vicinity of regionally specified nuclear groups[7] (similar to the organized axonal arrays demonstrated in spinal cord explants by Sobkowicz and co-workers) (see section A; Figs. IV-8;9).] It will be of interest to analyze the degree to which the observed phasic spike firing patterns are mediated by synaptic network activities under these *in vitro* conditions where close correlations with hormonal release can be concomitantly determined. Cultures of dissociated fetal mouse hypothalamic cells may also be useful for these studies since they have been shown to form monolayers of organized reaggregated cells, including many mature neurons with cytologic features characteristic of neurosecretory cells of hypothalamic tissue *in situ* (Benda et al., 1975). Electron microscopy revealed that abundant synapses and characteristic dense-core vesicles in nerve terminals had formed by 10 days *in vitro* (see also Masurovsky et al., 1972).

Another interesting limbic tissue culture model has been developed using supraoptic nucleus tissue from neonatal puppies (Sakai et al., 1974). Although little or no spontaneous spike activity was detected during intracellular microelectrode recordings in these explants (cf. Geller, 1975), the neurons could be excited to initiate activity by bath exposure to glutamate and nicotine, and these effects were concentration-dependent. Spike frequency increased from approximately 2/sec to 10/sec as the glutamate level was raised from 10^{-7} to 10^{-5} M. Glutamate-excited cells, moreover, could be depressed by exposure to GABA, and 10^{-6} to 10^{-5} M concentrations produced dose-dependent decreases in spike frequency as well as membrane hyperpolarization (cf. Gähwiler, 1975) (see section E; Chap. VI-B). Finally, norepinephrine as well as the β-adrenergic agonist isoproterenol also inhibited spiking activity that had been initiated either by glutamate or nicotine, but these depressant effects appeared to be mediated by ionic mechanisms different than those involved in the GABA effects (Sakai et al., 1974; see also Marks et al., 1973). These studies demonstrate that supraoptic neurons in long-term explants maintain marked selective chemosensitivity properties to their *in situ* counterparts (e.g., Barker et al., 1971); and although initial attempts to detect vasopressin release were negative (Sakai et al., 1974), this tissue culture model may be valuable for further analyses of mechanisms regulating neurosecretion in hypothalamic nuclei.

---

[7] Addition of testosterone at explantation resulted in an intense neuritic proliferation radiating out from the margins of some portions of the preoptic/anterior hypothalamus and mammillary regions, accompanied by enhanced neuronal maturation and myelinogenesis (Toran-Allerand, 1975). Explants of nearby medial regions of the hypothalamus showed no such growth-stimulating effects in testosterone. Moreover, the presence of antibodies to estradiol and testosterone produced the exact opposite developmental effect only in regions previously shown to be stimulated. These findings suggest that the maturation of certain hypothalamic regions are selectively advanced by the addition of androgen at birth. The selective effects of testosterone on the growth and maturation of specific types of neurons in hypothalamus explants provide a significant extension of the well-known selective growth stimulation of sensory and sympathetic ganglion cells, and catecholaminergic CNS neurons, by NGF (Chaps. III-B and IV-B1).

B. Olfactory Bulb

Explants of olfactory bulb from 18- and 19-day fetal mice have been cultured in Maximow slide chambers for periods up to 5 weeks (Corrigall et al., 1975). During the first few days *in vitro,* compound spike potentials representing conductile activity are the only bioelectric responses that can be evoked. By the end of the first week in culture, however, characteristic synaptically generated negative slow-wave potentials can be evoked, and in older cultures these slow-wave discharges may also occur spontaneously.

Although young cultures (3 to 7 days *in vitro*) show no evidence of synaptic slow waves in BSS, these complex network discharges are readily elicited after addition of GABA antagonists, e.g., bicuculline or picrotoxin, (10^{-5} M) or after substituting propionates for the chlorides in BSS, as in 18-day fetal neocortex and hippocampal explants at 3 days *in vitro* (Figs. IV-31;32). Furthermore, in older cultures slow waves occurring in BSS are depressed by the addition of GABA (10^{-4} M) as in cerebral explants (Chap. VI-B).[8] The data suggest development of GABA-mediated inhibitory synaptic circuits in these isolated olfactory bulb explants as well as complex excitatory synaptic networks, resembling organized bioelectric activities observed during maturation of cerebral neocortex and hippocampus explants in culture (see above) (Crain and Bornstein, 1974; Crain, 1975*a,c*). In these relatively simpler bulbar cultures, moreover, it may be possible to identify the granule-to-mitral synapse as a specific component of the inhibitory network.

In addition to slow-wave activities, positive or positive-negative unit spikes with amplitudes reaching several millivolts have been recorded extracellularly (via saline-filled micropipettes with ca. 3-μm tips) from presumptive mitral cells in the olfactory bulb explant. These large unit spikes may occur spontaneously by 1–2 days *in vitro,* well before the first slow-wave network discharges can be detected; and they may also be evoked, at 3- to 10-msec latency, following stimulation of the explant or the neuritic outgrowth. The spikes frequently exhibit an inflection on the rising phase, resembling A-B fragmentation seen in giant extracellular spikes recorded from

---

[8] Strychnine, on the other hand, was ineffective (up to 3×10^{-5} M) in enhancing slow-wave activity in olfactory bulb explants and glycine produced no depressant effects at levels as high as 3×10^{-3} M (see Chap. VI-A,B). This is consistent with observations *in situ* which have demonstrated that the inhibition of mitral cells following lateral olfactory tract stimulation is not affected by strychnine, applied intravenously (Green et al., 1962; Nicoll, 1971) or iontophoretically (Felix and McLennan, 1971), in contrast to the potent effects of bicuculline and GABA. Furthermore, in contrast to the maintenance of evoked spike activity in 10 mM Mg^{++}, the slow-wave potentials were reversibly blocked in this concentration of Mg^{++}, even in the presence of 10^{-5} M bicuculline. Addition of 1 mM EGTA to the BSS to chelate free Ca^{++} also reversibly blocked the slow-wave responses without affecting spike potentials (see Chap. VI-E). Slow-wave discharges similar to those elicited in bicuculline could also be evoked after introduction of 10^{-5} M picrotoxin or 10^{-4} M *d*-tubocurarine (see also Chap. VI-C) (Corrigall et al., 1976).

mitral cells of the olfactory bulb *in situ* (Phillips et al., 1963).[9] The large positive (or positive-negative) unit spikes in the bulb explants are in marked contrast to the smaller, predominantly negative spikes that are generally recorded from other types of CNS tissues under similar experimental conditions in culture. Since these spikes have been seen even in the youngest cultures, olfactory bulb explants provide a valuable model system in which the development of synaptic network activity may be analyzed in relation to an identified type of cerebral neuron. Furthermore, introduction of olfactory epithelium (Farbman and Gesteland, 1974) to these deafferented olfactory bulb explants should permit direct *in vitro* studies of the effects of sensory innervation on this specialized cerebral tissue, in extension of our analyses of DRG innervation of sensory target neurons in spinal cord and brainstem (see sections B, C) (Crain and Peterson, 1974*b*, 1975*a–c*).

E. CEREBELLUM

Although extra- and intracellular microelectrode recordings from explants of neonatal rat and cat cerebellum by Hild and Tasaki (1962) failed

---

[9] Unusually large amplitude (up to 70 mV) extracellular spikes have also been seen in recordings from other CNS neurons *in situ* (e.g., Granit and Phillips, 1956) and from dorsal root ganglion cells in culture (Crain, 1956) when the tip of the micropipette is critically positioned in intimate relation to the nerve cell membrane. The large amplitudes in the latter studies over those observed in the bulb explants are probably due to the finer tips of the micropipettes used (ca. 1 μm or less).

Paired-stimulus analyses of the large unit spikes in olfactory bulb explants indicate the development *in vitro* of an inhibitory system analogous to that seen to suppress the activity of mitral cells *in situ* following antidromic or orthodromic activation (Shepherd, 1972). Neurons in young cultures showed relatively uniform spike amplitude in response to test stimuli as the test interval following a conditioning stimulus was progressively shortened (Corrigall et al., 1976). Attenuation of spike amplitude at test intervals less than 15 msec merely indicated relative refractoriness characteristic of conductile membranes. In older cultures, on the other hand, the test stimulus to a neuron failed, at times, to evoke a spike even when applied as long as 70 msec after a conditioning stimulus, suggesting involvement of processes that are much longer-lasting than the usual postspike refractoriness.

In preliminary pharmacologic studies on the neurons generating large positive unit spikes, introduction of GABA (5×10^{-4} M) completely, but reversibly, blocked all spontaneous activity. In bicuculline (10^{-5} M), the unit spike firing rates, which normally ranged up to 20/sec in BSS, were now seen to occur at rates as high as 200/sec for short intervals. These high frequency bursts generally began during the rising phase of typical negative slow-wave potentials (spontaneous or evoked) and their amplitudes were rapidly and progressively attenuated, suggestive of spike inactivation mechanisms. As the unit spikes gradually returned to normal amplitudes during the final phase of the slow-wave potential, the spike discharge rates were observed to remain significantly higher than in BSS for more than 1–2 sec.

In view of the characteristic depressant effect of GABA on spontaneous activity of the mitral cells in culture and the enhancement of these spike discharges in bicuculline, it may be that the GABA-ergic properties observed in both the slow-wave and single-unit recordings are due to the same system, namely the granule-to-mitral synapse which appears to utilize GABA as transmitter *in situ* (McLennan, 1971; Nicoll, 1971). Kim (1972) has demonstrated that reciprocal synapses do, indeed, occur in cultures of olfactory bulb (and these might well be the dendrodendritic synapses between mitral and granule cells).

to detect evidence of synaptic activity, significant data were obtained demonstrating propagation of action potentials in directly visualized dendritic processes as well as the capacity of these neurons to generate spontaneous repetitive action potentials (Chap. I). On the basis of electrophysiologic studies of explants obtained from various regions of the CNS, it seemed probable that the absence of synaptic functions in Hild and Tasaki's cultures was due to technical details rather than to an inability of cerebellar tissue to form synaptic networks after isolation *in vitro* (Crain, 1966). More recent extracellular microelectrode recordings from neonatal rodent and cat cerebellar explants have provided evidence that complex synaptic interactions

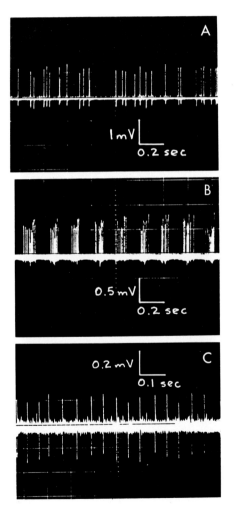

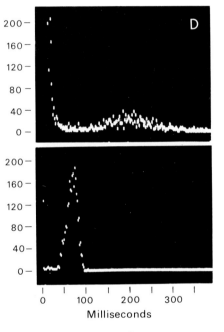

FIG. IV-43. Extracellularly recorded spontaneous action potentials of neuron somas from neonatal rat cerebellar cultures. **A:** Sample of the most frequently observed discharge pattern. **B:** Sometimes spikes occur in trains, with silent periods between the bursts. **C:** Nerve cells in peripheral areas of cultures exhibit regular discharge patterns. D_1: Interspike interval distribution of Purkinje cell recorded in Hanks' BSS (0.9 mM Mg^{2+}). D_2: Interspike distribution recorded from the same neuron in a solution with 8 mM Mg^{2+}. Time between the two measurements, 10 min. Bin width, 4 msec. Total counts, 3,000. (From Gähwiler, Mamoon, and Tobias, 1973.)

can indeed also occur in these cultures (Gähwiler et al., 1972, 1973; Schlapfer et al., 1972; Leiman and Seil, 1973; Calvet, 1974; Lumsden et al., 1975;
see also Walker and Hild, 1972; Walker, 1975). Irregular spike firing patterns were generally observed, including high-frequency bursts (up to 50/sec)
followed by long silent intervals [Figs. IV-43;44A; see also the elegant intracellular recordings by Nelson and Peacock (1973) from arrays of dissociated cerebellar neurons after formation of complex excitatory and inhibitory synaptic connections in culture (Figs. V-10;11)]. Increasing the
Mg^{++} concentration from 1 to 8 mM led to significant regularization of firing
in about half of the treated Purkinje cells, whereas bioelectric discharges
ceased in the others (Fig. IV-43D) (Gähwiler et al., 1973). Pentobarbital
(20 μg/ml) produced similar effects. These results suggested that the component of spontaneous cerebellar discharges which involved a regular pattern of spike firing, as observed in normal as well as high Mg^{++} media, was
not synaptically mediated (see also Chap. VI-B). Microiontophoretic application of GABA and glycine decreases spike firing rates of Purkinje cells
in cerebellar explants, and the GABA effects in some of the cells were antagonized by bicuculline and picrotoxin, as *in situ* (Geller and Woodward,
1974). [Similar, but apparently more reproducible and more selective, effects of GABA antagonists have been observed with bath application of
these and related agents (Gähwiler, 1975, 1976a) (Chap. VI-B).] Microiontophoresis of glutamate and homocysteate, on the other hand, produced
a characteristic increase in firing rates.

In contrast to the highly synchronized EEG-like slow-wave activity that
generally occurs in cerebral explants concomitant with spike barrages (Figs.
IV-37–39) (see section D), cerebellar explants showed only repetitive spike
bursting patterns when recordings were made from both types of tissues
with the same electrophysiologic techniques (Calvet, 1974) (cf. Figs. IV-
44A and IV-40). Even when complex discharges lasting up to 5 sec were
evoked by electric stimuli, involving spike bursts interspersed with "inhibitory pauses," no prominent slow-wave potentials were observed (Leiman and Seil, 1973).[10] On the other hand, when an antimitotic agent (methylazoxymethanol acetate; MAM) was added to the culture medium to prevent
multiplication of granule cells, synchronized sequences of spikes and slow
waves began to occur for the first time (Fig. IV-44D) (Calvet et al., 1974).

---

[10] In more recent studies of neonatal rat cerebellum explants in which a piece of underlying
brainstem was left attached to provide extracerebellar pathways, simultaneous recordings from
several cerebellar sites showed an unusual degree of synchronized burst activity (Calvet and
Lepault, 1975), in contrast to the asynchrony characteristic of spike bursts in cerebellum explants disconnected from brainstem (e.g., Fig. IV-44A). However, even in the case of spike
synchronization in combined brainstem + cerebellum explants, no slow wave potentials could
be detected in the cerebellar tissue, in contrast to clearcut synchronized negative slow waves
which were recorded in the nearby brainstem regions. These data suggest that the Purkinje
cell burst synchronization is triggered by a common source in the brainstem nuclei.

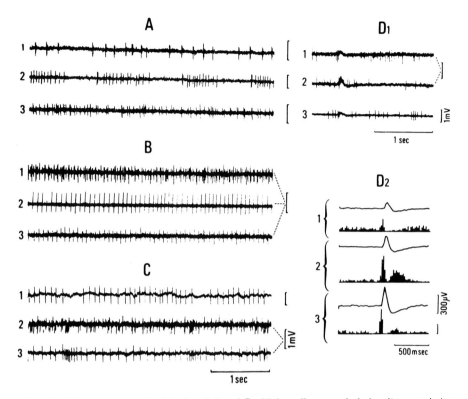

FIG. IV-44. Spontaneous electrical activity of Purkinje cells recorded simultaneously by three extracellular microelectrodes 100–120 μm apart. **A:** Rat cerebellum; 27 days *in vitro*(DIV); standard medium. Trains of 5–15 spikes occur repetitively without any evident correlation between the three traces. Note that the bursts of the third sweep are not clearly individualized, as may occur in approximately 25% of the neurons recorded in standard cultures. **B,C:** Rat cerebellum; 28 DIV; medium with antimitotic agent (MAM). Neurons fire regularly at a rate of approximately 15/sec. This regular pattern of firing of one Purkinje cell may be inhibited (**C,** first sweep) while one or two nearby neurons are excited (**C,** second and third sweeps). **D:** Rat cerebellum; 31 DIV; medium with MAM. The synchronized inhibitory slow waves are recorded as an extracellular positivity of each active electrode close to each hyperpolarized Purkinje cell soma and are accompanied by a spike inhibition (**D$_1$**). In **D$_2$**, 25 waves have been averaged and the spikes counted in samples of 20 msec duration. Note that the third trace is the first to be involved in the brief spike increase preceding the onset of the wave. (Negativity downward, as in Fig. IV-40. Vertical bar: probability of occurrence of 1.2 spike during the 20 msec sample duration.) (From Calvet, Drian, and Privat, 1974.)

Electron microscopic analyses of these MAM-treated cerebellar explants showed unusual numbers of special types of large-bouton synapses on the spines and shafts of Purkinje cell dendrites which appear *in situ* to be associated with recurrent collateral endings of Purkinje cell axons (Privat, 1975). The latter "form closed loops and are probably responsible for large positive slow-wave potentials accompanied by a silencing of the spike generation" (Calvet et al., 1974), as may occur in cerebral explants (see section D and

Chap. VII-C). In addition to this unusual enhancement of synchronized bioelectric activities in cerebellar explants, the deficit in granule cells pro-duced by the antimitotic agent also led to decreased spike bursting patterns and more regular spike firing rates, except for intermittent onset of synchro-nized excitatory or inhibitory slow-wave potentials (Fig. IV-44B,C). These studies of cerebellar explants growing under experimentally altered culture conditions provide another interesting demonstration of the potentialities of this model system for analyses of mechanisms underlying development of specific types of CNS networks.[11]

A series of valuable morphologic analyses of organized fetal rodent cere-bellar explants have, in fact, already been carried out with both selective silver techniques and electron microscopy (Wolf, 1964, 1970; Wolf and Dubois-Dalcq, 1970; Seil, 1972); but aside from the above experiments by Calvet et al. (1974),[10] most electrophysiologic studies have not yet attempted systematic analyses of the functional correlates of the highly ordered arrays of Purkinje cells, granule cells, and other characteristic cerebellar neurons that can be identified by their unusual cytologic features (similar to the elegant morphologic analyses of organotypic spinal cord, hippocampal, and hypothalamic explants noted in sections B–D).

Techniques for extension of electrophysiologic studies of freshly isolated adult brain slices from the usual ca. 300 μm thick slices to much thinner ones (ca. 70–80 μm) were developed by Yamamoto (1975). He showed that during microelectrode recordings in thin slices of guinea pig cere-bellum, where Purkinje cell perikarya and some dendrites could be directly observed under the microscope, synaptic functions and characteristic chemo-sensitivity could be retained for several hours. This technique should be valuable for correlative studies with cerebellar tissue cultures, and it may also facilitate renewed attempts to maintain slices of adult brain in long-term culture (Chap. II-A1).

F. INVERTEBRATE CNS

1. Insect Ganglia

Complex bioelectric discharges have also been observed to occur spon-taneously in explants of cockroach embryo CNS ganglia cultured for many weeks in a chemically defined medium (Provine et al., 1973; Seshan et al., 1974). In some cases there were rhythmic oscillatory bursts that resembled patterns characteristic of mammalian CNS explants (see sections A, D;

---

[11] The prominent slow-wave potentials that appear in MAM-treated cerebellar explants may be related to the large synchronous spike bursts and long-lasting depolarization shifts which have been recorded intracellularly in networks of dissociated fetal mouse cerebellar neurons (Nelson and Peacock, 1973). In both types of cultures, deficits in granule cells may lead to relatively unusual bioelectric discharge patterns.

Chap. VII-A). Furthermore, spontaneous discharges occurred synchronously between different types of ganglia after formation of neuritic bridges in culture (Provine et al., 1973), as in mammalian CNS explant arrays (see section C; Chap. VII-B). All complex bursting and interganglionic transmission were blocked by raising the Mg^{++} concentration, suggesting synaptic mediation of these activities. Cultures of cockroach ganglia should therefore provide a useful model system for studies of invertebrate CNS development and for comparative analyses of basic CNS functions shared by widely divergent phyla (Levi-Montalcini and Seshan, 1973). The capacity of these insect tissues to form complex synaptic networks during long-term maturation in a completely synthetic culture medium (Chen and Levi-Montalcini, 1969) offers another advantage over existing mammalian CNS culture which still require serum, or other undefined nutrients, for normal development and long-term maintenance *in vitro* (Chap. II-A).

Cultures of dissociated embryonic *Drosophila* cells have also been studied during early stages of differentiation of neurons and muscle cells *in vitro* (Seecof et al., 1971). Electrophysiologic recordings demonstrated development of functional neuromuscular junctions (Seecof et al., 1972), and formation of ganglion-like clusters *in vitro* has also been observed (Seecof et al., 1973). Cultures of *Drosophila* neurons should be of great value for systematic analyses of genetic factors in the development of neural circuits, in correlation with the elegant studies of neurologic mutants *in situ* (e.g., Ikeda and Kaplan, 1970; see also review by Hoyle, 1974).

2. Leech and Aplysia Ganglia

Isolated leech ganglia have been maintained for long periods *in vitro,* and characteristic action potentials and postsynaptic potentials can be recorded intracellularly even after 2 months in culture (Nicholls and Van Essen, 1974; Nicholls et al., 1976). Relatively normal reflexes can be evoked by mechanical stimulation of sensory endings in the ganglion preparation isolated *in vitro,* but significant changes in the sensory-evoked synaptic potentials occur (increases in amplitude, duration, and pattern) which may be due to denervation supersensitivity, accessory sprouting of collateral nerve fibers, or the formation of new synaptic contacts both in the neuronally isolated ganglion *in situ* as well as in culture (Nicholls and Van Essen, 1974; Nicholls et al., 1976). The unusually large size of many leech neurons and glial cells should greatly facilitate electrophysiologic analyses during development and regeneration of the neural circuits in cultures of these well-characterized CNS tissues (Nicholls and Baylor, 1968; Jansen and Nicholls, 1972).

Organ cultures of *Aplysia* ganglia have also been maintained for long periods *in vitro,* and normal action potentials as well as spontaneous or evoked postsynaptic potentials can be recorded intracellularly for 4–5 weeks in culture (Strumwasser, 1971, 1974). Although no growth or regeneration seems to occur after explantation of these ganglia (in a nutrient medium containing 20% *Aplysia* serum), spontaneous unitary spikes can be recorded from the nerve trunks for up to 6 weeks (utilizing platinum wires embedded in a special sterile culture chamber). The wave forms of these axonal spikes are quite stable from day to day, and some of the units have shown clear-cut circadian rhythms (Strumwasser, 1974).

These organ culture techniques will undoubtedly also be applied fruitfully to many other types of invertebrate neurons that have become classic test objects for basic neurophysiologic analyses because of the unusually large size of their perikarya, dendrites, or synaptic regions (e.g., squid giant axon, crayfish stretch receptor, etc.) (see also lobster CNS cultures: Chap. II-A2).

V

Formation of Functional Synaptic Networks in Cultures of Dissociated Neurons

Although major emphasis in this volume is on cultures of organized neural tissue explants, this chapter reviews some of the exciting electrophysiologic experiments carried out during the past few years with cultures of dissociated neurons. Attention is focused on studies related to development of functional synaptic relationships between isolated arrays of neurons in culture. Many other physiologic and biochemical properties of dissociated neurons, glia, and neuroblastoma cells in culture were recently reviewed (Sato, 1973; Nelson, 1975; Varon, 1975; see also Chap. I). Some types of neuroblastoma cells can indeed be cultured under conditions where they sprout axons, generate characteristic action potentials, and show depolarizing or hyperpolarizing responses to various neuropharmacologic agents (Nelson, 1975). Since large quantities of membrane can be obtained from these rapidly growing cells, the cultures may be useful for characterization of critical chemical factors associated with the development of conductile membranes in these clones (for review see Schrier et al., 1974; Richelson, 1975). These cells do not, however, appear to be capable of forming normal synaptic relationships with a wide variety of target nerve and muscle cells tested so far under various culture conditions (for review see Giller et al., 1975). On the other hand, recent experiments with somatic hybrids formed between certain neuroblastoma cells and glial tumor cells showed that functional cholinergic synapses can indeed develop between these dissociated hybrid cells and skeletal muscle fibers (Nelson et al., 1976), analogous to connections between rodent sympathetic ganglion cells and skeletal muscle (Crain and Peterson, 1974a; Nurse and O'Lague, 1975; see below). These cultures may be valuable for correlative electrophysiologic, biochemical, and genetic analyses of developing synaptic membranes.

A. PERIPHERAL GANGLIA

1. Dorsal Root Ganglion Cells

Cytologic studies of completely dissociated chick embryo dorsal root ganglion (DRG) neurons growing in culture (Fig. III-8) were first reported by Nakai (1956) in Pomerat's laboratory after preliminary development of this technique by Levi-Montalcini (see also Levi-Montalcini and Angeletti,

1963). It was not until 1969, however, that characteristic action potentials were demonstrated by Scott et al. after dissociation of 10-day chick embryo DRG neurons and reaggregation in culture into organized layers overlying a connective tissue substrate. Scott's intracellular recordings of the membrane resting and action potentials of dissociated DRG neurons and their general excitability properties studied after 4–7 weeks *in vitro* were quite comparable to those observed in cultures of intact ganglia (Crain, 1956) (Chap. III-A). The range of conduction velocities of the neurites was estimated to be approximately 0.1–0.6 meters/sec. The upper limit is comparable to the velocity of 0.5 meters/sec obtained in freshly isolated preparations of 10-day chick embryo sciatic nerve (Carpenter and Bergland, 1957), but this indicates that relatively little increase had occurred in culture even after 4–7 weeks of development. Measurements of conduction velocity in more organized (often myelinated) dorsal root fascicles connecting DRG perikaryal clusters to spinal cord (Figs. II-1, IV-20; Chap. IV-B) ranged well over 1 meter/sec (Crain and Peterson, 1964). Electrophysiologic studies of similar dissociated chick embryo DRG neurons were also carried out by Varon and Raiborne (1971) in collaboration with Marchiofava, and characteristic membrane action potentials could already be evoked during the first few days in culture (and occasionally even in cells which had not yet attached and grown neurites: Varon, 1975). Although no signs of synaptic functions were detected in the intracellular recordings from dissociated DRG neurons, correlative electron micrographs revealed the presence of axosomatic synapses in at least some of these cultures (Miller et al., 1970; see also Lodin et al., 1973). The electron microscopic data, however, are congruent with intracellular recordings from some of the DRG neurons in cultures of intact chick ganglia, which showed depolarizing potentials resembling excitatory postsynaptic potentials (EPSPs) in addition to characteristic spike potentials (Chap. III-A; Fig. III-7) (Crain, 1971*a*). Furthermore, in more recent intracellular studies of dissociated chick DRG neurons, "on rare occasion . . . depolarizing potentials [were recorded] in one sensory ganglion cell after stimulating another" (Fischbach and Dichter, 1974; see also evidence noted from intracellular recordings of dissociated fetal mouse DRG neurons by Peacock et al., 1973). These studies suggest that under appropriate environmental conditions DRG neurons may indeed make functional synaptic connections with one another (see also Chap. III-A), as occurs between principal sympathetic ganglion neurons in culture (section 2).

Extracellular recordings of action potentials evoked in dissociated DRG neurons (from chick and mouse embryos) were studied by Okun (1972) after removal of most of the culture medium and replacement by an oil overlay (Chap. II-B). This technique facilitated analysis of impulses propagating through the complex neuritic arborizations of these dispersed DRG neurons growing in a monolayer array. Propagated action potentials were detected as early as 20 hr *in vitro* (after explantation from 7- to 10-day chick embryos) and could be recorded within 50–100 μm of newly growing neurite terminals in tests made during the first few days *in vitro*. Conduction velocities ranged from 0.05 to 0.3 meters/sec. Furthermore, complex spike-burst patterns evoked in some of these dissociated DRG networks (involving as many as 10 spikes and lasting up to 50 msec) led Okun to suggest that they may involve synaptic interactions, but this evidence is less compelling than that obtained with intracellular recordings in other DRG studies (noted above). Of particular interest was Okun's claim that most of the Schwann and connective tissue cells had been removed from these DRG cultures by differential adhesion procedures carried out during dissociation prior to explantation (Chap. II-A). Such cell fractionation experiments need to be extended more thoroughly and systematically to evaluate the degree to which the development and maintenance of neuronal functions may be dependent on critical associations with various non-neuronal supporting cells (see also sections B and C).

The effect of γ-aminobutyric acid (GABA) on dissociated newborn rat DRG neurons was studied by Obata (1974) during intracellular recordings after several days in culture. Microiontophoretic application of GABA near DRG perikarya produced a characteristic depolarization and a decrease in membrane resistance of the cultured DRG neurons, as occurs *in situ* (DeGroat, 1972; DeGroat et al., 1972; Feltz and Rasminsky, 1974) (Chap. IV-B). Similar depolarizations were produced by superfusion of 0.1–0.5 mM GABA (whereas glutamic acid, acetylcholine, and norepinephrine had no effect). These studies provide valuable data on the chemosensitivity properties of sensory ganglion cells that may be useful for analyses of mechanisms underlying the role of GABA in primary afferent depolarization and presynaptic inhibition (Chap. IV-B). On the other hand, application of GABA to cultures of dissociated spinal cord and cerebral neurons by microiontophoresis or superfusion produced membrane *hyper*polarizations as occurs *in situ* (Ransom et al., 1974; Godfrey et al., 1975) (see sections B,C; Chaps. IV-B, VI-B).

Introduction of tetrodotoxin (TTX), a drug that selectively blocks active Na^+ channels (Chap. IV-A), at concentrations which abolish all spikes in cord neurons (see Fig. V-5D; section B), did not block the action potential of dissociated chick DRG neurons; it merely decreased the rate of rise of the spike (Dichter, 1975). In fact, removal of all extracellular Na^+ from the bathing solution did not abolish these DRG cell spikes. However, if all external Ca^{++} was also removed, or if an inhibitor of Ca spikes (e.g., $CoCl_2$) was added to the Na-free or TTX medium, the DRG spike was abolished. These and related data indicate that the chick DRG perikaryon action potential is produced by both Na and Ca mechanisms together. The spike-generating mechanism in the axons of these DRG neurons, on the other hand, appears to be primarily mediated by Na^+ (Dichter, 1975; Dichter and

Fischbach, in preparation). Action potentials in one population of neurons in guinea pig Auerbach's plexus have also been shown to be resistant to TTX and in this case too the perikaryal spike appears to be generated by Ca mechanisms (Hirst and Spence, 1973). On the other hand, TTX (10^{-7} to 10^{-6} g/ml) blocked action-potential generation in dissociated sympathetic ganglion cells without altering the resting potential (Chalazonitis et al., 1974) or the ACh-evoked depolarizing potentials of these neurons (Obata, 1974; O'Lague et al., 1976; see also section 2), as occurs *in situ* (Koketsu and Nishi, 1969).

2. Sympathetic Ganglion Cells

Pharmacologic studies have also been made during intracellular recordings of characteristic resting and action potentials of dissociated sympathetic ganglion cells (from 1-day rat superior cervical ganglia) after 1–4 weeks in culture (Obata, 1974). GABA produced depolarizations of sympathetic neurons similar to those of dissociated DRG neurons—and as occurs in sympathetic ganglia *in situ* (DeGroat, 1970). On the other hand, although acetylcholine (ACh) had no effect on the DRG neurons, it produced marked depolarizations of sympathetic ganglion cells[1] by iontophoretic or bath (0.1 mM) application. These effects are to be expected in view of the transmitter role of ACh in the superior cervical ganglion *in situ* (e.g., Koketsu, 1969). Similar depolarizations were produced by iontophoretic application of ACh to trypsin-dissociated chick paravertebral sympathetic ganglion cells (from 11-day embryos) after 3–22 days in culture (Chalazonitis et al., 1974). The dissociated chick sympathetic neurons showed characteristic action potentials as well as ACh sensitivity, but no signs of synaptic potentials were noted. [Primary mediation of the sympathetic ganglion cell spikes by a Na^+ conductance mechanism was demonstrated by their blockade in TTX (ca. 10^{-7} to 10^{-6} g/ml) (Chalazonitis et al., 1974; Obata, 1974), in contrast to the resistance of DRG spikes to TTX (Dichter, 1975; see section 1).]

On the other hand, an unexpected formation of excitatory cholinergic synapses was observed among mechanically dissociated (Chap. II-A2) rat superior cervical ganglion cells after several weeks in culture (O'Lague et al., 1974). The functional properties of these synapses were elegantly analyzed during microelectrode impalements of pre- and postsynaptic neurons under direct visual observation [Fig. V-1; see also similar experi-

---

[1] Iontophoretically applied ACh also depolarized dissociated chromaffin-like cells from adult human and gerbil adrenal medulla maintained up to 1 week in culture (Biales et al., 1975). The cells exhibited formaldehyde-induced fluorescence characteristic of catecholamine-containing cells and generated characteristic resting and action potentials. It will be of interest to determine whether electrical excitability is involved in hormonal secretion by these adrenal (and related tumor) cells (Tischler et al., 1976), analogous to that which may occur in hypothalamic neurosecretory cells (see Chap. IV-D5a).

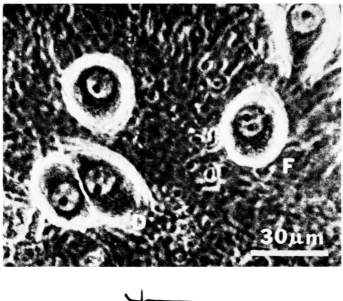

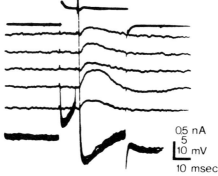

FIG. V-1. Synaptic interaction between sympathetic neurons in culture. **Top:** Phase-contrast micrograph showing a "driver-follower" pair of neurons (D,F); culture of dissociated rat superior cervical ganglion cells, 20 days *in vitro*. **Bottom:** Intracellular recordings from "driver" and "follower" neurons. **Top oscilloscope trace:** Stimulating current supplied to cell D, five sweeps superimposed. **Bottom trace:** The resulting action potentials in D, five sweeps superimposed. **Middle five traces:** EPSPs evoked in cell F; beam displaced between sweeps. (From O'Lague, Obata, Claude, Furshpan, and Potter, 1974.)

ments with central nervous system (CNS) neurons in section B]. Approximately 1–3 msec after the peak of an action potential in a "driver" neuron, a characteristic EPSP occurred in a nearby "follower" neuron (Fig. V-1). In some cases the delay was as long as 20 msec, indicating long conduction paths that possibly involved multisynaptic circuits. These EPSPs were markedly attenuated after increasing the Mg^{++}/Ca^{++} ratio (Figs. V-2,4), as occurs at chemical synapses generally (see Figs. V-8C, VI-7; Chaps.

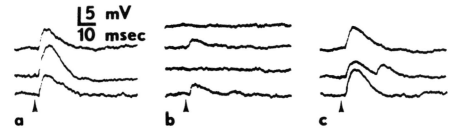

FIG. V-2. Effect of Ca^{++} and Mg^{++} concentrations on synaptic transmission between sympathetic neurons (Fig. V-1). **a** and **c:** EPSPs recorded in a 33-day-old culture perfused with 0.18 mM Mg^{++} and 2.8 mM Ca^{++} (standard concentrations), before and after 3.5 mM Mg^{++} and 0.15 mM Ca^{++} **(b)**. *Arrowheads* indicate the time at the peak of the action potential in the "driver" cell. (From O'Lague, Obata, Claude, Furshpan, and Potter, 1974.)

IV-A1, VI-E). Furthermore, the EPSPs were selectively depressed by nicotinic blocking agents (e.g., *d*-tubocurarine or hexamethonium) at concentrations (10^{-5} M) comparable to those effective in intact sympathetic ganglia of adult mammals (e.g., Perri et al., 1970). Of special interest was the demonstration that in older cultures where abundant synapses had developed iontophoretic application of ACh was often as much as 5–25 times more effective in depolarizing these sympathetic neurons compared to the sensitivity of the immature ganglion cells studied by Obata (1974) during the first week *in vitro*. "The regions of high sensitivity appeared to be sharply circumscribed and at such spots the ACh response could be made to mimic closely the appearance of an EPSP . . . [leaving] little doubt that under these conditions principal [ganglion] cells form cholinergic synapses with each other" (O'Lague et al., 1974). Since cholinergic synapses do not seem to occur between principal ganglion cells *in situ,* it will be of interest to investigate the mechanisms leading to their abundant formation in these cultures. Similarly unexpected signs of functional cholinergic synapses were observed between mouse sympathetic ganglion cells and some skeletal muscle fibers under special conditions in explant cultures (Chaps. III-B, IV-A, VIII-B) (Crain and Peterson, 1974*a*) and between dissociated rat sympathetic neurons and skeletal myotubes (Nurse and O'Lague, 1975). Are these simply due to the survival in culture of a small population of cholinergic sympathetic neurons (e.g., Yamauchi et al., 1973), or do these experiments provide clues to complex "plastic" properties of normally adrenergic sympathetic neurons under altered environmental conditions?[2]

---

[2] Patterson and Chun (1974) demonstrated that ACh-synthesis in dissociated sympathetic ganglion cell cultures was increased 100- to 1,000-fold in the presence of non-neuronal cells from sympathetic ganglia, and electrophysiologic analyses by O'Lague et al. (1974, 1976) showed that abundant cholinergic synapses had developed concomitantly in these cultures (in contrast to the low ACh synthesis and sparse evidence of excitatory synapses in cultures deficient in appropriate non-neuronal cells). Recent studies by Patterson et al. (1976) indicate, moreover, that exudates from cardiac muscle tissue cultures can produce similar enhancement of ACh synthesis in dissociated sympathetic ganglion cell cultures grown in the absence of

Alternatively, principal sympathetic ganglion cells may simultaneously synthesize both catecholamines and ACh, as suggested by Burn and Rand's (1965) dual transmitter hypothesis. This would be more compatible with the cytochemical and electron microscopic analyses of similar dissociated rat superior cervical ganglion cells, by Rees and Bunge (1974), which demonstrated that the synapses which form abundantly in their cultures are clearly adrenergic. It will be of interest to determine if the adrenergic synapses in Rees and Bunge's cultures also show cholinergic functions when tested with electrophysiologic and pharmacologic techniques similar to those used by O'Lague et al. (1974).[3] A significant related study was carried out on

---

appropriate non-neuronal cells. Correlative electrophysiologic studies of the latter cultures, and analyses of various fractions of the heart-conditioned media, may provide valuable insights into regulatory mechanisms associated with cholinergic synaptogenesis. It is of interest, in this regard, that under a different set of culture conditions where dissociated sympathetic ganglion cells are grown in the relative absence of non-neuronal cells by use of mitotic inhibitors instead of low-CO_2 media (cf. Bunge et al., 1974 versus O'Lague et al., 1974), abundant cholinergic synapses can, nevertheless, develop and show characteristic functions (Burton et al., 1975; Ko et al., 1976*b*). In the latter case, however, spinal cord explants were present in the culture and many of the dissociated sympathetic neurons were also innervated by cord neurons (Ko et al., 1975, 1976*a,b;* see below). Perhaps some component in the nutrient medium used by Bunge et al. (or exuded by the spinal cord tissue?) enhanced synaptogenesis among their dissociated sympathetic neurons, involving a similar mode of action as provided by addition of heart-conditioned medium to the cultures studied by O'Lague et al. (1974, 1976) (see also section B: footnotes 3,4).

[3] These correlative electrophysiologic tests were performed by Ko et al. (1976*b*) and they demonstrate that although the intrinsic synaptic connections in 3-week cultures have the cytochemical characteristics of noradrenergic endings all of the synapses analyzed by intracellular recordings in older ($>$ 4 weeks) cultures showed cholinergic properties (blocked by 10^{-4} M mecamylamine or hexamethonium). Since cholinergic synapses between principal neurons have not been observed *in situ*, the results suggest that the culture system may induce a change in transmitter production (see also footnote 2).

The paradox has been heightened by recent evidence that these same cultured superior cervical ganglion neurons (3–7 weeks *in vitro*) retain the ability to take up norepinephrine from the bathing fluid and show Ca^{++}-dependent release of this transmitter when the neurons are depolarized by high K^+ or exposed to tyramine (Burton and Bunge, 1975). Since iontophoretic or bath application of norepinephrine did not elicit any change in the resting or action potentials of similar sympathetic neurons in culture (Obata, 1974; see above), as *in situ* (e.g., Christ and Nishi, 1971), noradrenergic receptors may be absent in the cultures studied by Bunge and co-workers even though noradrenergic presynaptic terminals have been identified by electron microscopy and have been shown to release this transmitter, as noted above. Although the presence of noradrenergic receptors has not been excluded in the latter cultures, Burton and Bunge (1975) conclude that the "most reasonable explanation . . . would appear to be that the synapses, as initially formed during the first weeks in culture, store and release norepinephrine but, in response to the culture environment . . . the cells may be induced to add acetylcholine synthesis to their continuing catecholamine production. The cells thus retain the ability to take up and release norepinephrine and add to this the production and release of acetylcholine." This view is similar to the earlier hypothesis proposed by Burn and Rand (1965) (see above).

In explants of sympathetic ganglia presented with cardiac muscle, on the other hand, characteristic noradrenergic functions appeared to develop *in vitro* as evidenced by the transient increase in rate of cardiac muscle contractions within about 1 sec after a brief volley of sympathetic ganglion stimuli (Crain, 1968; Purves et al., 1974; see Chap. III-B). Nevertheless, as noted above, when sympathetic ganglia are co-cultured with skeletal muscle at least some of the ganglion cells can develop cholinergic synaptic functions (Crain and Peterson, 1974*a;* Nurse and O'Lague, 1975; Chaps. III-B, VIII-B).

synapses forming between spinal cord neurons and similar mechanically dissociated sympathetic ganglion cells (Bunge et al., 1974) (Fig. V-3A). Two types of synapses were observed by electron microscopy of these cultures. One type showed similar adrenergic dense-core vesicles as in isolated ganglion cell cultures (Rees and Bunge, 1974). The other type contained only clear vesicles, and these cholinergic-like synapses (Fig. V-3B) degenerated selectively 2–3 days after extirpation of the spinal cord explant. Intracellular recordings from the dissociated sympathetic neurons showed characteristic membrane resting and action potentials, comparable to the studies by O'Lague et al. (1974); but in ganglion cells grown near spinal cord explants, small local depolarizations frequently occurred spontaneously, sometimes associated with the generation of action potentials (Fig. V-3B). No such spontaneous activity was detected in superior cervical ganglion cells cultured in the absence of spinal cord. The synaptic nature of the local potentials was suggested by increases in their amplitude during hyperpolarization of the postsynaptic membrane and their reduction in amplitude and frequency when the Mg^{++} concentration was increased to 15 mM (see

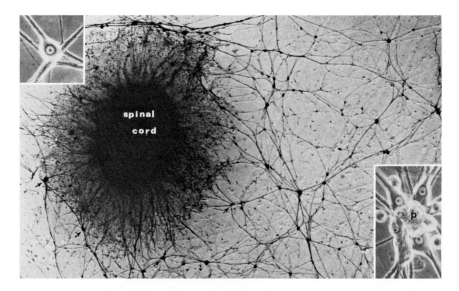

FIG. V-3A. Photomicrograph of a spinal cord (SC) explant (15-day fetal rat) providing both neuritic and cellular outgrowth which interacts with the cells (examples at *arrows*) and fibers of a network of dissociated superior cervical ganglion neurons (SCGN; from 19- to 21-day fetal rat). Note particularly the lower region where SC neurites can be seen separate from cellular components of the outgrowth. **Inset** (left): A single SCGN neuron in a network. **Inset** (right): A cluster of neurons accompanied by both single and clumps of phagocytes (p) as is common when a mitotic inhibitor is not used. This preparation was grown for 6 days in culture without a mitotic inhibitor, then fixed with OsO$_4$ and stained with Sudan black. ×21. Insets are phase-contrast pictures of living cells. ×170. (From Bunge, Rees, Wood, Burton, and Ko, 1974.)

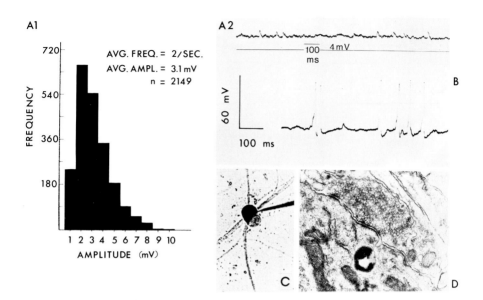

FIG. V-3B. Spontaneous local potentials recorded intracellularly from a dissociated superior cervical ganglion neuron (SCGN) in culture with spinal cord (SC) 2–4 weeks (Fig. V-3A). **A₁**: Frequency distribution of the amplitudes of 2,149 small local potentials recorded from a SCGN grown with SC for 2.5 weeks. **A₂**: A 1-sec sample from the record used for the histogram in **A₁**. More than six small depolarizations are shown in the upper trace. **B**: Spontaneous activity from another SCGN grown with SC for 4 weeks. In this cell action potentials occurred at an average rate of 3.41 imp/sec. The discharges, however, generally occurred in bursts of 2–4 imp, and the intervals between bursts frequently contained small local depolarizations. The modal frequency during the bursts was above 25 imp/sec. **C**: Injection of fast green dye into another SCGN. Current levels and pulse durations were adjusted to yield intense staining within 5–15 min. ×130. **D**: Electron micrograph of a cholinergic, axosomatic synapse found on or in the vicinity of the cell whose responses are shown in **B**. Localization of the cell was aided by the technique of dye injection shown in **C**. ×22,000; note lysosomal body in postsynaptic cell. (From Bunge, Rees, Wood, Burton, and Ko, 1974.)

also Fig. V-4). The spontaneous depolarizations of the sympathetic neurons generally occurred at rates below 5/sec, but at times bursts of 25/sec were observed. Bunge et al. (1974) suggest that these depolarizations may have been due to spontaneous discharges generated in the spinal cord explants (Chaps. IV-A, VII-A) leading to chemical transmitter activity at the cord-ganglion synapses, as *in situ*. These interpretations were recently confirmed by electrically stimulating ventral horn regions of the spinal cord explant with extracellular microelectrodes (Ko et al., 1975, 1976a) and recording intracellular EPSPs in the dissociated superior cervical ganglion neurons (Fig. V-4). These synaptic potentials could be mimicked by iontophoretic application of ACh. Both the ACh-evoked potential and the EPSP elicited by spinal cord stimuli were shown to be blocked by nicotinic blocking agents (*d*-tubocurarine or hexamethonium at 10^{-4} M) and the EPSPs could be se-

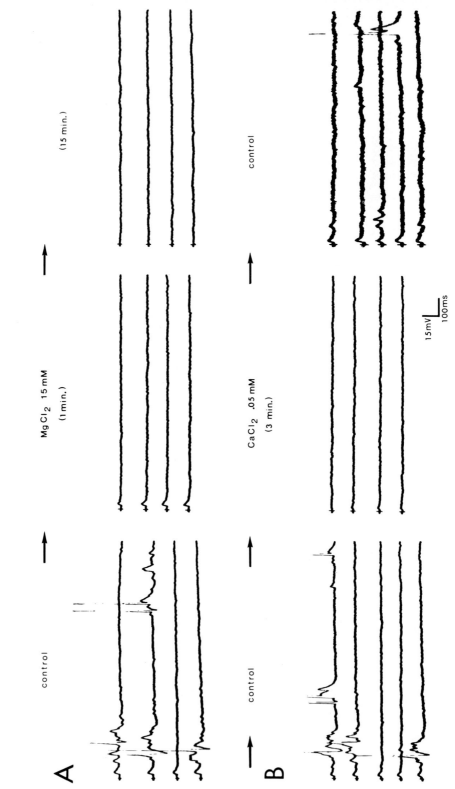

lectively depressed by increasing the Mg^{++} concentration (Fig. V-4). These results suggest that the spinal cord explants form a cholinergic nicotinic synapse *de novo* in culture on the sympathetic neurons that is functionally similar to the synapse made in the intact animal.

The experiments with dissociated sympathetic ganglion cells presented to explants of spinal cord demonstrate the potentialities of combining the advantages of the two types of culture techniques, i.e., the enhanced visibility and accessibility of dissociated neurons with the regionally organized neuronal arrays in CNS explants. Introduction of dissociated DRG cells, muscle cells, etc. near spinal cord explants should also provide valuable preparations for correlative cytologic and electrophysiologic analyses of specific types of synapses during development in culture.

B. SPINAL CORD AND BRAINSTEM

Although dissociation techniques were successfully applied to peripheral ganglion cells during the 1960s (see section A), application of this method to CNS tissues lagged far behind (Varon and Raiborn, 1969). As Varon (1970) noted in a review: "The field of dissociated neural *cell cultures* is presently undergoing the same growth pains as did the field of explant cultures some decades ago. . . . Dissociated nerve cells do survive *in vitro* and, at least in the case of ganglionic ones, can mature functionally as well as morphologically (Scott et al., 1969; Varon and Raiborn, 1971). . . . Neurites growing out of an explant (Crain et al., 1968b) can connect functionally with other neurons that were not part of the same pre-laid tissue pattern. Finally, newly formed synaptic connections have been identified by electron microscopy (Stefanelli et al., 1967) in cultured reaggregates of neuroretinal cells. It remains to discover (I hope in the near future) under what conditions two initially isolated nerve cells will produce in culture a mature and functional synapse and, in so doing, generate the basic link of the simplest model for a

---

FIG. V-4. Synaptically mediated potentials recorded intracellularly from dissociated sympathetic (SCGN) cells in response to selective stimulation of nearby spinal cord explant (similar cell array as in Fig. V-3A). **A:** in control solution (Eagle's minimum essential medium; MEM), four successive traces of potentials include an early EPSP with constant delay, followed by a series of additional EPSPs and action potentials (plus an occasional spontaneous barrage; second trace in frame on left). Introducing a solution containing 15 mM $MgCl_2$ blocks, within 1 min, both the complex late responses and the spontaneous activity but not the short-latency unitary EPSP (middle frame). In 15 min, all the evoked synaptically mediated potentials are eliminated (right frame), whereas action potentials can still be elicited by direct current passage across the ganglion cell membrane (see also Figs. V-2;8C; VI-7;8;10B,D). These effects are reversible and all the responses, including spontaneous potentials (e.g., first trace in left frame in **B**), reappear in control MEM. **B:** Similar blockade of all responses also occurs after reducing the Ca^{++} concentration to 0.05 mM (middle frame) and the effects are again reversible (right frame) (see also Fig. VI-10F,G). All the traces within each frame are consecutive. (From Ko, Burton, and Bunge, 1976a.)

neuronal network." Shortly thereafter, Fischbach (1970) did indeed report characteristic intracellularly recorded action potentials and EPSPs in studies of dissociated cells from spinal cord and skeletal muscle of chick embryo after formation of interneuronal as well as neuromuscular synapses in culture. Furthermore, the postsynaptic potentials (PSPs) in some neurons "occurred in definite patterns and at regular intervals" (Fig. V-5). (Excellent reviews are available on the extensive electrophysiologic analyses of neuro-muscular interactions carried out with cultures of dissociated muscle cells, e.g., Nelson, 1973, 1975; Shimada and Fischman, 1973; Fischbach, 1974, 1976; Fischbach et al., 1974*a,b;* see also Chap. IV-A2).

A more dramatic demonstration of intrinsic self-organizing properties of CNS neurons soon followed, utilizing small clusters of neurons after reaggregation *in vitro* of dissociated cells obtained from 13- to 14-day fetal mouse spinal cord and brainstem ("presynaptic" stages) and also from 18-day fetal mouse neocortex (see Section C). After enzymatic treatment with

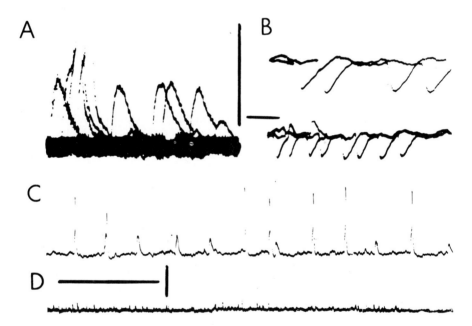

FIG. V-5. Spontaneous synaptic potentials recorded intracellularly from chick embryo spinal cord neurons (2–3 weeks *in vitro*). **A** and **B:** Superimposed traces showing depolarizing potentials (EPSPs) in one cell **(A),** hyperpolarizing potentials (IPSPs) in another cell **(B,** upper record), and both in a third cell **(B,** lower record). Vertical bar = 10 mV for **A,** 12 mV for **B.** Horizontal bar = 5 msec for **A;** 10 msec for **B,** upper; 20 msec for **B,** lower. **C:** A continuous record showing regularly occurring, large EPSPs that often trigger action potentials. Note the few small PSPs. **D:** Small PSPs recorded in the presence of tetrodotoxin (10^{-7} g/ml). (All spontaneous and evoked action potentials were abolished at this concentration.) Vertical bar = 10 mV for **C,** 5 mV for **D.** Horizontal bar = 1 sec for **C,** 5 sec for **D.** (From Fischbach and Dichter, 1974.)

0.25% trypsin in Ca^{++}- and Mg^{++}-free balanced salt solution (BSS) and repeated pipetting, cell suspensions (approximately 10^6 cells per milliliter of normal culture medium) were explanted onto collagen-coated coverglasses and incubated in Maximow depression slides, using the same procedures as for standard CNS explant cultures (Bornstein and Model, 1971, 1972). Microscopic observation immediately following explantation confirmed that the cells had been completely dissociated prior to culture. Cytologic studies indicated development of characteristic neurons and glial cells, both within the clusters as well as in the neuropil and neuritic bridges connecting many of the discrete clusters (Fig. V-6). Formation of abundant axodendritic and axosomatic synapses was demonstrated by electron microscopy of these reaggregated neuronal networks (Bornstein and Model, 1972; see also Bird and James, 1973; Fischbach and Dichter, 1974), in an extension of ultrastructural studies of synaptogenesis and maturation in undissociated fetal CNS explants (Chap. IV-A,D).[4]

After 2–4 weeks *in vitro*, complex repetitive spike discharges were recorded, spontaneously as well as in response to electric stimuli, from dozens of discrete neuronal clusters that had become attached to the collagen-coated coverglass over an area of approximately 1 cm^2 (Fig. V-7) and which appeared to be connected to one another by complex neuritic bridges (Crain and Bornstein, 1971, 1972). In the larger clusters containing dozens of neurons, characteristic long-lasting potentials were often observed in association with the spike barrages. The complex bioelectric potentials recorded in each cluster were clearly generated *within* the cell cluster, and they were not merely indications of impulses propagating along neurites passing through the cluster (as might occur between the two large cord explants in Figs. V-6;7$C_{1,2}$). Similar bioelectric discharges were also obtained from CNS reaggregates in cultures where no undissociated large explants had been included (Fig. V-8).

After introduction of strychnine (10^{-6} to 10^{-5} M) the amplitude of these

---

[4] Histofluorescence and electron microscopy studies of dissociated chick embryo spinal cord neurons cultured on previously established "feeder layers" of chick embryo liver cells (2–5 weeks *in vitro*) show a remarkable degree of catecholaminergic fluorescence in many of the perikarya and neurites and large numbers of dense-cored vesicles in the neurites (Bird and James, 1975). The catecholaminergic properties of these neurites were rarely observed in similar dissociated spinal cord cultures on collagen-coated coverslips or on feeder layers of kidney cells, and their occurrence in spinal cord *in situ* is generally considered to be due to axons from catecholaminergic neurons located in the brainstem (Chap. IV-C2). The authors suggest that "liver may stimulate catecholamine production in spinal cord cells [which may] in fact possess the synthetic pathways necessary for catecholamine production, albeit these pathways are ordinarily operative only to a minor degree" (Bird and James, 1975). This phenomenon may be analogous to the marked increase in cholinergic (but *not* in catecholaminergic) properties of dissociated sympathetic ganglion cells cultured in the presence of certain types of non-neuronal cells or in heart-conditioned media (Patterson and Chun, 1974; Patterson et al., 1976; section A2); also to the 10-fold increase in activity of choline acetyltransferase in cultures of dissociated spinal cord and skeletal muscle cells compared to spinal cord cells grown alone (Giller et al., 1973, 1975).

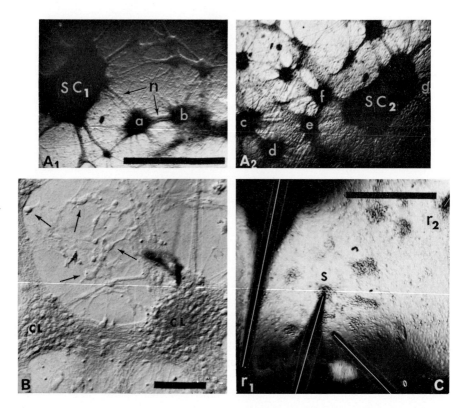

FIG. V-6. Photomicrographs of cultured reaggregates of fetal mouse spinal cord, brainstem, and cerebral cortex tissues, 2 weeks after complete cellular dissociation at explantation. $A_{1,2}$: Low-power montage of a culture showing clusters of reaggregated spinal cord and brainstem cells (a–g) which developed between (and in vicinity of) two undissociated fetal mouse spinal cord cross sections (SC_1 and SC_2) explanted 1 week earlier. (Discontinuities at junction between photomicrographs A_1 and A_2 are due to different angles of oblique illumination used to enhance salient features of the unstained array.) Fine bundles of arborizing neurites (n) connect these clusters to one another and to the large cord explants. Microelectrode recordings from this culture showed that clusters a–g and explants $SC_{1,2}$ were all functionally connected in a complex synaptic network (Fig. V-7). Scale: 1 mm. **B:** Higher-power view of a small region of this network including two reaggregated clusters (CL). Many neuron cell bodies can be seen both within the clusters as well as in a looser monolayer array (e.g., at *arrows*). Scale 100 μm. **C:** Photomicrograph of cultured reaggregates of fetal mouse cerebral cortex (2 weeks *in vitro*) obtained during electrophysiologic recordings (Fig. V-8). In this case the dispersed brain cells had reaggregated on a completely cell-free collagen-coated coverglass. Electric stimuli were applied via a pair of stimulating electrodes, with the cathode in the cluster (s); complex discharges were recorded with microelectrodes in clusters r_1 and r_2. (The white line was applied over the central axis of each micropipette shaft for clarity; cluster r_1 is not visible at this low magnification owing to optical distortion produced by micropipettes dipping into the overlying culture medium.) Scale: 1 mm. (From Crain and Bornstein, 1972; Crain, 1974*a*.)

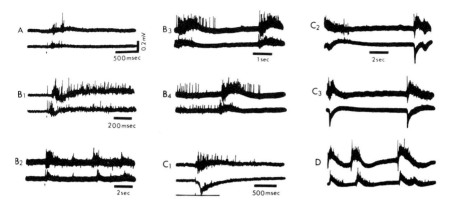

FIG. V-7. Complex evoked and spontaneous bioelectric discharges in cultured reaggregates of fetal mouse brainstem and spinal cord tissues, 2 weeks after random dispersion at explantation. **A:** Simultaneous microelectrode recordings of repetitive spike barrages and long-lasting negative slow-wave responses in two clusters of reaggregated neurons (Fig. V-6A, a, g) located 3 mm apart, elicited by single stimulus applied to the intervening large cord explant (Fig. V-6A, SC_2). **B:** After introduction of strychnine (10 μg/ml), evoked discharges became greatly enhanced in amplitude, duration, and complexity ($B_{1,2}$), and similar repetitive-spike and slow-wave potentials now occur spontaneously and *synchronously* between these distant regions ($B_{3,4}$) of the reaggregated neural network. C_1: One recording electrode (lower sweep) relocated from a cluster (g in Fig. V-6A) to nearby large cord explant (SC_2); the stimulus is now applied to another cluster (d in Fig. V-6A) midway between the two recording sites. Note the relatively long latency of the positive slow-wave response from the large explant (lower sweep). $C_{2,3}$: Discharges also occur spontaneously and synchronously between the cluster (a in Fig. V-6A) and the cord explants (SC_2 in Fig. V-6A). **D:** Simultaneous recordings of spontaneous discharges from two reaggregated clusters (ca. 3 mm apart) in another culture of dissociated brainstem and cord tissues after introduction of strychnine. Note the marked similarity of these complex repetitive spike and slow-wave sequences to those recorded in the first culture (cf. $B_{3,4}$ and $C_{2,3}$, upper sweeps). (From Crain and Bornstein, 1972; Crain, 1974a.)

slow waves and the duration and complexity of the discharge sequences were greatly enhanced (Figs. V-7B,D;8B). On the other hand, all of the complex bioelectric activities were rapidly blocked by raising the Mg^{++} concentration of the medium from 1 to 5 mM (Fig. V-8C_1), although short-latency spike potentials could still be evoked (Fig. V-8C_2). The sensitivity of these reaggregated CNS neurons to pharmacologic agents is clearly similar to that observed in larger intact CNS explants (Chaps. IV-A, VI), and the data indicate that functional synaptic networks have developed even after this more traumatic dissociation procedure. Furthermore, it is of great interest that the spontaneous and evoked activities in the neuronal reaggregates were often clearly synchronized, even between clusters separated by distances greater than 3 mm (Figs. V-7B,D;8B), as well as between reaggregates and larger intact cord explants (Fig. V-7C). The marked variation in latencies of the discharges between clusters reflect delays due to slow propagation of impulses in these fine-diameter neurites and to complex

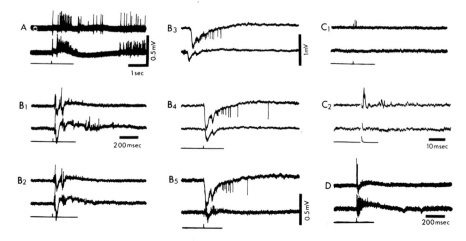

FIG. V-8. Organotypic spike barrages and oscillatory afterdischarges in cultured re-aggregates of fetal mouse cerebral cortex, 2 weeks after complete cellular dissociation. **A:** Long-lasting intermittent bursts of repetitive spikes in two clusters of reaggregated neurons (Fig. V-6, $r_{1,2}$) located 2 mm apart, evoked by single stimulus applied to another cluster (s) midway between them. **B:** After the introduction of strychnine (10 μg/ml), slow-wave components become greatly enhanced in amplitude and rhythmic positive potentials (ca. 15/sec) appear superimposed on a long-lasting negativity ($B_{1,2}$, especially in lower sweeps). B_3: Similar repetitive sequences also occur spontaneously and synchronously between the two clusters. Note the large amplitude of these slow waves and associated repetitive spike potentials. Also note the sequential increase in amplitude of spikes during later stages of the spontaneous barrage sequence (upper sweep). This is even more evident in the discharges triggered shortly afterward by single stimuli ($B_{4,5}$). Note the striking stereotyped, yet quite complex, pattern of these evoked and spontaneous discharges (B_{3-5}, upper sweeps; cf. Fig. IV-37). C_1: After increasing the Mg^{++} concentration from 1 to 5 mM, all complex discharges are completely blocked, and only brief, short-latency spike potentials can be evoked (C_2: cf. Figs. V-4; VI-7). **D:** Return of complex discharges after return to 1 mM Mg^{++}. (From Crain and Bornstein, 1972; Crain, 1974a.)

polysynaptic transmission. Synchronization was greatly enhanced after introduction of strychnine, and even some of the small clusters containing only a few neuron perikarya showed patterned, long-lasting repetitive spike bursts occurring synchronously with more complex discharges in larger clusters.

These experiments demonstrate that completely dissociated immature mammalian CNS neurons not only are able to form synaptic connections after reaggregation in culture, they can also organize from a state of random dispersion into functional synaptic networks capable of generating complex organotypic discharge patterns indicative of inhibitory as well as excitatory components. Since these dissociated neurons can now be studied with cyto-logic and bioelectric techniques during the entire period of regeneration and reaggregation in culture (Chap. II-B), this method should greatly facilitate analysis of the role of each of the cells in these experimental networks in generating characteristic CNS discharge patterns. Furthermore, since histologic studies have not yet been made to determine the degree of patterned cellular organization in our neuronal reaggregates (cf. DeLong, 1970), it remains a moot question if these organotypic CNS discharges can be generated by synaptic circuits with relatively unspecific neuronal connections (Crain, 1966; Székely, 1966; Nelson, 1967; Crain et al., 1968b), or even by cell assemblies of randomly connected neurons with appropriate biophysical properties, as in computer models of CNS networks (Farley, 1962; Andersen and Andersson, 1968).

Intracellular recordings were recently obtained from similar cultures of trypsin-dissociated embryonic spinal cord neurons (mouse: Peacock et al., 1973; chick: Fischbach and Dichter, 1974), in which the neurons were arrayed rather sparsely (and connective tissue was minimized by use of antimitotic agents: Chap. II-B) so as to facilitate visualization and microelectrode manipulation (Fig. V-9). After 2–3 weeks *in vitro*, clear-cut EPSPs often occurred spontaneously (Fig. V-5) and could be evoked by selective

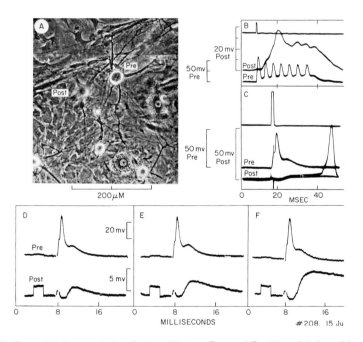

FIG. V-9. A: Synaptically coupled cells identified as Pre and Post in a 34-day-old culture of dissociated fetal mouse spinal cord neurons. **B:** Summated EPSP (middle trace) in Post to a burst of action potentials (lower trace) elicited in Pre by short current pulse (upper trace). **C:** A postsynaptic action potential in Post (lower trace) following a presynaptic action potential (middle trace) response to current stimulation (upper trace). The recording was obtained on the second penetration of the cell. **D, E, F:** During hyperpolarization of the Post cell below its action potential threshold. EPSPs of varying amplitudes (lower traces) follow presynaptic action potentials (upper traces). Upper calibration marker holds for Pre and lower calibration marker for Post. (From Peacock, Nelson, and Goldstone, 1973.)

stimulation of specific neurons under direct visual control (Fig. V-9B,D–F, as in Fig. V-1). Repetitive presynaptic impulses led to the development of more complex summated EPSPs, which in turn triggered action potentials (Fig. V-9B). Furthermore, IPSPs were also recorded in these cultures of dissociated cord neurons (Fig. V-5B). The IPSPs showed characteristic inversion to depolarizing potentials when the membrane was hyperpolarized by 10–20 mV and typical chloride ion dependence (Fischbach and Dichter, 1974; see also Chap. VI-D). Introduction of TTX rapidly abolished spontaneous and evoked action potentials in all cord neurons tested (Fig. V-5C,D), in contrast to the ineffectiveness of this agent on the action potentials of DRG neurons (section A-1). Small PSPs, however, were not blocked by TTX (Fig. V-5D) and they are probably due to spontaneous release of transmitter from the presynaptic neuron, i.e. they are miniature PSPs. During simultaneous intracellular stimulation and recording, direct electrotonic spread of current between two neurons was never observed even when the two cell bodies appeared continuous. Electron micrographs of such "touching" neurons showed that their membranes were not separated by intervening connective tissue cells or glia. This does not, however, preclude occurrence of electrically coupled gap junctions at the earliest stages of synaptogenesis (e.g., Potter et al., 1966; Furshpan and Potter, 1968) since intracellular microelectrode tests have been limited so far primarily to older dissociated CNS cultures. Furthermore, by simultaneously recording from two neurons while stimulating several others in turn, it was possible to show that one neuron could receive synaptic input from more than one cell and that one neuron could innervate more than one cell. Contiguity was not a good criterion for functional contact. In fact, immediately adjacent cells were rarely synaptically connected, suggesting that synapse formation may have involved some degree of specificity (Fischbach and Dichter, 1974).

These elegant experiments provide a valuable extension of the studies of synaptic network discharges recorded extracellularly in reaggregated neuronal clusters (Figs. V-7;8). They demonstrate, moreover, the potentialities of correlative extra- and intracellular microelectrode studies in such "simple" neuronal arrays in culture. With the use of the Nomarski interference microscope, it may indeed soon become possible to visualize synaptic boutons and other physiologically significant cell structures in long-term cultures of mammalian CNS networks during highly localized microelectrode stimulation and recordings (e.g., Fischbach et al., 1973; Fischbach and Dichter, 1974; see also Ransom and Nelson, 1975, and below), as was recently achieved by Kuffler et al. (1971) with these new optics while studying synapses on freshly isolated frog parasympathetic ganglion cells. Application of these techniques to the synapses on dissociated rat sympathetic ganglion cells in culture (Bunge et al., 1974; O'Lague et al., 1974) should be equally fruitful (see section A).

Microiontophoretic application of glutamate, GABA, and glycine in similar low-density cultures of dissociated mouse spinal cord neurons produced characteristic membrane conductance changes (Ransom et al., 1974; Ransom and Barker, 1975; Ransom and Nelson, 1975). The cells in these thinly dispersed arrays showed similar synaptic potentials as observed in previous studies (see above) and PSPs were blocked in 10 mM Mg^{++} (Ransom and Barker, 1975). In some innervated cells glutamate sensitivity was particularly high near dendritic terminals, whereas noninnervated cells showed low sensitivity. The reversal potential for glutamate was substantially more negative than that for the EPSP. GABA produced a marked increase in membrane conductance in many cells with the equilibrium potential for the GABA response being between −20 and −60 mV in different cells. Glycine produced no responses when tested in the complete culture medium, which contained 0.4 mM glycine (Chap. VI-A), but glycine conductance increases and hyperpolarizations were readily obtained in glycine-free medium. Characteristic GABA hyperpolarizations could be elicited, however, in the complete culture medium. These data suggest that chronic application of high concentrations of glycine causes complete desensitization to this amino acid. Furthermore, since spinal cord cells still respond to GABA in cultures desensitized to glycine, the GABA receptor appears to be distinct from the glycine receptor (Ransom and Nelson, 1975). The reversal potentials for the GABA and glycine responses were, moreover, close to the reversal potential for the IPSPs recorded in response to presynaptic stimulation.

These experiments illustrate the depth of the significant data on electrophysiologic and pharmacologic properties of CNS neurons that can now be achieved with improved dissociated culture techniques. Of special importance is the feasibility of detailed topographic analyses of the chemosensitivity of entire CNS neurons in these low-density cultures using accurate microelectrode positioning under direct visual observation. The paucity of non-neuronal cells not only facilitates detailed cytologic study, it also permits more intimate and accurate localization of the iontophoresis pipette tip at selected sites on the nerve cell membrane (Ransom and Nelson, 1975), analogous to the elegant topographic chemosensitivity studies at synaptic-bouton sites by Kuffler et al. (1971), as noted above. This experimental approach will become even more valuable as methods are developed to identify more clearly the specific types of neurons which survive in these dissociated CNS cultures (e.g., Fischbach, 1976) (Chap. II-A2. See also review by Ransom and Nelson, 1975; Chap. IX-A).

C. CEREBRAL CORTEX AND CEREBELLUM

In small reaggregates of dissociated 18-day fetal mouse cerebral cortex tissue (Fig. V-6C), remarkably organotypic oscillatory (ca. 10–15/sec) afterdischarges also occurred spontaneously as well as in response to stimuli (Fig. V-8B; cf. Figs. IV-37;38). These stereotyped complex repetitive discharge sequences have heretofore been observed only in well-organized undissociated CNS explants. All of the other electrophysiologic properties observed in the reaggregates of dissociated cord neurons (see section B) could also be demonstrated in these dissociated cerebral cultures (Crain and Bornstein, 1972).[5]

Intracellular microelectrode studies by Nelson and Peacock (1973) in cultures of dissociated fetal mouse (11- to 16-day) cerebellar neurons provide further evidence that dispersed CNS cells can develop organotypic synaptic networks *in vitro*. In addition to demonstrating characteristic EPSPs and IPSPs in these cerebellar neurons, Nelson and Peacock (1973) carried out a rather elaborate analysis of the complex patterned activities generated by a small group of neurons in a 1-month-old culture (Figs. V-10;11). This experiment provides a particularly dramatic illustration of the potentialities for quantitative electrophysiologic analyses of mammalian synaptic networks under culture conditions that permit concomitant microscopic observation of an entire group of neuronal perikarya and their neuritic arborizations.

Similarly impressive intracellular recordings were made more recently by Nelson and co-workers in thinly arrayed cultures of dissociated fetal rat (15–20 day) cerebral cells (Godfrey et al., 1975); see details of special fluorodeoxyuridine (FdU) exposure in Chap. II-A2. After 1–2 months *in vitro,* characteristic action potentials and bursts of spikes superimposed on depolarizing waves could be evoked by brief electric stimuli. IPSPs and EPSPs were elicited in many of the neurons, including evidence of reciprocal excitatory and inhibitory connections between one pair of cells.[6] Ionto-

---

[5] Reaggregates of dissociated fetal mouse cerebral cells cultured in rotating-shaker flasks may develop a high degree of histologic organization including laminar arrays of cortical neurons (DeLong, 1970; see also Levitt et al., 1975) (Chaps. II-A2 and IV-C3). However, no electrophysiologic studies have been reported as yet on these interesting preparations.

Correlative biochemical analyses have been carried out by Seeds (1971, 1973) and others on similar brain cell reaggregates (see reviews in Nelson, 1975; Richelson, 1975). The activities of three neuronal enzymes showed marked increases during the first 3 weeks after explantation as occur during normal maturation *in situ*. Choline acetyltransferase increased 20-fold to an activity 70% of adult mouse brain *in situ*, acetylcholinesterase activity increased 10-fold to 40% of adult brain (see Chap. VI-C), and glutamate decarboxylase (GAD) activity increased five-fold to 33% of adult brain (Seeds, 1973). The GAD level increased more than twofold during the first 4 days in culture and then rose much more slowly during the following 2 weeks. These GAD analyses are consonant with preliminary data obtained on explants of 18-day fetal mouse hippocampus (Lehrer et al., *in preparation*) and correlate well with electrophysiologic evidence of early onset of GABA-mediated tonic inhibition (see Chap. IV-D3).

[6] Similar EPSPs and IPSPs have been observed during intracellular recordings in cultures of trypsin-dissociated cerebral cortical neurons (from 18-day fetal rat) by Dichter (1975). In these experiments, the dissociated cerebral neurons developed mature cytologic and bioelectric properties in relatively routine culture media without the FdU treatment utilized by Godfrey et al. (1975).

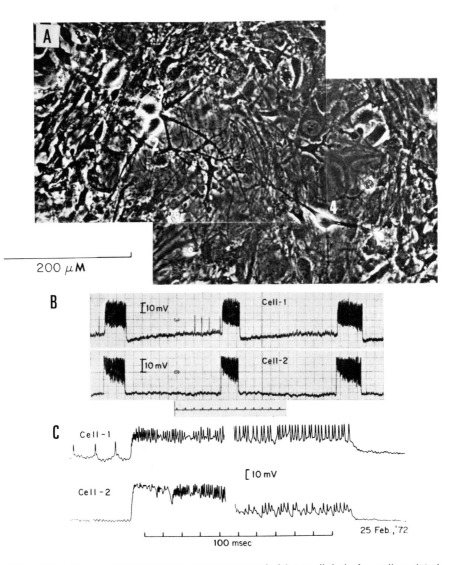

FIG. V-10. Action potential bursting patterns recorded intracellularly from dissociated fetal mouse cerebellar neurons. **A:** Phase-contrast photomicrograph of four neurons in a 32-day-old culture. **B:** Synchronous bursts of action potentials recorded from cells 1 and 2, which had resting potentials of −56 and −60 mV, respectively. **C:** Recording of bursts at a faster time base to show synchrony of burst onset and termination. The prolonged period (ca. 1–2 sec) was deleted during the middle of the burst. Note the similarity to paroxysmal depolarizing shift (PDS) discharges in hippocampal explants (Fig. IV-42). (From Nelson and Peacock, 1973.)

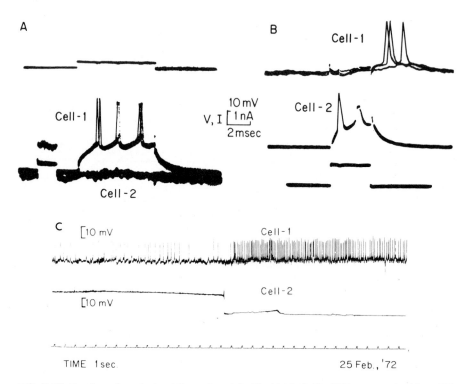

FIG. V-11. Continued analysis of the network in Fig. V-10. **A:** No PSPs are evoked in cell 2 by action potential firing of cell 1 in response to direct electric stimulation (upper trace). **B:** PSPs and action potentials are evoked in cell 1 (upper trace) by presynaptic firing of cell 2 (middle trace) to direct stimulation (lower trace). **C:** After cell 3 was eliminated, cell 2 was repenetrated (middle trace, at center of trace). The bursting pattern is no longer present in either cell 1 or 2. Penetration of cell 2 is accompanied by an acceleration of firing rate in cell 1. (From Nelson and Peacock, 1973.)

phoretic application of glycine and GABA was carried out on these cerebral neurons in correlation with similar experiments by Ransom and Nelson (1975) on dissociated spinal cord neurons (see above). Similar results were obtained with both types of neurons, except that the glycine response in the brain cells was not desensitized in 0.5 mM glycine as had been observed with the cord neurons (see above; also Chap. VI-A,B). This remarkable demonstration of characteristic synaptic activities and membrane responses to applied neurotransmitters in such a *thinly arrayed* group of mammalian cerebral neurons maintained for 1–2 *months* in culture marks the culmination of the strenuous attempts to achieve this goal in many laboratories during the past decade or more. The hopes expressed by Varon in his 1970 review (see section B) have now been successfully achieved, and correlative cytologic and physiologic analyses of dissociated CNS neurons during development in culture will undoubtedly provide valuable new insights into neural functions during the coming decade.

VI

Characteristic Sensitivities of CNS Explant Discharge Patterns to Selective Pharmacologic and Metabolic Agents

A. STRYCHNINE versus GLYCINE

The potent effect of strychnine in enhancing complex evoked and spontaneous discharges in CNS explants shortly after onset of synaptogenesis (Chap. IV-A,D) suggests that inhibitory synaptic circuits may begin to function rather early in development of the central nervous system (CNS) (Crain and Peterson, 1967; Crain, 1974a; Crain and Bornstein, 1974). Still more dramatic effects attributable to development of inhibitory circuits in CNS explants are observed in many older cultures where few signs of complex bioelectric activity can be detected in the normal culture medium. Even with large single or repetitive electric stimuli, the responses may be limited to brief series of spike potentials, often followed by a simple positive wave (e.g., Fig. IV-4D; see also Figs. VI-2A;9A, VII-4A). Introduction of strychnine (ca. 10^{-6} M) reveals, however, that these explants have indeed retained their capacity to generate elaborate, organotypic, synaptically mediated discharges consisting of long-lasting negative slow waves and repetitive spike barrages (e.g., Fig. VII-1; see also Fig. IV-4E–L).[1] The thresholds for activating these complex network discharges are often reduced under strychnine to levels that lead to spontaneous activity. In normal culture media, however, inhibitory circuits effectively quench activation of these networks following initial generation of action potentials in some of the neurons.

On the other hand, application of 10^{-3} M glycine to those spinal cord explants that can generate complex discharges in normal culture medium leads to rapid depression of most of the complex slow-wave and repetitive-spike activities, and only brief spike bursts or simple negative slow-wave responses can then be evoked (Fig. VI-1B,D,F) (Crain, 1972b,c; 1974b). The glycine depression can be prevented by adding a low concentration of

---

[1] Strychnine (up to 3×10^{-5} M) had no significant effects on fetal mouse olfactory bulb explant responses even though 10^{-6}–10^{-5} M bicuculline generally led to onset of prominent negative slow-wave discharges in this type of CNS tissue (Corrigall et al., 1976). These data provide additional evidence regarding the relative specificity of action of strychnine (at levels of 10^{-6}–10^{-5} M) on cerebral neocortex, hippocampus, and spinal cord explants [and on cerebellar explants at even lower concentrations (Gähwiler, 1976a)].

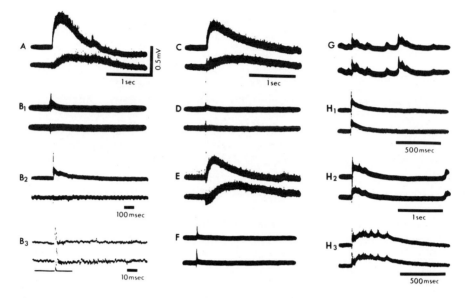

FIG. VI-1. Selective depression of major components of complex synaptic network discharges of fetal spinal cord explants in high-glycine BSS and complete recovery after addition of strychnine. **A:** Complex slow-wave and spike-barrage responses evoked in two regions of cord explant in BSS, by a single stimulus to another cord site (1 month *in vitro*). (Many of the individual spike potentials are obscured or only faintly visible in the records at slow sweep rates. **B**$_{1,2}$: Rapid disappearance of most components of the complex afterdischarge following introduction of 10^{-3} M glycine. Almost complete block occurs after several minutes (**B**$_3$). **C:** Original complex responses are rapidly restored after return to BSS. **D:** Sustained depression occurs again after return to 10^{-3} M glycine. **E:** Approximately 1 min after introduction of 10^{-6} M strychnine plus 10^{-3} M glycine, there is almost complete restoration of complex discharges (which are maintained in this solution as well as after return to BSS). Note the spontaneous spikes prior to the onset of the stimulus, as well as the long-lasting spike barrage during slow-wave responses. **F:** Similar block with 10^{-3} M glycine in another cord explant (2 weeks *in vitro*). **G:** Restoration of long-lasting rhythmic afterdischarge in BSS. **H**$_1$: Partial depression after return to 10^{-3} M glycine plus 10^{-7} M strychnine. Within 2 min, however, the complex afterdischarge pattern began to reappear (**H**$_2$) and became still more prominent after another minute (**H**$_3$). (From Crain, 1974*b*.)

strychnine (10^{-6} M: Fig. VI-1E; 10^{-7} M: Fig. VI-1H), whereas strychnine is ineffective against high-Mg^{++} or low-Ca^{++} blockades (Fig. VI-8; see also section E) (Crain and Pollack, 1973; Crain, 1974*b*). Introduction of 10^{-7} M strychnine to the culture medium is probably comparable to the 0.1 mg/kg dosage (intravenous) in the adult cat which produces selective reduction of synaptic inhibition in spinal cord neurons (Bradley et al., 1953; Curtis et al., 1971*a*). These data suggest that strychnine enhancement of bioelectric discharges of CNS explants may be due to selective interference with glycine-sensitive receptors, possibly related to inhibitory synaptic membranes, as occurs *in situ* (e.g., Curtis et al., 1971*a*). The depressant effects of glycine perfusion on synaptically mediated discharges of spinal cord explants are consonant with Hösli et al.'s (1971, 1973, 1975a) demonstration that micro-electrophoretic application of glycine produces characteristic hyperpolarization potentials and increased membrane conductance of neurons in similar rat spinal cord explants, as occurs *in situ* in mimicry of inhibitory synaptic transmitter effects (Curtis et al., 1967, 1968; Werman et al., 1968; Curtis, 1975) (see also the glycine effects on dissociated cord neurons in Chap. V-B,C).

The specificity of glycine depression of spinal cord explant discharges is further supported by the following evidence: (1) In cultures of cord-in-nervated skeletal muscle (Figs. II-1, IV-10;13) (Crain et al., 1970; Crain and Peterson, 1974*a*) coordinated muscle contractions can still be evoked by ventral cord stimuli during this glycine blockade of internuncial CNS activity. (2) Explants of cerebral neocortex show little or no depression in 10^{-3} M glycine (Fig. VI-3G), whereas 10^{-4} M γ-aminobutyric acid (GABA) produces marked cerebral and cerebellar blocking effects (Fig. VI-3B; see also section B). (3) GABA (10^{-3} M) also produces serious depression of ventral spinal cord discharges, but 10^{-7} M strychnine is ineffective in pre-venting this blockade; even 10^{-6} M strychnine produces only transient re-covery (Crain, 1974*b*). (4) Bicuculline, picrotoxin, and penicillin, on the other hand, which appear to antagonize GABA receptor sites *in situ* (Curtis et al., 1971*b,c,* 1972; Davidoff, 1972*a,b*), can produce sustained recovery from GABA blockades of ventral cord discharges at concentrations that are ineffective against glycine depressions (see section B). (5) No depression of cord discharges occurs with 10^{-3} M levels of α-aminobutyric acid, γ-guanidinobutyric acid, serine, leucine, threonine, tryptophane, and other amino acids. (6) A series of peptides including glycyl-γ-aminobutyric acid, glycyltryptophane, and glycylglycylglycine show no depressing effects at 10^{-3} M, and some may even produce excitatory effects on cord and cerebral explants. The latter data are in agreement with earlier observations of Purpura (1960) indicating that topical application of the dipeptide γ-amino-butyryl-γ-aminobutyric acid on adult cat cerebral cortex *in situ* markedly augmented surface-negative cortical evoked responses, in contrast to the powerful depressant effects of GABA. The absence of depression and the possible excitatory effects of these peptides provide further support for specificity of action of the component amino acids, and the data also sug-gest that enzymatic control of the formation and breakdown of simple peptides at synapses may be a significant mechanism for regulating CNS excitability (Crain, 1975*c,* 1975*d;* see also Reichelt and Kvamme, 1973).

Although high glycine concentrations (10^{-3} M) are used in the bathing fluid to produce these profound depressions of synaptically mediated dis-charges in CNS explants, the controls noted above suggest that the effects may nevertheless be of physiologic significance. Effective microelectrophoretic application of glycine and other putative transmitters (e.g., Curtis et al., 1968) probably produces concentrations of approximately 10^{-4} to 10^{-3} M near the neuronal cell surface (Curtis, *personal communication*). Moreover, although normal glycine levels in cerebrospinal fluid (CSF) are of the order of 10^{-5} M (Dickinson and Hamilton, 1966), local concentrations in the vicinity of CNS neurons may reach much higher values. It is of interest in this regard that serum glycine levels are approximately 2×10^{-4} M, and some of the standard synthetic tissue culture media—e.g., Puck's medium N-16 (Puck et al., 1958)—contain 10^{-3} glycine (see Chap. V-B).

Intraventricular or intrathecal injections of 2.5–5 mg glycine in adult cats (3–4 kg) produce marked selective inhibition of flexor and crossed extension reflexes, and 4–15 mg abolishes the facilitation of these reflexes produced by 10 μg strychnine (Dhawan et al., 1972). The concentrations of glycine and strychnine which developed in the CSF following these injections may well be comparable to the levels used to bathe the CNS explants. Furthermore, the requirement of 1,000-fold higher concentration of glycine to neutralize strychnine effects in the cat is quite similar to the glycine/strychnine ratios obtained in the CNS cultures. These studies of exogeneous application of glycine and strychnine to CNS explants (and GABA-picrotoxin; see section B) do not preclude, of course, the possibility that glycine and GABA may simply mimic some unidentified inhibitory synaptic transmitter agents, and that their depressant effects may not necessarily be confined to inhibitory postsynaptic membranes (Chap. IV-D).

It should be emphasized that diffuse introduction of pharmacologic and transmitter agents into the solution bathing CNS explants provides, in contrast to microiontophoretic application, a relatively controlled concentration of the agent in the medium surrounding the entire neuron—including all of its extensively arborizing dendrites studded with synapses—not just the perikaryal zone as often occurs in CNS experiments *in situ* as well as with explants (e.g, Geller and Woodward, 1974). Furthermore, the effects of antagonists can be quantitatively measured by systematic "titrations" with the agonist, assuming that a reliable bioelectric parameter of synaptic network function is available (e.g., evoked repetitive-spike or slow-wave discharges, or spontaneous patterned spike firing sequences; see section B). Bath exposure to transmitters is limited, however, to agents that do not involve rapid desensitization effects; otherwise, iontophoretic application can be far more efficient for detecting transient alterations in excitability properties. On the other hand, microiontophoretic application of chemical agents in low-density monolayer cultures of dissociated CNS neurons (in contrast to its use on intact CNS explants) provides an extremely valuable opportunity to determine the topologic chemosensitivity of the entire neuron, from the perikaryon out to the dendritic and axonal terminal regions (e.g., Ransom and Nelson, 1975) (Chap. V-B).

B. BICUCULLINE versus GABA

1. Effects of Picrotoxin and Bicuculline

A similar selective antagonism occurs between picrotoxin (or bicuculline) and GABA in cerebral explants—as shown above (section A) between strychnine and glycine in spinal cord explants. Just as low levels of strychnine (10^{-7} to 10^{-6} M) can produce dramatic appearance or enhancement of complex discharges in older, strongly inhibited cord explants, introduction of similar concentrations of picrotoxin in cerebral neocortex and hippocampus explants leads to marked increases in amplitude and duration of evoked responses (Fig. VI-2B,D) (Crain, 1972b,c; 1975c). Furthermore, inversion of the polarity of early-latency positive slow-wave potentials occurs (cf. Fig. VI-2B versus VI-2 A$_2$, upper sweeps; Fig. VI-2D$_2$ versus VI-2 E$_1$), as observed with higher levels of strychnine in some cerebral explants (Crain, 1964a) or with lower levels in spinal cord. The positive slow-wave "population discharges" may represent extracellular recordings of summated inhibitory postsynaptic potentials (IPSPs), which can be selectively depressed by antagonists of the inhibitory transmitter agents involved in these synaptic networks. Excitatory postsynaptic potential (EPSP) components then dominate the network discharges and may account for the large negative slow-wave potentials observed during exposure of cerebral explants to picrotoxin, strychnine, etc. (Crain, 1966, 1969) (Chaps. IV-D, VII-D.)

Although 10^{-4} M GABA shows little depressant effect on spinal cord activity, this concentration produces marked blockade of complex discharges in previously active cerebral cortex explants (Fig. VI-3B). Introduction of 2×10^{-5} M picrotoxin prevents this GABA depression even when 10^{-3} M GABA is added (Fig. VI-3C), just as 10^{-7} M strychnine prevents a 10^{-3} M glycine depression in spinal cord explants (Fig. VI-1). GABA (10^{-3} M) may produce transient excitatory effects on some network components of cerebral explants (Fig. VI-3E$_1$), resembling the primary afferent depolarization potentials (PADs) evoked in dorsal spinal cord by dorsal root ganglion (DRG) stimuli (Fig. IV-19C). However, application of 10^{-3} M GABA generally leads to profound depression of most cerebral neocortex and hippocampus explant discharges, as occurs with almost all ventral spinal cord network discharges as well as long-latency dorsal cord responses (Chap. IV-B).

These pharmacologic data on cord and cerebral explants are compatible with the results of microelectrophoretic application of GABA and glycine in cat spinal cord *in situ*, which suggests that GABA may be the inhibitory transmitter at bicuculline- and picrotoxin-sensitive axodendritic and axo-axonic synapses mediating "prolonged inhibition" of spinal motoneurons,

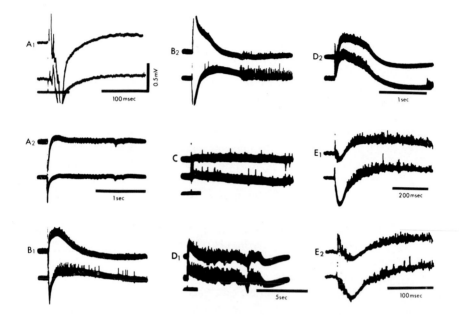

FIG. VI-2. Enhancement of the complex synaptic network discharge of fetal mouse cerebral neocortex explants by low levels of picrotoxin (1 month in culture). **A₁**: Simultaneous recordings of a brief spike burst and a large positive slow-wave potential (ca. 50 msec in duration) evoked at two sites in a cerebral explant in regular BSS, in response to a brief stimulus applied at a third site. **A₂**: At a slower sweep rate, a negative slow wave of small amplitude can be seen following early positivity, and after a much longer latency an oscillatory (ca. 10/sec) afterdischarge is barely discernible above the noise level. An increase in stimulus strength does not elicit any additional increment in these network responses. **B₁**: After introduction of picrotoxin at 2×10^{-7} M, the amplitude and duration of the negative slow-wave response at one site is greatly increased (upper sweep), even with a single weak stimulus. A still-longer-duration (ca. 1 sec) negative slow wave now appears at the other site (lower sweep); it is of small amplitude and is accompanied by a long-lasting barrage of spike potentials. **B₂**: Increasing the picrotoxin level to 2×10^{-6} M further enhances these effects. **C:** Asynchronous low-frequency spike barrages evoked at two sites of another cerebral explant in regular BSS, in response to a stimulus applied at a third site. **D₁**: After introduction of picrotoxin at 2×10^{-6} M, much more elaborate responses could be elicited at the same or smaller stimulus strength (and these also occurred spontaneously). Note the complex sequence of slow waves and high-frequency spike barrages lasting for nearly 10 sec. **D₂**: Increasing the picrotoxin level to 2×10^{-5} M further enhanced the amplitude of the initial negative slow-wave response. **E₁**: After return to regular BSS, an early-latency positive potential of large amplitude appears (similar to that in **A**) and is now followed by a negative slow wave and a high-frequency spike barrage (as in the explant in **A**; see also Fig. IV-42A). **E₂**: A faster sweep shows that the early positive slow wave is preceded by short but clear-cut spike bursts. (From Crain, 1975c).

whereas glycine is probably the transmitter at strychnine-sensitive, axo-somatic synapses mediating "direct" inhibition of motoneurons (Curtis et al., 1971*b;* Curtis and Johnston, 1974; Curtis, 1975). The tissue culture experiments are also consonant with *in situ* studies suggesting that GABA is an important inhibitory transmitter in cerebral cortex (Curtis et al., 1971*c*).

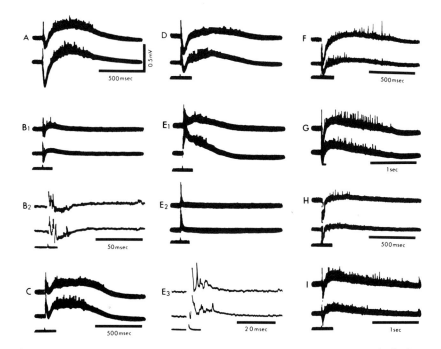

FIG. VI-3. Selective depression of major components of the synaptic network discharges of a fetal mouse cerebral neocortex explant in high GABA, and antagonism by picrotoxin. **A:** Simultaneous recordings of complex discharges evoked at two sites in a cerebral explant by a stimulus applied at a third site, in regular BSS after recovery from picrotoxin (same culture as in Fig. VI-2, after records E). **B:** Disappearance of most components of complex responses within 2 min after introduction of 10^{-4} M GABA. Only a short spike burst and a small positive slow wave can be evoked, even with very large stimuli (cf. ventral spinal cord explants, which generally require 10^{-3} M GABA to produce this degree of depression, e.g. Fig. IV-19E_1). **C:** After recovery in regular BSS, introduction of picrotoxin at 2×10^{-5} M together with 10^{-3} M GABA produces no significant depression. Elaborate responses can still be evoked with small stimuli even though the GABA concentration is 10 times the level required to produce the blockade in **B**. **D:** Restoration of the characteristic response pattern after return to regular BSS (note recovery of the early-latency positive slow wave as in **A**). **E_1:** There is a transient shift to a large negative slow-wave response immediately after introduction of 10^{-3} M GABA (see text). **E_2:** Within 1 min, however, complete depression develops, and only simple spike bursts can be evoked, even with large stimuli (**E_3**). **F:** Restoration of characteristic complex discharges after thorough rinsing in regular BSS (as in **A** and **D** where picrotoxin was used to expedite recovery). **G:** Introduction of 10^{-3} M glycine produces no significant depression (in contrast to the strong block which generally occurs in spinal cord explants, e.g., Fig. VI-1). **H:** Taurine at 10^{-3} M, on the other hand, depresses part of the cerebral network discharge but is less effective than 10^{-4} M GABA (**B**). **(I):** Restoration of characteristic responses after return to regular BSS. (From Crain, 1975c.)

Furthermore, the lack of depressant effects of 10^{-3} M glycine on cerebral explants (Fig. VI-3G; cf. glycine block in cord: Fig. VI-1B) agrees well with the "very weak effects of glycine on [cerebral] neurons" (Curtis et al., 1971c; Curtis, 1975). Finally, the moderate depressant effects of 10^{-3} M taurine (Fig. VI-3H versus VI-3G) may be related to data *in situ,* suggesting taurine as a possible inhibitory transmitter in rat brain (Curtis and Watkins, 1965; Davison and Kaczmarek, 1971; cf. Lahdesmaki and Oja, 1972). The relatively potent excitant effect of strychnine on cerebral explants (although generally requiring higher concentrations than in spinal cord cultures) is evidently not related to antagonism of glycinergic synapses as in cord. It may instead be due to antagonism of other cerebral inhibitory pathways, and it is of interest that the depressant effects of taurine (as well as of several other amino acids) are also blocked by strychnine (Curtis and Johnston, 1974).

Our studies of the effects of GABA versus bicuculline and picrotoxin on evoked potentials in cerebral explants are also consonant with analyses (Gähwiler, 1975, 1976a) of the effects of these agents on the spontaneous firing patterns of neonatal rat cerebellar explants. As described above (Chap. IV-E), Gähwiler et al. (1973) utilized Mg^{++} and other pharmacologic agents to characterize prominent components of the spontaneous spike discharges in their cerebellar explants which appeared to be mediated by synaptic network activity (e.g., irregular spike firing patterns, etc.). These baselines have now been utilized to study the effects of GABA and other presumptive transmitter agents and their antagonists on synaptic activities in cerebellar cultures. Addition of low concentrations of GABA (10^{-6} M) to the bathing medium rapidly reduced the normal spontaneous firing rate of Purkinje cells; and complete (but reversible) block occurred at 10^{-5} M (Fig. VI-4; see also Fig. IV-43). No tests were made to determine if 10^{-5} M GABA also suppressed evoked synaptic network discharges in cerebellar explants. It may well be that somewhat higher concentrations would be required — approaching 10^{-4} M as in our cerebral explants. Glycine, on the other hand, produced no significant depression of the characteristic cerebel-

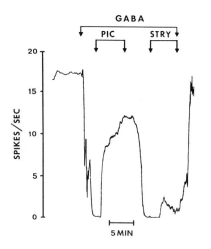

FIG. VI-4. Depressant effect of GABA on the spontaneous firing rate of Purkinje cells in cerebellum explant, and antagonism by picrotoxin (neonatal rat; 15 days *in vitro*). Note the block of spontaneous activity shortly after introduction of GABA (10^{-5} M) and the rapid recovery after addition of picrotoxin (10^{-5} M). Block occurs again in GABA after withdrawal of picrotoxin, but strychnine (10^{-5} M) leads only to a small transient increase in the firing rate. Note the reversibility of the actions of all three drugs and the similarity to their effects on cerebral explant discharges (Fig. VI-3). (From Gähwiler, 1975.)

lar neuron discharges at concentrations approaching 10^{-3} M, and blocking effects at higher concentrations were apparently nonspecific since they were not prevented by concomitant application of 10^{-6} to 10^{-5} M strychnine (Gähwiler, 1976a). Introduction of strychnine alone, however, elicited significant excitatory effects on cerebellar spike firing patterns at low concentrations (10^{-8} to 10^{-6} M), suggesting other modes of action in addition to glycine antagonism (as in our cerebral cultures; see above).

Introduction of bicuculline (10^{-8} M) or picrotoxin (10^{-5} M) during blockade of spontaneous discharges of cerebellar neurons by 10^{-5} M GABA rapidly reversed this depression, whereas strychnine (10^{-7} to 10^{-5} M) was ineffective (Fig. VI-4). These data on cerebellar network activities are also remarkably congruent with our observations in cerebral explants (Figs. VI-2;3). Finally, Gähwiler (1975) demonstrated powerful excitatory effects of bicuculline (10^{-10} to 10^{-6} M) and picrotoxin (10^{-7} to 10^{-4} M) when added alone to cerebellar explants. In view of the selective antagonism of these agents to exogeneously applied GABA (in contrast to strychnine), the data suggest the "existence of functional synapses in cultures of rat cerebellum in which endogenous GABA is used as transmitter" (Gähwiler and Stähelin, 1975), in agreement with our earlier conclusions based on analogous studies in cerebral explants (Crain, 1972a,b; 1974b).

Geller and Woodward (1974) also studied the effects of GABA and its antagonists on neurons in cerebellar explants using microiontophoretic techniques (Chap. IV-E). Although "picrotoxin blocked the action of GABA in two instances it had no effect in three instances. Bicuculline blocked the action of GABA on two cells in which it did not alter the pattern of firing. On seven other cells, bicuculline evoked cyclic bursts of firing, and may have obscured a blocking of GABA action" (Geller and Woodward, 1974). These data are ambiguous regarding synaptic effects, but they are useful for comparison with similar iontophoretic studies in cerebellum *in situ,* where the focus is primarily on the chemosensitivity of Purkinje neuron perikarya to locally applied putative neurotransmitters. Relatively high local concentration gradients of GABA may be produced by microiontophoretic application near the neuron perikaryon; and some of the negative results with picrotoxin, for example, may have been due to the development of unduly high local concentrations of GABA producing nonspecific hyperpolarization of the cerebellar neurons, as observed by Gähwiler (1976) with bath application of high concentrations of glycine to cerebellar explants. In contrast, the low concentrations of bicuculline (10^{-8} M) and picrotoxin (10^{-6} M) which rapidly reversed GABA blockade of cerebellar network discharges in Gähwiler's (1975) perfusion experiments (Fig. VI-4) demonstrate the sensitivity of this relatively simple experimental method for quantitative pharmacologic studies of synaptic network functions. Extension of these studies by the use of electrically evoked (Leiman and Seil, 1973) as well as spontaneous discharges should provide significant additional insights into the effects of pharmacologic agents on cerebellar explants.

2. Excitatory Effects of Penicillin

As noted above (see section A), penicillin produced sustained recovery from GABA blockade of ventral spinal cord discharges at concentrations (ca. 1,000 units/ml; sodium penicillin G) that were ineffective against glycine depressions — similar to the GABA antagonist effects observed with bicuculline and picrotoxin (Crain, 1974*b*). These data on spinal cord explants are consonant with *in situ* studies which suggest that the convulsive effects of penicillin may be mediated by specific antagonism to GABA (Curtis et al., 1972; Davidoff, 1972*c*). Enhancement of evoked network discharges in spinal cord and cerebral explants have been observed after introduction of penicillin concentrations as low as 100 units/ml (i.e., less than 100 μg/ml). The excitatory effects during exposure to higher concentrations of penicillin (1,000–5,000 units/ml) have been quite variable in different CNS explants; some show spontaneous convulsive discharge sequences (as in Fig. VI-11; see also Leiman et al., 1975), whereas others are often limited to marked enhancement of evoked slow-wave discharges with little evidence of sustained spontaneous activity. The factors underlying the wide variations in susceptibility of CNS explants to convulsive agents such as penicillin need to be investigated more systematically and may include degree of maturation, metabolic state of the explant, presence of specific types of pacemaker neurons, etc. (Crain, 1966, 1969, 1972*a*) (see also section E1; Chap. VII-B).

C. *d*-TUBOCURARINE versus ACETYLCHOLINE

Complex oscillatory afterdischarges are often dramatically enhanced in spinal cord and cerebral explants after introduction of *d*-tubocurarine (ca. 10^{-4} M in Fig. VI-5; see also Fig. IV-38) (Crain, 1964*a*, 1969; Crain and Bornstein, 1964). The amplitudes of the rhythmic, repetitive slow-wave potentials elicited in curare may become unusually large (up to 2 mV with our usual 3- to 5-μm electrodes). These excitatory effects are in sharp contrast to the potent blockade of cholinergic neuromuscular synapses in cord-innervated skeletal muscle fibers ($< 10^{-5}$ M) in the same cultures (Crain, 1970*a;* Crain et al., 1970).[2] The curare-induced paroxysmal activities show interesting similarities to repetitive bursts of large positive waves obtained by Chang (1953) from rabbit cerebral cortex after intravenous injec-

---

[2] *d*-Tubocurarine (10^{-5} to 10^{-4} M) also blocks the nicotinic-cholinergic synapses in cultures of dissociated sympathetic ganglion cells (O'Lague et al., 1974, 1976; Ko et al., 1976*a,b*) (Chap. V-A2).

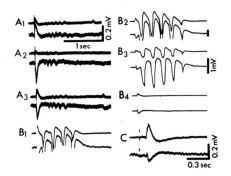

FIG. VI-5. Intermittent appearance of paroxysmal waves elicited under *d*-tubocurarine, and the large shift in latency of evoked responses produced by local neuropil stimulation. **A₁**: Sudden restoration of the preparoxysmal response pattern in the cerebral explant in Fig. IV-38, several minutes after record IV-38C₂ (culture still contained *d*-tubocurarine at 100 μg/ml). The deep recording electrode (lower sweep) was moved to within 100 μm of the superficial recording electrode. Note the resulting reversal of polarity (cf. Fig. IV-38B₂). **A₂**: Deep recording electrode restored to the original site. Note the return of positivity in depth (lower sweep), as in Fig. IV-38B₂. **A₃**: The superficial recording electrode was advanced slightly to make better contact with the excitable tissue. Note the restoration of negativity, as in record **A₁** (upper sweeps). **B₁**: Sudden return, again, of the large paroxysmal-wave response (cf. Fig. IV-38C). **B₂,₃**: Lower amplification reveals the unusually large amplitude of these waves. **B₄**: Restoration of normal response amplitudes, several minutes afterward, as in record **A₃**, but at the same amplification as used for record **B₃**. **C**: The amplification was increased to that used for record **A₃**, and the stimulating electrode was withdrawn approximately 5–10 μm away from the neuron soma layer into overlying neuropil. Note the marked increase in latency of both superficial and deep responses to ca. 100 msec (see also Fig. VI-9B₂,D₃). (From Crain and Bornstein, 1964.)

tion of this drug, and by Feldberg and Fleischauer (1962, 1963) from cat hippocampus after intraventricular perfusion. They may be partly due to selective blockade of cholinergic inhibitory receptor sites in the cerebral explants, as has been suggested to account for these phenomena *in situ* (Phyllis and York, 1968*a,b;* Bhargava and Meldrum 1969, 1971; cf. Hill et al., 1972; Daniels and Spehlmann, 1973). Preliminary experiments with cerebral and hippocampus explants suggest that introduction of low concentrations of acetylcholine into the medium may antagonize these curare convulsions, similar to the attenuation by eserine of cortical paroxysmal responses produced by topical application of *d*-tubocurarine or strychnine (Bhargava and Meldrum, 1971). On the other hand, the increased threshold for triggering these paroxysmal discharges which develops during sub-stained exposure to *d*-tubocurarine (Crain and Bornstein, 1964) may reflect curare depression of cholinergic excitatory receptors on other neurons in these cerebral synaptic networks (Crain, 1969) (see Chap. IV-D4a). Moreover, relatively low concentrations of acetylcholine and eserine (ca. 0.1 μg/ml) may produce enhancement and unusual prolongation of evoked potentials in some cerebral explants as well as generation of long series of rhythmic sharp waves of gradually increasing repetition rate (Crain, 1969).

CNS explants therefore provide a useful preparation for systematic studies with more selective anticholinergic agents to clarify some of the complex cholinergic inhibitory as well as excitatory synaptic systems which appear to be functioning in these cultures. The apparent antagonism by d-tubo-curarine of the inhibitory influence of endogenous GABA (Hill et al., 1972) also requires further analysis.

Biochemical analyses during development *in vitro* of spinal cord and cerebral tissues, as explants or in dissociated cell cultures, show significant increases in enzymes associated with cholinergic transmission, i.e., choline-acetylase and acetylcholinesterase (e.g., Seeds, 1971, 1973; Kim et al., 1972, 1974; for review see Richelson, 1975).[3] Cytochemical studies in chick embryo spinal cord cultures show that the activity of both enzymes increases concomitantly with synaptogenesis, and the enzymes become widely distributed throughout the perikaryal regions, dendrites, and axons (Kim et al., 1972, 1974). On the other hand, the abundant distribution of acetyl-cholinesterase within the perikarya of DRG neurons (as well as of moto-neurons) in cultures of fetal rat cord and DRG explants (Tischner and Thomas, 1973) suggests that its presence may not be directly related to synaptic functions (e.g., Pannese et al., 1971).

D. CHLORIDE-FREE MEDIA

After transfer of cerebral neocortex, hippocampus, and spinal cord explants to chloride-free BSS [by replacing all chlorides with propionates, or other large anions which cannot penetrate the activated inhibitory synaptic membrane: (Ito et al., 1962)], the usual negative slow-wave responses suddenly become remarkably larger (up to 10-fold), often reaching amplitudes of 3 mV with our usual 3–5 μm electrodes (Fig. VI-6) (Crain, 1974c, *in preparation*). These paroxysmal discharges are probably due to summated EPSPs generated by the synaptic networks in the CNS explants after release from *all* types of chloride-dependent inhibitory synaptic restraints. In chloride (Cl$^-$) deficient media, IPSPs generated by increased membrane Cl$^-$ conductance mechanisms will tend to depolarize—instead of hyper-polarize—the neurons, since their membrane will be driven towards a new Cl$^-$ equilibrium potential which approaches zero as the extracellular Cl$^-$ concentration is reduced towards the low intracellular Cl$^-$ concentration characteristic of many types of neurons (Eccles, 1964; Yamamoto and Kawai, 1968). The explant discharges in Cl$^-$-free BSS are much larger than observed in strychnine, bicuculline or other drugs, but they are still suppressed by raising the Mg^{++} level to 10 mM. The hyperexcitability of CNS

---

[3] Biochemical and electrophysiologic studies of dissociated sympathetic ganglion cell cultures have demonstrated a marked increase in ACh-synthesis concomitant with increasing development of functional cholinergic synapses (Patterson and Chun, 1974; O'Lague et al., 1974, 1976; see Chap. V-A2).

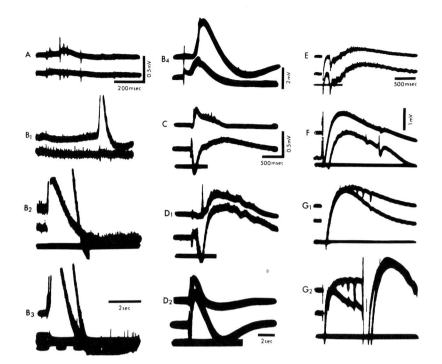

FIG. VI-6. Excitatory effects on bioelectric activities of fetal mouse spinal cord and cerebral explants following removal of chloride ions from the culture medium. **A:** Simultaneous recordings of simple spike bursts and small-amplitude slow-wave responses at two sites in a spinal cord explant (15 days *in vitro*) in response to a stimulus applied at a third site, in regular BSS. **B₁:** Within 1 min after replacing regular BSS with a chloride-free BSS (propionate substituted for all chloride ions), a large-amplitude negative slow-wave potential occurred spontaneously, concomitantly with the appearance of high-frequency spike barrages. **B₂:** Negative slow-wave responses evoked by single stimuli in chloride-free BSS are remarkably large in amplitude (peak of response on upper sweep was way off the oscilloscope screen); they are followed by long-lasting positive phases. **B₃,₄:** Addition of 10^{-3} M glycine to the chloride-free BSS is ineffective in depressing complex cord discharges (as occurs with this level of glycine in regular BSS; cf. Fig. VI-1). Note the five-fold reduction in gain in **B₄**, indicating that the cord population responses in chloride-free medium reach amplitudes of more than 3 mV. (The third and fourth sweeps in **B₃** were left intact since the unusually large potentials in the upper two sweeps led to complex overlapping. The third stimulus-monitoring sweep is also seen in **B₂**, and the fourth sweep shows a 1-sec time calibration.) **C:** Typical complex, evoked responses recorded at two sites in a cerebral neocortex explant (7 days *in vitro*). **D:** After replacement of regular BSS by chloride-free (propionate) BSS, the amplitude of the negative slow-wave component of response at one site becomes approximately three times larger (lower sweep), and the negative slow-wave potential at the other site becomes much longer in duration as well as larger in amplitude. **E:** Small-amplitude responses evoked in another explant of cerebral neocortex (15 days *in vitro*). **F:** Removal of chloride ions (propionate BSS) again produces marked augmentation of negative slow-wave responses (note lower gain in **F** versus **E**). **G₁:** Hippocampal explant (on the same culture coverglass as the neocortex in records **E** and **F**) shows similar dramatic enhancement in evoked responses after replacement of regular BSS with chloride-free BSS (amplitudes in regular BSS had been comparable to those in **E**). **G₂:** After several minutes in propionate BSS, the evoked responses became somewhat smaller; but huge diphasic (positive-negative) slow-wave potentials occurred at times during the course of the more common oscillatory (ca. 5/sec) afterdischarge sequences. Note the peak of the large spike potential which occurred midway during the initial positive slow wave (the remainder of this spike potential could not be resolved at this slow sweep rate). (From Crain, *in preparation*.)

explants after transfer to chloride-free media provides further evidence that these organized synaptic networks in culture are under tonic inhibitory controls, as previously shown in freshly isolated brain slices where inhibition was selectively blocked in chloride-free media (Yamamoto and Kawai, 1968). Similar enhancement of negative slow-wave responses occurs even during early stages of synaptogenesis in cerebral neocortex and hippocampus explants (Fig. IV-31C,F) (Chap. IV-D). Preliminary experiments indicate that the concentrations of glycine and GABA that normally block synaptic network discharges in spinal cord and cerebral explants (sections A, B) are no longer effective after removal of chlorides from the medium (Fig. VI-6B$_{3,4}$), as observed by Kawai and Yamamoto (1967) in fresh slices of superior colliculus and by Kudo et al. (1975) in frog spinal cord.

The unusual GABA-mediated EPSPs on DRG terminals which appear to underlie the primary afferent depolarization (PAD) potentials in explants of dorsal spinal cord and dorsal column nuclei (Chap. IV-B,C) might be produced by a similar GABA-initiated increase in membrane Cl$^-$ conductance *if* the intracellular Cl$^-$ concentration of DRG axon terminals were actually higher than the normal extracellular Cl$^-$ concentration (Nishi et al., 1974; Kudo et al., 1975).

E. CAFFEINE AND CYCLIC AMP versus MG^{++} AND LOW CA^{++}

Previous experiments had shown that caffeine (10^{-3} M) elicited convulsive discharges in cerebral cortex explants (Crain, 1966; see also Fig. VI-7F) resembling the characteristic hyperexcitability produced by caffeine in the CNS *in situ* (Ritchie, 1970). Since this methylxanthine inhibits cerebral cyclic AMP-phosphodiesterase (Butcher and Sutherland, 1962; Cheung, 1970; see below), the possibility arose that the excitatory effects in cultured cerebral tissues could be due to an increased level of endogenous cyclic AMP (adenosine 3',5'-cyclic monophosphate) following interference with its normal rate of hydrolysis by this enzyme. Although in several biochemical studies with brain slices and muscle sarcoplasmic reticulum fractions, caffeine, theophylline, and other methylxanthine effects do not appear to be mediated by cyclic AMP (Weber, 1968; Kakiuchi et al., 1969; Breckenridge, 1970), these data do not preclude involvement of cyclic AMP in caffeine enhancement of CNS excitability in organotypic cultures or *in situ* (Ritchie, 1970).

1. Experimental Data in CNS Cultures

Increasing the Mg^{++} concentration of the culture medium from 1 to 5–10 mM produces selective depression of complex discharges mediated by poly-

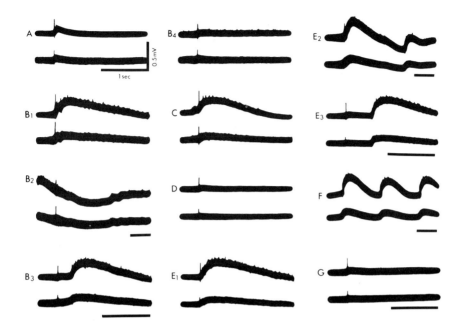

FIG. VI-7. Restorative effects of caffeine on complex discharges in fetal mouse spinal cord explant after acute depression in high-Mg^{++} BSS (13 days *in vitro*). **A:** Almost complete depression of characteristic complex discharges of cord explant (in response to single cord stimuli) several minutes after increasing the Mg^{++} concentration from 1 to 5 mM (10^{-6} M strychnine was present during the entire experiment). **B:** Long-lasting negative slow-wave and spike-barrage responses are restored (**B$_1$**) approximately 1 min after adding 10^{-3} M caffeine to the 5 mM Mg^{++} BSS. Similar large-amplitude discharges also begin to occur spontaneously (**B$_2$**) and continue for about 5 min. By 7 min, the latency of evoked responses increases markedly to approximately 300 msec (**B$_3$**), and complete depression ensues about 1 min later (**B$_4$**). **C:** Complex discharges are restored after return to regular BSS. **D:** Sustained block occurs within 1 min after increasing the Mg^{++} level again to 5 mM. **E:** Within 2 min after adding 10^{-3} M caffeine to the 5 mM Mg^{++} BSS, responses are even larger than those in regular BSS (cf. **E$_{1,2}$** versus **C**). By 7 min, however, response latencies again become very long (500 msec in **E$_3$**), and complete blockade develops soon afterward (as in **B$_{3,4}$**). **F:** A convulsive series of discharges occurs shortly after return to BSS. **G:** Nevertheless, increasing the Mg^{++} level to 5 mM still results in rapid and complete depression. (From Crain and Pollack, 1973.)

synaptic circuits without blocking propagated spike potentials[4] (Figs. VI-7A, D;8B$_2$;10B$_2$; also Figs. V-2,4,8C) (Crain et al., 1968*a*). Similar effects can be produced by removing Ca^{++} from the medium (Fig. VI-10F) or by adding the chelating agent EGTA (10^{-3} M) or the anesthetics Xylocaine (10^{-4} M) and procaine (10^{-3} M) (Fig. VI-9). The first three procedures decrease the

---

[4] Similar selective block of synaptically mediated responses in high Mg^{++} concentration has been demonstrated in adult frog CNS *in situ:* spinal cord (Katz and Miledi, 1963) and cerebellum (Hackett, 1975); and similar effects have been obtained in freshly isolated frog spinal cord bathed in low Ca^{++} solutions (Dambach and Erulkar, 1973).

availability of Ca^{++} to the CNS tissue, and Xylocaine may act similarly (Blaustein and Goldman, 1966; Kuperman et al., 1968; Dettbarn, 1971). Although introduction of strychnine along with these blocking agents does not prevent the Ca^{++}-deficit depressions, caffeine (10^{-3} M) produces within a few minutes a transient (up to 15 min) restoration of the original complex bioelectric discharges after complete blockade in high Mg^{++} (Fig. VI-7B) (Crain and Pollack, 1973). Furthermore, introduction of low concentrations (ca. 10^{-6} M) of cyclic AMP (or its dibutyryl derivative) to Ca^{++}-deprived spinal cord and cerebral cortex explants produces restorative effects similar to those of 10^{-3} M caffeine — not only during high-Mg^{++} blockade but also during Ca^{++}-free and 10^{-4} M Xylocaine blockades (Figs. VI-8F;10C$_1$,G$_1$) (Crain and Pollack, 1973).[5] Similar dramatic restorative effects during high-Mg^{++} blockades have also been produced with a much lower concentration (ca. 10^{-6} M) of another phosphodiesterase (PDE) inhibitor, SQ 66,442. [This agent is approximately 100-fold more potent than caffeine as an inhibitor of cerebral PDE (M. Chasin, *personal communication*); see also data on similar PDE inhibitors in Beer et al. (1972) and Chasin et al. (1972).] On the other hand, addition of 5'AMP (10^{-6} M) or ATP (10^{-6} M) to Mg^{++}-blocked cultures did not restore complex bioelectric activity (Fig. VI-8C), whereas subsequent introduction of dibutyryl cyclic AMP in the same cord explants did indeed restore activity (Fig. VI-8F). These experiments provide support for specificity of action by cyclic AMP in relation to its precursor (ATP) and primary breakdown product (AMP).

In some CNS explants monitored over periods of several hours in a regular balanced salt solution (BSS), introduction of cyclic AMP or dibutyryl cyclic AMP at low concentrations (ca. 10^{-6} M) often produced convulsive bioelectric effects (as may also occur with caffeine), but the degree of excitation was quite variable, both in regard to enhancement and prolongation

---

[5] Selective blockade of synaptic transmitter release may require careful control of the Mg^{++} concentration to which a CNS explant is exposed. In our cyclic AMP experiments the *minimal* concentration of Mg^{++} required to block the complex network activity reliably was used (Crain and Pollack, 1973). This critical Mg^{++} level was determined at the beginning of each experiment since it generally varied from 5 to 10 mM in different explants. The restorative effects of cyclic AMP were far less evident, or absent, if the Mg^{++} concentration was substantially higher than this critical value. As soon as the complex activity was blocked, the high-Mg^{++} BSS was replaced by the solution to which dibutyryl cyclic AMP or caffeine had been added. This resulted in partial or complete restoration of the baseline-type complex slow-wave discharges within a few minutes (Figs. IV-7;8). These data are consonant with recent experiments in mouse cerebellar explants where 10 mM Mg^{++} produced a generalized depression of antidromically conducted spike potentials in addition to synaptic blockade (Marshall et al., 1975). Concerns were expressed that "even low levels of Mg^{++} cannot be used as a test for synaptic activity unless careful controls of neural excitability are also performed" (Marshall et al., 1975). On the other hand, 8 mM Mg^{++} appeared to produce more selective depression of synaptically mediated activity in cerebellar explants studied by Gähwiler et al. (1973), as noted in Chap. IV-E (Fig. IV-43D). The excitability properties of some types of CNS axons may, however, be unusually sensitive to depression by Mg^{++} concentrations that are required to block synaptic transmitter release. In these cases Co^{++} (0.5–2 mM) or Mn^{++} (0.1–1 mM) may produce more selective synaptic blockade (Hackett, 1975, *personal communication*).

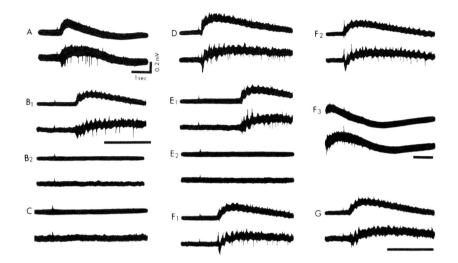

FIG. VI-8. Restorative effects of dibutyryl cyclic AMP on complex discharge activity of fetal spinal cord explant after acute depression in high-Mg^{++} BSS (13 days *in vitro*). **A:** Organotypic slow-wave and spike-barrage responses evoked in two regions of a cord explant by a single stimulus to another cord site during exposure to a low concentration of strychnine (10^{-6} M) in BSS. (The strychnine concentration was maintained at 10^{-6} M during the entire experiment.) **B$_1$:** Responses at both sites occur with much longer latency (ca. 400 msec) when a similar or larger stimulus is applied after increasing the Mg^{++} level from 1 to 5 mM. **B$_2$:** Approximately 2 min later, complex cord discharges can no longer be evoked even with very large cord stimuli (only an early-latency spike potential can be detected at a faster sweep). **C:** The block of complex activity continues after adding 3×10^{-6} M 5'-AMP to the 5 mM Mg^{++} BSS. **D:** Restoration of characteristic discharges after return to regular BSS. **E:** Similar partial (**E$_1$**) and complete (**E$_2$**) depression of complex responses within 1–2 min after increasing Mg^{++} again to 5 mM. Note the unusually long (1 sec) latencies in **E$_1$**. **F:** Within 1 min after adding 2×10^{-6} M dibutyryl cyclic AMP to the 5 mM Mg^{++} BSS, organotypic cord discharges can again be evoked with a single cord stimulus (**F$_1$**; cf. **B$_1$** and **E$_1$**). Soon afterward these complex responses occur with shorter latency (**F$_2$**; cf. **D**), and similar discharges begin to appear spontaneously at both cord sites (**F$_3$**; cf. **A**), occurring sporadically during the next 10 min, followed by complete depression as in **B$_2$** and **E$_2$**. **G:** Restoration of original responses after return to regular BSS. (From Crain and Pollack, 1973.)

of complex evoked responses as well as spontaneous discharges (Crain and Pollack, 1973). Long-lasting cyclic sequences of complex spike barrages and slow waves occurred in several of the 2- to 3-week-old cord explants during 1–2 hr of exposure to dibutyryl cyclic AMP (Fig. VI-11; cf. Fig. VI-7F). These convulsive effects were milder or absent in most of the younger or older explants tested. The excitatory effects of cyclic AMP were similar to those of dibutyryl cyclic AMP, but the latter generally resulted in a greater degree of complex activity and persisted for a longer time. It should be emphasized that these long series of repetitive discharges which appear after adding cyclic AMP to some CNS explants (Fig. VI-11) are not uniquely elicited by this chemical agent. Various CNS explants may show comparable

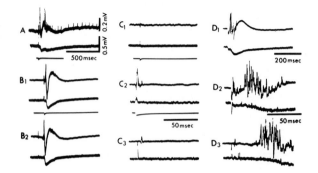

FIG. VI-9. Selective procaine block of characteristic evoked responses in newborn mouse cerebral neocortex explant (2 months *in vitro*). **A:** Simultaneous records at cortical depths of 50 μm (upper sweep) and 250 μm showing long-lasting responses following a single superficial stimulus applied approximately 500 μm away from the first recording electrode (Figs. IV-27;37). Note the complex, triphasic, predominantly negative potential at the superficial site (upper sweep) and the simpler positivity of similar duration recorded at a deeper site. Note also the large negative spikes superimposed on slow waves in the superficial response. The lowest sweep in this record (and in **B**$_1$, **C**$_1$, and **C**$_2$) shows the stimulus signal. **B**$_1$: After procaine (10 μg/ml) superimposed spikes are no longer seen. (Increased amplitude of positive potentials appeared earlier following preliminary application of *d*-tubocurarine.) **B**$_2$: Same recording conditions as in **B**$_1$, but the stimulus was applied to the subcortical region at a depth of about 1 mm. Note the large increase in response latency to approximately 60 msec. **C**$_1$: Several minutes after increasing the procaine concentration to 100 μg/ml. Note complete block of evoked long-duration responses (cf. **B**$_1$). **C**$_2$: A faster sweep rate reveals that early-latency spike potentials are still evoked (cf. **C**$_1$; as in high-Mg^{++} block, e.g., Fig. V-8C$_2$). **C**$_3$: After a stimulus to the subcortical region, only a small spike appears with a 5-msec latency at the superficial site (cf. **B**$_2$). **D**$_1$: Within 5 min after restoration of the control medium. Note the almost complete reappearance of characteristic evoked responses in both superficial and deep records following a superficial stimulus (cf. **A** and **B**$_1$). **D**$_2$: A faster sweep rate shows details of spike barrages which occur prior to slow waves (cf. **C**$_2$). **D**$_3$: After a subcortical stimulus, a 35-msec silent period occurs between the appearance of the first spike potential (cf. **C**$_3$) and the spike barrage preceding the slow waves (cf. **B**$_2$). (From Crain and Bornstein, 1964.)

sequences of convulsive activity even in regular medium (Fig. VII-2) (Corner and Crain, 1972), and many others become similarly hyperactive after introduction of strychnine (e.g., Fig. VII-1), picrotoxin, and other pharmacologic agents (see sections A-D). The cyclic AMP effects are significant primarily in view of the possibility that the *endogenous* distribution of this nucleotide may play an important role in regulating the excitability of neuronal systems.

During developmental studies of 18-day fetal mouse cerebral neocortex and hippocampus explants (Crain and Bornstein, 1974), introduction of caffeine (10^{-3} M) at stages shortly before the usual appearance of complex synaptically mediated discharges (3–4 days *in vitro*) (Chap. IV-D) sometimes led to precocious generation of long-lasting repetitive spike-barrage and slow-wave responses to electric stimuli instead of the usual simple spike potentials. Caffeine was generally most effective, however, when added

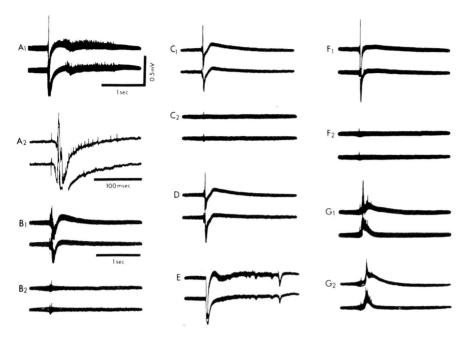

FIG. VI-10. Restorative effects of dibutyryl cyclic AMP on evoked potentials in mouse cerebral cortex explant after acute depression in high-Mg^{++} or Ca^{++}-free BSS (18-day fetus; 3 weeks *in vitro*). **A:** Complex long-lasting discharges (A_1) evoked in two regions of cerebral explant by a single stimulus at a third site (in BSS). Initial phases of these elaborate slow-wave and spike-barrage responses are seen more clearly at a faster sweep (A_2). **B:** Partial depression of these complex responses several minutes after increasing the Mg^{++} concentration from 1 to 10 mM (B_1), and complete block (except for a small, early-latency spike) within 5 min (B_2). **C:** After addition of 2×10^{-6} M dibutyryl cyclic AMP to the 10 mM Mg^{++} BSS, the primary phases of the original complex evoked discharges are restored (C_1; cf. A_1, B_1). Within 5 min, however, complete depression develops again (C_2). **D:** Second restoration of complex evoked responses in 2×10^{-6} M dibutyryl cyclic AMP plus 10 mM Mg^{++}, after an interim return to regular BSS and subsequent blockade in 10 mM Mg^{++} for 10 min. Responses could again be elicited for about 5 min. **E:** Restoration of original long-lasting discharges after return to regular BSS (cf. **A**). **F:** Partial depression of evoked discharges within 2 min after introduction of Ca^{++}-free BSS (F_1) and complete block shortly thereafter (F_2). **G:** Prominent negative slow-wave discharges can be elicited within 30 sec after addition of 2×10^{-6} M dibutyryl cyclic AMP to the Ca^{++}-free BSS. Latency of these responses increases within 1 min (G_2), and complete block soon occurred (reversible after return to regular BSS, as in **E**). (From Crain and Pollack, 1973.)

along with strychnine, picrotoxin, or bicuculline (see section E4), leading to the onset or a marked reduction in threshold of these precocious synaptically mediated discharges (Figs. IV-31;32; Chap. IV-D). Similar precocious, synaptically mediated bioelectric discharges have also been evoked under caffeine (10^{-3} M) in 14-day fetal mouse spinal cord explants after 2–3 days *in vitro* (Crain and Peterson, *in preparation*) (Fig. IV-2). In both types of CNS explants these caffeine effects could sometimes be produced at stages prior to the characteristic onset of strychnine sensitivity. These preliminary

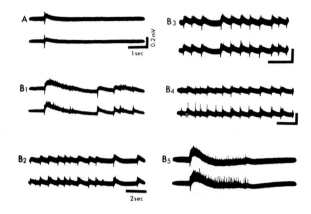

FIG. VI-11. Excitatory effects of dibutyryl cyclic AMP on bioelectric activity of mouse spinal cord explant in regular BSS (14-day fetus; 3 weeks *in vitro*). **A:** Simultaneous recordings of typical diphasic slow-wave responses evoked in two regions of a spinal cord explant by a single stimulus to another cord site during a 30-min observation period in BSS. **B:** Within 1 min after introduction of dibutyryl cyclic AMP (2×10^{-6} M), negative slow-wave potentials become larger in amplitude and much longer in duration ($\mathbf{B_1}$), and they also begin to occur spontaneously. After 20 min a long series of repetitive slow waves occur at 1–2/sec ($\mathbf{B_{2,3}}$), lasting for periods of approximately 30 sec and resuming in cyclic sequences after silent periods of 2–3 min ($\mathbf{B_4}$). $\mathbf{B_5}$: During a subsequent quiet period, a single cord stimulus triggers an elaborate slow-wave and a repetitive-spike response lasting more than 5 sec. (From Crain and Pollack, 1973.)

data suggest that low Ca^{++} or low cyclic AMP levels may be a significant factor underlying the high thresholds and extreme lability of synaptically mediated discharges shortly after synaptogenesis in the CNS (Crain, 1974*b*), and that strychnine-sensitive inhibitory circuits (Crain and Peterson, 1967) may become functional after an additional brief period of maturation (Chap. IV-A,D). These data are consonant with studies of convulsive activity produced by topical application of dibutyryl cyclic AMP to 6-day-old kitten cerebral neocortex (Purpura and Shofer, 1972), indicating that elaborate excitatory synaptic networks are already well organized but not normally active at this neonatal stage.

The low level of cyclic AMP (10^{-6} M) that produced direct functional effects in these experiments is of particular significance, since this appears to be the first demonstration of excitatory effects on vertebrate CNS tissue at concentrations approaching the physiologic range (Hardman et al., 1971). In other CNS preparations where significant excitatory and convulsive phenomena have been observed with exogenous cyclic AMP (topical or intraventricular application), concentrations of 10^{-4} to 10^{-3} M have generally been required (Gessa et al., 1970; Purpura and Shofer, 1972; Auerbach and Purpura, 1972) presumably because of greater diffusion barriers *in situ* (see also Forn et al., 1972).[6] Intracellular microiontophoresis of cyclic AMP into *Helix* neurons resulted in a depolarization for several seconds after the injection, during which period the frequency of spontaneous spike activity increased (Liberman et al., 1975). Similar injections of 5'AMP or 5'-ATP were ineffective. Furthermore, intracellular injection of dibutyryl cyclic AMP into sensory neurons in *Aplysia* ganglia produced heterosynaptic facilitation effects lasting for several minutes (Kandel et al., 1976b). These intracellular studies in invertebrate neurons provide further clues to presynaptic modes of action of cyclic AMP (section 2).

2. Presynaptic Mechanisms of Cyclic AMP Action

The effects of cyclic AMP on rat neuromuscular junctions provide a useful model for analysis of mechanisms underlying the mode of action of this agent at CNS synapses (Goldberg and Singer, 1969; Singer and Goldberg, 1970). Partial blockade of neuromuscular transmission was produced by appropriate concentrations of Mg^{++} (22 mM) or *d*-tubocurarine. Addition of dibutyryl cyclic AMP (4×10^{-3} M) clearly enhanced the amplitude of the endplate potentials at these depressed junctions. The cyclic AMP effects were interpreted as a facilitation of the release of acetylcholine from the presynaptic neuron since intracellular recordings showed an increase in frequency of miniature endplate potentials (MEPPs) without an increase in their average amplitude (see also Breckenridge and Bray, 1970), resembling epinephrine enhancement of neuromuscular transmission (Krnjevic and Miledi, 1958; Jenkinson et al., 1968). Furthermore, the same enhancement in MEPP frequency was obtained at these depressed junctions after adding the methylxanthine PDE inhibitors theophylline and caffeine ($0.2–2 \times 10^{-3}$ M), in agreement with similar observations by Elmqvist and Feldman (1965) after application of caffeine (5×10^{-3} M) to neuromuscular preparations blocked in calcium-free solutions. In both studies it was suggested that caffeine may act in the nerve terminal by mobilizing bound calcium stores,

---

[6] Superfusion of fetal mouse hippocampal deplants *in oculo* with cyclic GMP (guanosine 3',5'-cyclic monophosphate) produced marked excitatory effects on pyramidal cell spike discharges (Olson et al., 1976). The 8-bromo analogue of cyclic GMP was used in this study (at 10^{-3} M) since it is more resistant to hydrolysis by PDE. Superfusion of the deplants with the PDE inhibitor, isobutyl methyl xanthine (10^{-3} M), led to similar excitatory actions on pyramidal cells and also potentiated the excitatory effects of iontophoretically applied cyclic GMP and acetylcholine (Olson et al., 1976). Although the authors suggest that the excitatory effects of isobutyl methyl xanthine may be due to elevation of endogenous cyclic GMP levels in the hippocampal neurons, this PDE inhibitor may also increase cyclic AMP levels as proposed in our CNS explant studies (see above). However, since Olson et al. (1976) did not report on comparative effects of cyclic AMP on the hippocampal deplants *in oculo*, their suggestion that cyclic GMP and cyclic AMP may mediate a mutually antagonistic system of hippocampal afferents controlling the excitability of pyramidal neurons requires more direct evidence (see, however, Goldberg et al., 1973; Segal and Bloom, 1974; Stone et al., 1975).

but the more recent data obtained by Singer and Goldberg (1970) permitted additional speculation that the methylxanthine effects might be mediated by enhanced levels of endogenous cyclic AMP following PDE inhibition.

The present experiments extend these neuromuscular studies to CNS tissues *in vitro,* and they may provide significant clues to mechanisms underlying cyclic AMP effects on synaptic transmission in the CNS *in situ.* Following blockade of complex, synaptically mediated bioelectric activity in CNS explants by four different modes of acute Ca^{++} deprivation (low Ca^{++}, high Mg^{++}, EGTA, and Xylocaine), a low concentration of exogenous cyclic AMP is capable of promoting a temporary restoration of that activity. As reviewed by Rasmussen (1970), cyclic AMP has been demonstrated to mobilize membrane-bound calcium in a variety of cellular systems so that Ca^{++}-dependent secretory and related functions can be restored in Ca^{++}-free media, e.g., protein synthesis and catecholamine release in the adrenal gland (Farese, 1971; Peach, 1972), parathyroid gland function (Bell et al., 1972), and salivary gland secretion (Prince et al., 1972). It is tempting to speculate that this may also be the mechanism of action of exogenous cyclic AMP in restoring Ca^{++}-dependent, synaptically mediated bioelectric activity in CNS explants following depression by Ca^{++} deprivation (see also Breckenridge and Bray, 1970; Singer and Goldberg, 1970; Torda, 1972). The similar restorative effects obtained with PDE inhibitors (caffeine and SQ 65,442) in the cultures might then be interpreted as due to the resulting increase in endogenous levels of cyclic AMP, leading to mobilization of membrane-bound calcium in presynaptic terminals and thereby facilitating neurotransmitter release. Direct chemical evidence has recently been obtained of enhanced stimulation-induced release of norepinephrine and dopamine β-hydroxylase by sympathetic nerves innervating guinea pig vas deferens following exogenous application of dibutyryl cyclic AMP (10^{-4} M) or theophylline (10^{-3} M) in a freshly isolated preparation (Wooten et al., 1973). Furthermore, stimulus-induced release was restored by these agents after complete block in a Ca^{++}-free medium. These biochemical data on peripheral autonomic nerves are consonant with our electrophysiologic observations on cultured spinal cord and cerebral cortex (Crain and Pollack, 1972, 1973), and both groups have independently suggested that cyclic AMP may indeed play a significant role in mobilizing intracellular bound calcium so as to enhance neurotransmitter release at presynaptic nerve terminals, even in the absence of extracellular sources of calcium ions.

Since the cyclic AMP-enhanced network discharges of CNS explants in Ca^{++}-deprived media generally require triggering by an electric or neural stimulus, depolarization of the presynaptic terminals by invading nerve impulses probably still plays a major role in transmitter release under these experimental conditions. It is unlikely that the Ca^{++}-deprivation paradigms used in these tissue culture studies completely eliminated extracellular Ca^{++} in the interstitial spaces within the explants, so that at least some

Ca^{++} could probably still enter the presynaptic terminals during each impulse-produced depolarization. This subthreshold Ca^{++} influx could then summate with the cyclic AMP-mobilized intracellular Ca^{++} to reach levels necessary for effective transmitter release. A similar cyclic AMP mechanism might be involved in post-tetanic potentiation in Ca^{++}-free media—e.g., at frog neuromuscular junctions in 10^{-3} M EGTA, where Miledi and Thies (1967) suggested that: "calcium could still be responsible for the increase in MEPP frequency if one assumes that in Ca-free solutions the nerve impulse mobilizes some Ca from bound sites in the membrane, making it available for reactions that lead to transmitter release; and that the increase in ionized Ca within the membrane decays slowly."

Ample supplies of bound calcium for translocation to synaptic vesicles are probably present in membranes of axonal endoplasmic reticulum (Henkart, 1972) and mitochondria (e.g., Rasmussen, 1970; Baker et al., 1971; Llinás et al., 1972) in presynaptic terminals of CNS neurons (Birks, 1966; Korneliussen, 1972; Teichberg and Holtzman, 1973). Furthermore, cyclic AMP, adenyl cyclase, and PDE activity have been demonstrated in synaptic vesicle fractions from *pre*synaptic nerve endings of mammalian brain (Cheung and Salganicoff, 1967; Johnson et al., 1972b), as well as in post-synaptic membranes (Florendo et al., 1971). The remarkably long stimulus-response latencies (1–2 sec) of the synaptic network discharges in the CNS explants which occur during development of Ca^{++}-deprivation blockades (e.g., Fig. VI-8B_1,E_1,F_1) and the rapid restoration of normal latencies after adding cyclic AMP add further support to a mechanism involving facilitation of stimulus-secretion coupling through mobilization of calcium.

It is unlikely that decreased conduction velocity of nerve impulses in the CNS explants could account for much of this increased latency, since the lengths of the conductile neurites in the networks are quite short (ca. 1 mm) and propagation normally occurs at rates of approximately 0.1–1 meters/sec in these small-diameter (ca. 1 μm) fibers (Hild and Tasaki, 1962; Crain and Bornstein, 1964; Crain and Peterson, 1964, 1967). Conduction velocities would have to be far lower, of the order of millimeters per second, to account for the long (1–2 sec) response latencies in Ca^{++}-deprived media. It is more probable that these increased latencies are related to the effects of Ca^{++} deficits on complex multisynaptic circuits, since characteristic synaptic delays *in situ* appear to involve primarily the mechanism by which Ca^{++} triggers release of synaptic transmitter in axon terminals (Katz and Miledi, 1965a,b, 1968; Katz, 1969). [Similar long stimulus-response latencies have also been observed in immature CNS explants in normal medium, as well as in older ones when small, barely threshold stimuli are applied (Crain and Bornstein, 1964; Crain and Peterson, 1964; Crain et al., 1968b); see also alternative, but less-well-founded, "nerve net" interpretation proposed by Lumsden (1968) to account for the long response latencies in CNS explants.] Finally, the transient nature of these restorative periods (1–20 min) indicates that cyclic AMP is not simply substituting for Ca^{++} (since this should lead to more permanent restoration); it may indeed reflect limits to the releasable membrane-bound "calcium stores" in the terminals.

3. Postsynaptic Effects of Cyclic AMP

The electrophysiologic properties of these CNS explants, however, are quite complex, and extracellular recordings are relatively indirect indicators of the synaptic activities involved. It is therefore quite possible that the observed restorative effects of cyclic AMP may also involve direct transmitter-like depolarizing actions which enhance the sensitivity of *post*-synaptic or other neuronal membranes (e.g., Miller et al., 1971) independent of intracellular calcium mobilization [analogous to the hyperpolarizing effects of cyclic AMP on cerebellar Purkinje cells (Siggins et al., 1971*a,b*) and sympathetic ganglion cells (McAfee and Greengard, 1972; Rodnight, 1975)]. It should be noted, however, that even high concentrations of cyclic AMP (4×10^{-3} M) did not produce direct depolarizing effects in muscle (Singer and Goldberg, 1970). Iontophoretic application of cyclic AMP to cerebellar Purkinje cells produced only hyperpolarization (Siggins et al., 1971*a,b*), even when tested in neonatal rats before the onset of synaptogenesis (Hoffer, 1971).[7]

4. Cyclic AMP in Relation to Excitatory and Inhibitory Synapses

If cyclic AMP does in fact facilitate synaptic transmission by mobilization of membrane-bound calcium in presynaptic terminals, it should enhance inhibitory as well as excitatory synapses. Some of the variability in the

---

[7] Bath perfusion of 10^{-3} M cyclic AMP and dibutyryl cyclic AMP in rat cerebellar cultures produced moderate depressant effects on the spontaneous spike discharges of Purkinje neurons (Gähwiler 1976*b;* see also section B1). At concentrations up to 10^{-4} M, the rate of spike firing increased in some cells and decreased in others. PDE inhibitors were far more potent depressants of cerebellar spike firing, even in the absence of exogenous cyclic AMP. Papaverine (10^{-5} M), aminophylline (10^{-3} M) and caffeine (10^{-3} M) were all effective in abolishing the spontaneous discharges. These PDE inhibitors, moreover, strongly enhanced the depressant effects of exogenous cyclic AMP and noradrenalin on these cerebellar neurons. Gähwiler (1976*b*) interpreted the data as further support for the hypothesis that the inhibitory action of norepinephrine is mediated by a postsynaptic cyclic AMP mechanism (Siggins et al., 1971*a,b*). Alternatively, the PDE inhibitors may increase endogenous cyclic AMP levels in the presynaptic terminals, thereby enhancing release of norepinephrine or other inhibitory transmitters at the Purkinje cell synapses (see section E4). Although it is unlikely that noradrenergic synaptic inputs to the Purkinje neurons are present in these isolated cerebellar explants, clearcut GABA-ergic inhibitory synapses have been demonstrated (Gähwiler, 1975; section B1). It will therefore be of interest to extend these studies of PDE inhibitors to cultures containing Purkinje neurons which are devoid of synaptic inputs (see Chap. IV-E). This will provide a simpler preparation for direct analyses of the receptors on the postsynaptic neurons, similar to the studies by Hoffer (1971) of cyclic AMP effects on neonatal Purkinje cells before the onset of synaptogenesis (see above).

observed excitatory affects of cyclic AMP on CNS explants in normal media may thus be attributable to predominance of inhibitory circuits in certain explants. In the latter case, strychnine or picrotoxin could evoke marked excitatory effects by selective blocking of inhibitory receptor sites, whereas cyclic AMP might appear to be ineffective during tests for overt activity with extracellular electrodes. Furthermore, after more selective depression of the complex bioelectric activity of spinal cord explants by increasing the concentration of the postulated inhibitory synaptic transmitter glycine to 10^{-3} M, preliminary experiments indicate that cyclic AMP and caffeine do not overcome this type of blockade, whereas low concentrations of strychnine (10^{-7} M) can readily neutralize it (Fig. VI-1; see also section A) (Crain, 1974*b*, 1975*c*). These concentrations led to the use of strychnine as a means of enhancing the restorative effects of cyclic AMP during high-Mg^{++} and other Ca^{++}-deficit blockades (see section E1), even though strychnine alone was ineffective against these generalized synaptic depressions.

The sensitivity of organotypic bioelectric activities of spinal cord and cerebral cortex explants to cyclic AMP indicates that organized CNS tissue cultures can be utilized as a model system to investigate mechanisms underlying the complex effects of cyclic nucleotides on brain function. Furthermore, the restorative effects of cyclic AMP on synaptic activity during acute Ca^{++} deprivation of cultured neural tissues may provide a valuable experimental paradigm for studies related to CNS plasticity, e.g., synaptic facilitation and post-tetanic potentiation (Miledi and Thies, 1967; Breckenridge and Bray, 1970; Greengard and Kuo, 1970) (Chap. VIII-A) as well as to pathologic conditions involving Ca^{++} deficits in presynaptic nerve terminals (e.g., Lambert and Elmqvist, 1971; Takamori, 1972).

F. SERUM DEPRESSANT FACTORS

Initial electrophysiologic studies of sera from rabbits with experimental allergic encephalomyelitis (EAE) and humans with multiple sclerosis (MS) showed a reversible block of the complex bioelectric synaptic network discharges of rodent cerebral and spinal cord explants (Bornstein and Crain, 1965). Marked depression occurred within 5–20 min after exposure to these sera at concentrations of 10–25%, whereas spike potentials could often still be evoked (as in high-Mg^{++} or low-Ca^{++} blockades, e.g., Figs. VI-7–10). Abolition of depressant effects by preheating the sera, and restoration in some cases by adding fresh (unheated) guinea pig serum (10%), suggested that the effect was complement-dependent (see below). (More direct demonstration of complement dependence was difficult since many of the rabbit and human sera blocked bioelectric discharges even without addition of guinea pig serum.) Similar depression of complex bioelectric activity of mouse cerebellar explants by MS sera was reported by Lumsden (1972); and Cerf and Carels (1966) obtained remarkably similar electrophysiologic effects consisting of rapid, reversible, complement-dependent depression of polysynaptic reflex responses in freshly isolated adult frog spinal cord exposed to MS sera. Since depressant effects were not detected with sera from control animals and humans in any of these studies, the observations raised hopes that a sensitive electrophysiologic assay with isolated CNS tissue could avoid blood-brain barrier diffusion problems in analyzing the roles of antineuronal serum depressant agents as possible circulating pathogenic factors in EAE and MS (e.g., Bornstein, 1973*b;* McDonald, 1974).[8]

However, with improved and more standardized microelectrode recording techniques (Crain, 1973*a*), it became clear that many "normal" rabbit and human sera tested at concentrations of 10–25% also showed marked depressant effects on the bioelectric network activity of cultured CNS tissues. In all of these cases, antineuronal potency was blocked by heating the serum to 56°C for 15–30 min, but none of these heat-inactivated normal sera showed restoration of depressant potency after the addition of 10% fresh guinea pig serum, which was used as a source of complement (Crain, 1974*d*). Earlier data indicating that sera from normal animals and humans did not produce significant depressant effects on the bioelectric activity of CNS explants (Bornstein and Crain, 1965; Cerf and Carels, 1966; Lumsden, 1972) may have been due to limited sampling of sera that fortuitously contained low levels of "nonspecific depressants" (see below). Similar depression of evoked bioelectric discharges in mouse cerebral cultures was observed by Seil et al. (1975) within a few minutes after introduction of sera from normal rats as well as those with EAE at 25% concentrations. This report, however, did not indicate whether the depressant factors in rat sera

---

[8] These experiments suggested that serum depressant agents might, indeed, be causally related to the clinical manifestations of EAE and MS (Bornstein and Crain, 1965; Bornstein, 1973*b*). Paterson (1969) noted that this "would provide a handy explanation for the sudden appearance and disappearance of neurologic signs in both diseases and the waxing-waning, remittent course so characteristic of MS. Rapidly changing neurologic symptoms (hemiparesis or hypesthesia of an extremity appearing abruptly and then disappearing in a matter of hours) would be easy to understand in terms of altered transmission of electrical impulses across synaptic networks—a physiologic dysfunction resulting from antigen-antibody interactions. Such evanescent signs have always been difficult to understand in terms of histologic changes, i.e., perivascular cell infiltrates, demyelination, and plaque lesions."

Failure to transfer EAE passively by means of immune serum may reflect existence of blood-brain barriers and other obstacles that normally interfere with penetration of the active circulating agent into critical CNS regions *in situ*. During the acute phase of EAE and MS, the blood-brain barrier appears to become less effective, and it seems reasonable to hypothesize that serum proteins including antineuronal antibodies may then leak into certain regions of the CNS and locally produce rapid depression of neuronal network functions, as demonstrated in CNS cultures. Restoration of function *in situ* might then occur soon after resealing of the blood-brain barrier, just as CNS explants recover their bioelectric network properties shortly after removal of EAE serum. After return to normal culture medium, characteristic synaptic network discharges reappear even following prolonged exposure (for days or weeks) to high (25%) demyelinating concentrations of EAE serum. Functional recovery occurs long before any signs of remyelination, e.g., within hours or days following removal of the EAE serum (Bornstein and Crain, 1971; see below).

were thermolabile or complement-dependent, and no attempt was made to utilize possible differences in these physicochemical properties to distinguish between bioelectric depressant factors in normal and EAE sera (see below).

If the factors in EAE and MS sera regularly showed restoration of depressant potency following addition of fresh guinea pig serum to heat-inactivated samples, they could readily be differentiated from the nonspecific depressants, which appear to be irreversibly inactivated by heat exposure. However, addition of fresh guinea pig serum failed to restore depressant potency to more than half of the heated EAE sera which suggested that the hypothetical immunologic agents in these sera might themselves be thermolabile.

In order to investigate the nature of the bioelectric blocking factor(s) present in normal and EAE sera, γ-globulin fractions were prepared (by Dr. Vanda Lennon) from normal control rabbit sera and sera from rabbits inoculated intracutaneously with 1 mg human encephalitogenic basic protein in Freund's complete adjuvant. The rabbits developed clinical signs of EAE 3–4 weeks after inoculation, at which time serum samples were taken (Lumsden, 1972; Bornstein, 1973*b*). Proteins precipitated at 4°C by adding an equal volume of saturated ammonium sulfate were dialyzed against phosphate-buffered saline at 4°C, and the final "γ-globulin" fractions were concentrated to approximately normal serum protein concentration (ca. 10 mg/ml).

Direct exposure of fetal mouse hippocampal explants to γ-globulin serum fractions from rabbits with EAE as well as controls produced no signs of depressant effects on the synaptic network discharges (e.g., Fig. IV-42A; Chap. IV-D) during tests lasting 30–60 min, at concentrations (25%) comparable to those present in the tests of whole sera. However, within 5–20 min after addition of fresh guinea pig serum (10%) to cultures exposed to the γ-globulin fractions from control and EAE sera, bioelectric blockades developed (Crain et al., 1975*a*). Control tests showed that exposure of these CNS explants to fresh guinea pig serum alone at 5–10% concentration generally produced no significant depression of characteristic bioelectric activities (for periods of an hour or more). On the other hand, addition of preheated guinea pig serum to the γ-globulin fractions was ineffective. Furthermore, after heating the control and EAE γ-globulin fractions to 56°C for 30 min, addition of fresh unheated guinea pig serum no longer restored their depressant potency. These data demonstrate that both control sera and sera from rabbits with EAE contain depressant factors that appear to be complement-dependent, thermolabile, and precipitable with half-saturated ammonium sulfate. Although this preliminary series of serum γ-globulin tests did not differentiate between depressant factors in EAE versus control sera, it provided significant information regarding the complex properties of potent antineuronal factors present in all of these sera. These complex CNS depressant factors are distinct from the many simple, heat-stable serum constitutents that produce marked depression of bioelectric activity of CNS explants at concentrations approaching serum ranges *in situ,* e.g., glycine, GABA, and other amino acids related to inhibitory neurotransmitters (see sections A, B).

The complex variables involved in electrophysiologic assays of serum may account for failure to detect depressant effects in the earlier experiments with control sera: (1) variability in potency of the "nonspecific" depressant factors; (2) lability of these factors at room temperature; (3) differential susceptibility of particular types of synaptic networks to these depressant agents (Cerf and Carels, 1966), especially in view of the marked differences in pharmacologic sensitivities of explants from various CNS regions (Crain and Peterson, 1974*b,* 1975*a;* Crain, 1974*b,* 1975*b,c,d*): (4) varying degrees of glial diffusion barriers which may develop over CNS explants, resembling blood-brain barriers; (5) variations in the complement potency of the guinea pig sera.

These thermolabile, complement-dependent antineuronal factors in "γ-globulin" fractions of rabbit sera differ from the thermolabile factor recently reported by Ito et al. (1974) in normal rabbit serum that caused a massive transmitter release from frog motor nerve endings within 15–30 min at a 30% concentration, followed by gradual transmitter depletion and impaired neuromuscular transmission during the next few hours. Whereas the factor studied by Ito et al. appeared to be a component of complement, the thermolabile rabbit serum globulin factors that depress discharges of our CNS explants appear to be separable from but functionally dependent on complement. It should be noted that the concentration of guinea pig serum used as a source of complement in our tests was limited to 5–10% of the bathing medium (see above). Furthermore, preliminary experiments showed that, even if the globulin fraction was removed from the culture, after a 30 min exposure prior to introduction of guinea pig serum, depression of bioelectric activity of the explants still occurred within 5 min after exposure to the guinea pig serum alone. This provides additional evidence that the rabbit globulin fractions contain factors distinct from but dependent on complement.

In rabbits reaginic antibody (immunoglobulin E; IgE) is heat-labile (Zweifler and Robinson, 1969). It is possible that the neuronal blocking activity we have observed with certain normal rabbit sera may be due to the presence of antineuronal autoantibodies, which were shown by Nandy (1972, 1973) to develop progressively in the serum of aging mice starting around 6 months of age. Correlative studies of the effects of sera from immature versus aged rabbits and humans on the bioelectric discharges of CNS explants may provide insights into cerebral deficits associated with aging and may also help to clarify some of the ambiguities involved in analyses of serum factors related to more specific neurologic disorders such as EAE and MS.

Furthermore, in more recent tests where CNS explants were exposed to these γ-globulin serum fractions at greater dilutions, the fractions from rabbits with EAE could still produce strong depression at concentrations as low as 5–10% (in the presence of 5% fresh guinea pig serum), whereas the depressant factors in control fractions were ineffective under these conditions at concentrations of 10% or more (Crain et al., *in preparation*). Attempts are in progress to determine if the greater depressant potency of the EAE serum fractions is related to specific antibodies against encephalitogenic basic protein. Immunoadsorption of the serum fractions on columns containing this basic protein should selectively remove the depressant factor from the EAE serum.

Recent studies by Lumsden et al. (1975) with neonatal rat cerebellum explants exposed to sera from guinea pigs with EAE add further support to our original evidence of a reversible, complement-dependent bioelectric depressant factor in sera from rabbits with EAE (Bornstein and Crain, 1965). Under the bioassay conditions used by Lumsden et al. (1975), sera from normal guinea pigs had no detectable depressant effects on complex network discharges of their cerebellar explants even when tested at high concentrations (50%) for 1 hr (although they were readily blocked by raising the Mg^{++} level from 1 to 8 mM). In contrast, similar exposure to sera from guinea pigs with EAE resulted in marked depression of bioelectric discharges within 10–30 min. The absence of depressant effects with normal guinea pig sera suggests that sera from this species (or group) may contain lower concentrations of the nonspecific depressant factors observed in normal rabbit (Crain et al., 1975a) and rat sera (Seil et al., 1975). Lumsden et al. (1975) also reported that the depressant sera from guinea pigs with EAE were not effective on the complex network discharges of their cerebellum explants during the first few days after onset of synaptic activity, i.e., between 6 and 9 days *in vitro*. They interpreted this as evidence that the depression produced by EAE serum may be mediated by a primary destructive effect on myelin (which begins to form at approximately 9–10 days *in vitro*). Their data, however, do not preclude the alternative interpretation that "maturation effects [of the synaptic networks] may occur during which phase [6–9 days *in vitro*] sensitivity to the effects of the antibody is acquired independently of the concurrent events of myelination" (Lumsden et al., 1975). This ambiguity may be resolved by extension of these studies to cultures containing mature synaptic networks in the absence of myelin. Organized synaptic network discharges still develop in fetal mouse spinal cord explants where myelin formation is completely blocked during chronic exposure for months to low concentrations (1–3%) of serum from rabbits with EAE (Bornstein and Crain, 1971; Bornstein, 1973b). It will be of interest to determine if such mature synaptic networks (in the absence of myelin) are indeed insensitive to the depressant factors in sera from guinea pigs with EAE, as would be predicted by Lumsden et al.'s (1975) hypothesis. Preliminary tests with myelin-inhibited fetal mouse spinal cord explants (after maturation in low concentrations of EAE serum) suggest, however, that these synaptic networks are at least as sensitive to EAE sera as are normally myelinated explants (Crain and Bornstein, *in preparation*).

VII

Spontaneous Patterned Discharges in CNS Explants in Relation to Embryonic Motility, EEG, and Inhibitory Control Systems

A. SPONTANEOUS DISCHARGES AND EMBRYONIC MOTILITY

Most of the organotypic repetitive-spike barrages and complex slow waves evoked in CNS explants by electric stimuli have also been observed to occur spontaneously, either in normal culture media or after introduction of chemical agents (Chap. IV-A,D) (Figs. IV-5;39;40; VI-7;11). Analyses of the spontaneous discharge patterns in these and other types of cultured CNS tissues indicate that "pacemaker" neurons may generate spikes sporadically or rhythmically, and these spontaneous impulses can then trigger widespread network discharges throughout the explant, depending on the excitability threshold of the latter system (Corner and Crain, 1969, 1972). Although many of the older explants show few or no signs of spontaneous complex activity in normal culture media, they may be rapidly activated after introduction of strychnine, bicuculline, or other agents which selectively interfere with CNS inhibitory mechanisms *in situ* (Chaps. IV and VI). Exposure of quiescent CNS explants to low concentrations of strychnine or bicuculline often leads to the appearance of spontaneous discharge patterns similar to those observed in more active explants in normal culture medium (e.g., Fig. VII-1). Systematic recordings have been made of the temporal patterning of spontaneous complex discharges in a fairly large number of fetal rodent spinal cord and medulla explants in normal physiologic salt solution (Corner and Crain, 1972). These discharges last for periods of the order of 0.1 sec (up to several seconds), and they may occur at regular intervals of 1–10 sec, although activity patterns are often quite irregular (Fig. VII-2). Some explants also show clear periodicity in the recurrence of phases of relative activity and inactivity, with cycle times as long as 10 min or more (see also Walker, 1975).

The complex, yet stereotyped, spontaneous bioelectric discharge patterns in cultures of organized CNS tissues show remarkable mimicry of rhythmic activities which occur in the embryonic CNS *in situ,* as determined by electrophysiologic and behavioral motility studies in the intact animals. The parallels between our tissue culture model and recent microelectrode recordings of rhythmic polyneuronal burst discharges in the chick embryo

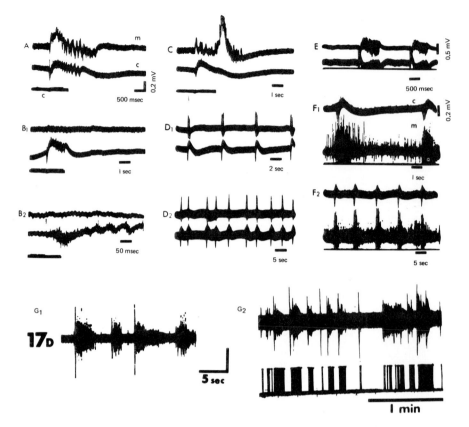

FIG. VII-1. Complex evoked and spontaneous discharges in coupled fetal rodent cord and adult rodent muscle explants (6- to 7-week cultures: see Fig. II-1). **A:** Simultaneous recordings of complex oscillatory (ca. 10/sec) afterdischarge evoked in mouse spinal cord (second sweep, c) and in mouse muscle (first sweep, m) by single cord stimulus (third sweep, c); in 10^{-5} M strychnine (as in isolated cord explants, e.g., Fig. IV-4). **B_1:** After introduction of *d*-tubocurarine (10 µg/ml), the entire cord-evoked muscle response disappears whereas the characteristic repetitive discharge still occurs in cord. At a faster sweep rate (**B_2**), the primary spike barrage in cord can be seen more clearly, followed by a secondary oscillatory (15/sec) afterdischarge. **C:** After return to normal medium, a complex repetitive discharge appears again in the muscle, lasting more than 4 sec following a cord stimulus, which now evokes a simpler, but still-longer-lasting response in the cord. **D:** Similar complex spontaneous discharges occurring rhythmically (at 3- to 5-sec intervals) and synchronously in another pair of coupled mouse cord and muscle explants (in 10^{-5} M strychnine). **E:** Similar spontaneous discharges in coupled explants of mouse cord and rat muscle. **F:** Similar spontaneous discharges in coupled explants of rat cord and mouse muscle. Note the repetitive fibrillatory potentials continuing in muscle during intervals between synchronized cord and muscle discharges. (Muscle spikes have been retouched during the first 4 sec of the second sweep in **F_1**: spikes during remainder of this record are barely visible at this slow sweep rate, but their amplitude and temporal patterns are actually similar. In **F_2** the muscle spike bursts that occur synchronously with cord discharges have been reinforced; spikes also continue to occur, at a lower frequency, during intervals between periodic discharges of cord and muscle, as in **F_1**.) **G_1:** Spontaneous burst discharges recorded in a 17-day chick embryo spinal cord *in ovo* (amplitude scale: 0.1 mV). **G_2:** Simultaneous recordings of similar cord burst discharges (17-day chick embryo *in ovo*) and visually observed body movements (lower trace). (**A–F** from Crain, Alfei and Peterson, 1970. **G_1** from Provine, 1972. **G_2** from Ripley and Provine, 1972.)

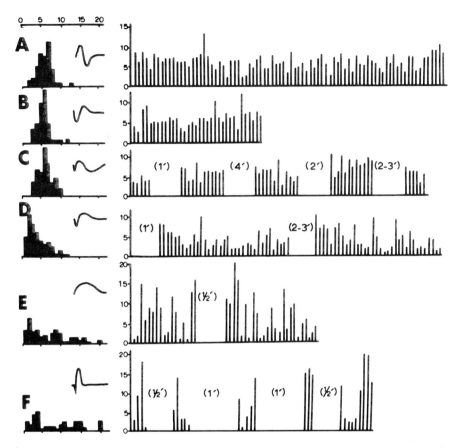

FIG. VII-2. Temporal patterning of several types of spontaneous complex discharges in mouse cord and medulla explants, studied for periods of 15 min to 3 hr. In each case the stereotyped complex waveform is illustrated (with a 1-sec sweep duration) in the insert between an "interdischarge interval histogram" (at left) and an "interdischarge interval tachogram" (at right). An interdischarge interval was defined as the time elapsed between the end of one complex discharge sequence and the onset of the next one. In the histograms **(A–F),** the number of occurrences is plotted against the duration (in seconds) of the interdischarge interval. In the tachograms the duration (in seconds) of the interdischarge interval is plotted against a series of consecutive interdischarge intervals, with arbitrary gaps indicating exceptionally long intervals ranging from 0.2 to 4 min. **A:** Explant that showed continuous and relatively regular discharges (mouse cord, 19 days *in vitro*). **B:** Same as **A** (mouse medulla, 27 days *in vitro*). **C:** Equally regular discharges as in **A** and **B** but with cyclic interruption of the complex periods, in each of which the first five or so intervals last 5–10 sec, whereas for the rest of the active phase intervals shorter than 5 sec predominate (mouse medulla, 15 days *in vitro*). **E:** More continuous but extremely irregular pattern of spontaneous potentials (mouse cord, 13 days *in vitro*). **F:** Irregular succession of intervals but with frequent, longer interruptions in this preparation than in record **E** (mouse cord, 13 days *in vitro*). (From Corner and Crain, 1972.)

spinal cord *in ovo* (Fig. VII-1G$_1$) (Provine et al., 1970; Provine, 1971, 1972) are striking. Provine's (1971) conclusion that these "polyneuronal burst discharges are neural correlates of motility . . . [in] the embryonic spinal cord" (Fig. VII-1G$_2$) provides strong support for the relevance of the CNS tissue culture model for studies of mechanisms underlying early behavioral development (see also Ripley and Provine, 1972; Provine, 1973). The culture model has been further strengthened by the demonstration of a similar relationship *in vitro* between spontaneous rhythmic, patterned bio-electric discharges in fetal rodent spinal cord explants and coordinated contractions of innervated skeletal muscle fibers (Crain, 1970*a*; Crain et al., 1970; Crain and Peterson, 1974*a*) (Chap. IV-A). Parallel cord-muscle rela-tions have also been observed in microelectrode studies of larval amphibian cultures (Corner and Crain, 1965). Further analyses of the cellular and molecular mechanisms involved in the "spontaneous" generation and spread of excitation through organotypic embryonic CNS explants may therefore provide valuable insights into problems associated with early behavioral development.

   The rhythmic muscular discharges and contractions triggered in some of these explants by complex oscillatory afterdischarges in the coupled cord tissue also show remarkable resemblance to repetitive muscle activity pat-terns observed by Tower (1937*a*) after chronic neuronal isolation of lum-bosacral spinal cord in the dog *in situ*. A single electric stimulus to this deafferented cord "often excited rhythmic action at a rate of 5 to 20 cycles per second lasting for several minutes . . . [indicating maintenance of] a high degree of functional organization . . . showing some of the phenomena of reciprocal innervation" (see also Crain, 1966).

B. EEG MODELS

1. Experimental Observations

   Our developmental studies of CNS explants demonstrate that small fragments of embryonic cerebral and other CNS tissues, isolated *in vitro,* have the intrinsic capacity to organize neural networks requiring only a brief electric stimulus to trigger long-lasting rhythmic activities which mimic some of the important patterns of the electroencephalogram (EEG). Whether these organotypic, repetitive discharges occur continuously — as in normal CNS *in situ* — depend on a variety of environmental variables, as shown by their "spontaneous" appearance after introduction of pharmacologic agents into the culture medium (Crain, 1966, 1972*a*; see also, for example, marked enhancement by eserine and acetylcholine of spindle-like activity in neuro-nally isolated slabs of adult cat cerebral neocortex: Kristiansen and Courtois, 1949). Moreover, application of a relatively small number of brief electric stimuli per minute to a small fraction of the cells in a cerebral explant (or occasional generation of spontaneous spike potentials in a few neurons) would suffice to trigger some of these organized cultures into a state of continuous, widespread, EEG-like activity [resembling Burns' (1958) observations of neuronally isolated cortical slabs *in situ;* see also Andersen and Anderssen (1968)].

More continuous spontaneous activity has been obtained by Cunningham and co-workers (1961, 1962) with large metal electrodes (ca. 100 μm) embedded at explantation in cultures of chick embryo spinal cord and cerebrum maintained up to 2 weeks *in vitro* (Fig. VII-3). The culture technique used in these experiments precluded microscopic observation of the cells in the living state, and no histologic data of sectioned explants

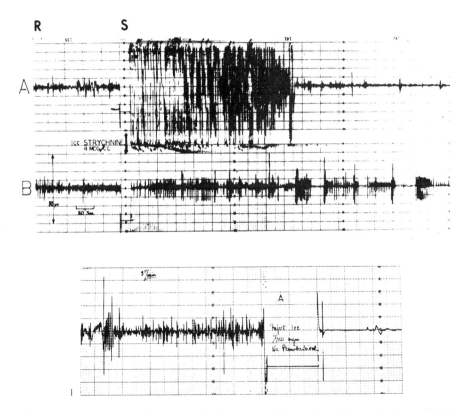

FIG. VII-3. Spontaneous slow-wave discharges in chick embryo telencephalon explants (15 days *in ovo;* 2–3 days *in vitro*) and effects of strychnine and barbiturates. **Top record:** Characteristic spontaneous potentials are recorded from two explants (**A** and **B**) in normal culture medium (R to S). Strychnine (4 μg/ml) is added at S. The increase in magnitude of the potentials in both explants is obvious as is the subsequent inhibition of the potentials in explant **A. Bottom record:** Similar spontaneous activity recorded from another cerebral explant. Sodium phenobarbital (1.3 μg/ml) is introduced (A) and rapidly suppresses spontaneous discharges. Time and amplitude calibrations: 10 sec and 4 μV per major division, respectively. (From Cunningham and Stephens, 1961; Cunningham, 1962.)

have been reported. Strychnine enhanced and anesthetics blocked these spontaneous waves, although the data were difficult to interpret since no attempt was made to utilize microelectrode techniques and electric stimulation to demonstrate characteristic neuronal responses (Chap. IV-D). Evaluation of these data was further complicated by the small amplitude of the spontaneous potentials recorded by Cunningham with these large metal electrodes (due to serious shunting of the bioelectric signals generated at substantial distances from the tip of the embedded wire). Although the amplitudes recorded under these inefficient conditions were less than one-tenth of the potentials routinely observed with 5-μm electrodes carefully positioned near the excitable neural elements (cf. Figs. VII-3 versus VII-4–6), the low resistance of the large metal electrodes resulted in a favorable signal/noise ratio (Chap. II-B2). With careful "calibration" of such wire electrodes embedded within or near an explant [by correlative recordings with manipulator-positioned microelectrodes (Cunningham et al., 1966, 1970) and by comparing spontaneous and electrically evoked potentials recorded with the large wire electrodes], this relatively simple mode of monitoring bioelectric activity of CNS explants may indeed be useful for certain types of long-term studies where "crude EEG-like" activity levels could suffice for correlation with other properties of these cells.

Use of a grid of finer-diameter wires attached to the culture dish would of course provide much more significant information (Chap. II-B1). Shtark et al. (1974) in fact obtained EEG-type recordings from late fetal or neonatal rat cerebral explants attached to the surface of a special multielectrode matrix — prepared by vacuum deposit and microetching techniques (Chap. II-B1) — during development for several weeks *in vitro*. Although use of metallic electrodes needs to be controlled since they may have produced additional foci of chronic irritation in the vicinity of the electrodes, it is of interest that the sustained rhythmic bioelectric activity obtained in CNS cultures by Cunningham (1962) resembles that seen in a number of neuronally isolated, embryonic CNS preparations (e.g., Weiss, 1941*a,b;* 1950; Hamburger and Balaban, 1963). Perhaps sustained spontaneous activity tends to be damped out in many of our long-term cord and cerebral explants by development of inhibitory neural networks (see sections C, D). One must also consider whether normal "pacemaker" properties are limited to specific elements of the CNS (which may not have regularly survived or been included in these explants). Bioelectric studies of cerebral cultures in which a substantial amount of subcortical gray matter has been included along with cortical tissue may help to clarify the role of subcortical centers in modifying or generating spontaneous activity of the cortical regions (Crain, 1965*b;* see below). Even in the much larger, chronic, neuronally isolated cerebral cortical slabs *in situ,* Echlin (1959) and Grafstein and Sastry (1957) noted the "unstable" and "intermittent" character of the spontaneous electrical activity in these tissues, in spite of the fact that marked hyperexcitability develops to electric and chemical stimuli (see also Burns, 1958; Morrell, 1961). Furthermore, although spontaneous activity resembling the EEG was still detected after chronic neuronal isolation of cat spinal cord *in situ,* the amplitude of these potentials were markedly attenuated (Ten Cate, 1950; Mark and Gasteiger, 1953).

Moreover, evaluation of the evidence favoring spontaneous activity in "isolated" CNS slabs *in situ* is subject to indeterminant factors introduced by maintenance of connections with the circulatory system. Marked alterations in activity of such slabs can be produced by selective stimulation of distant regions of the CNS after long latencies attributable to hormonal mediation (Ingvar, 1955; Aladjalova, 1964). In addition, Morrell (1963) pointed out that "it is never possible to be sure that the . . . neuronal . . . isolation is really complete . . . it is certain that a few fine nerve twigs accompany the pial vessels into the slab." These neurites may, indeed, constitute a sufficient anatomic pathway to permit triggering of discharges within an "isolated" slab from surrounding normal CNS if the slab tissue is in a hyperexcitable state. This view is supported by the demonstration of long-lasting, widespread afterdischarges in strychninized spinal cord and cerebral explants following a brief stimulus to a single peripherally located neurite (Crain and Bornstein, 1964; Crain and Peterson, 1964).

Explants of the medial portion of the rostral medulla have been paired with cerebral neocortex in an attempt to develop a model for studies of the effects of the "reticular activating system" on cerebral tissues (Crain et al., 1968*b*). Neuritic bridges grew across gaps between these explants, similar to those between cord and brainstem (Fig. IV-20) (Chap. IV-C). Not only could medulla discharges trigger characteristic cerebral evoked potentials (Figs. VII-4B$_3$,C;6), but repetitive stimulation of the medulla explant sometimes appeared to produce a *sustained* increase in the excitability of the cerebral explant (Fig. VII-4C$_1$). Similar changes in the cerebral tissue, lasting for at least several minutes after repetitive stimulation of a coupled medulla or spinal cord explant, have also been observed without the application of strychnine (see also Crain, 1966) (Chap. VIII-A).

In addition to the evidence described above for excitatory interactions between coupled CNS explants, the patterning of spike barrages recorded from the medulla concomitantly with cerebral afterdischarges suggests that *inhibitory* impulses may also be transmitted from one explant to the other. Although the data supporting this interpretation are still fragmentary, they indicate that a remarkable degree of complex interaction can occur between these two types of CNS explants. The "silent periods" in the records from the medulla after a local cerebral stimulus (Fig. VII-4C$_{3,4,6}$), for example, may be due merely to variations in the latency of triggering medulla spike activity, but the sudden onset of the latter activity at the same time as the appearance of a large positive cerebral slow-wave response is most intriguing. Of further interest in this regard is the observation that a less effec-

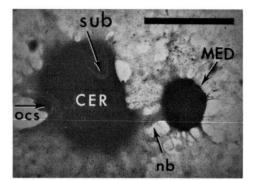

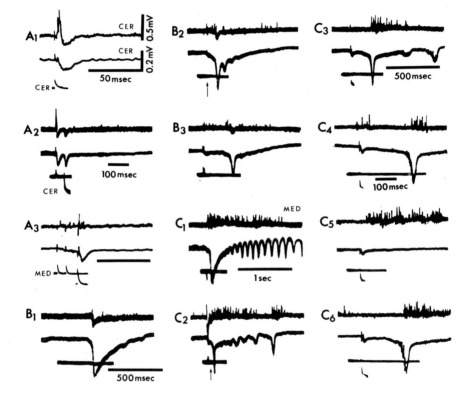

FIG. VII-4. Functional connections between separate explants of fetal mouse cerebrum (CER) and medulla (MED) after growth and maturation in culture. **Top:** Actual array of explants (from 14-day fetus; 3 weeks *in vitro*). Note that a neuritic bridge (nb) has formed between the medulla and the subcortical edge (sub) of the cerebral explant (Figs. IV-27;28). Scale: 1 mm. **Bottom: A₁:** Evoked potentials of relatively short duration at two superficial cerebral sites after a deep cerebral stimulus. **A₂:** The application of paired stimuli at two deep cerebral sites indicates no evidence of facilitation effects. **A₃:** Spike potential of brief duration and small amplitude is evoked by a stimulus to the medulla explant; and little sign of facilitation occurs when test stimuli are then applied at medulla and cerebral sites. (Note that stimulus signals to medulla and cerebral explants appear on the third

tive cerebral stimulus — one which failed to trigger a long-lasting cerebral afterdischarge — nevertheless evoked a sustained spike barrage in the medulla after a much *shorter* latency (cf. Fig. VII-4C_5 and VII-4$C_{3,4,6}$). Even when a repetitive spike discharge began spontaneously in the medulla explant *before* the application of a cerebral stimulus (Fig. VII-4C_4), it appeared to be rapidly quenched and did not develop again until the onset of the cerebral positive slow wave. These data suggest that local cerebral stimuli can activate neurons which may interfere with generation of spike barrages from the medulla.

Furthermore, spontaneous recordings obtained in this (and another) culture (after return from strychnine to control medium) showed rhythmic series of *positive* cerebral slow waves arising shortly after each prominent spike burst in the medulla explant (Figs. VII-5A–F;6). It has been suggested that the positive and negative slow waves generated by these cerebral explants represent extracellular records of summated inhibitory (IPSPs) and excitatory (EPSPs) postsynaptic potentials, respectively (Crain and Bornstein, 1964; Crain, 1966) (Chap. IV-D). The present data might then be interpreted as indicating the periodic generation of impulses in medulla "pacemaker" neurons, which in addition to producing cerebral excitatory effects also propagate through inhibitory neurites to cerebral neurons, where they generate large IPSPs. The medulla spike barrage may then be periodically self-quenched (possibly by local recurrent inhibitory networks), thereby attenuating the inhibitory activity to the cerebral explant. In some cases these repetitive sequences of spike bursts alternating with silent periods in the medulla have been seen even when cerebral activity disappeared for various intervals. In other cases, however, spike barrages in the medulla appeared to become longer-lasting and less sharply interrupted by silent

---

and fourth sweeps, respectively.) **B:** Onset of more complex discharges of larger amplitude and longer duration after application of strychnine (10 μg/ml), occurring spontaneously (**B**$_1$) and after a cerebral stimulus (**B**$_2$). **B**$_3$: Complex cerebral potentials evoked for the first time by medulla stimuli (cf. **A**$_3$), after a relatively long latency (cf. **B**$_2$). **C**$_1$: Much longer-lasting characteristic cerebral oscillatory (about 10/sec) afterdischarges evoked by a single cerebral stimulus a few minutes after a series of medulla stimuli (cf. **B**$_2$). Simultaneous recording from medulla explants shows the rapid onset of a long-lasting, repetitive spike barrage (at high frequency). **C**$_2$: Similar medulla and cerebral afterdischarges following paired medulla and cerebral stimuli. Note that medulla spikes tend to occur in bursts that are somewhat synchronized with the positive phases of the cerebral oscillatory sequences. **C**$_5$: Positive cerebral potential of small amplitude and long duration evoked by a single cerebral stimulus. This may be followed by a positive slow wave of much larger amplitude (**C**$_{3,4,6}$), with a latency of approximately 200 msec. Note that the onset of high-frequency spike barrages in the medulla tends to be delayed during the interval between the onset of early and late cerebral evoked potentials. On the other hand, when a cerebral stimulus is ineffective in triggering a later cerebral slow wave (**C**$_5$), a spike barrage in the medulla begins shortly after cerebral stimulus and continues unabated for a long period (cf. **C**$_{3,4,6}$). Even when a repetitive spike discharge begins spontaneously in the medulla explant before application of a cerebral stimulus (**C**$_4$), it appears to become rapidly quenched and does not develop again until a later cerebral slow wave occurs. (From Crain, Peterson, and Bornstein, 1968*b*.)

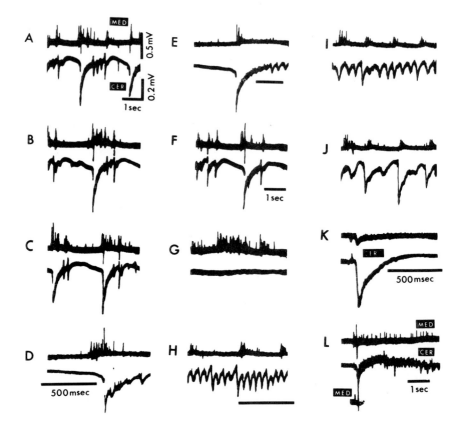

FIG. VII-5. Excitatory and "inhibitory" interactions between paired cerebrum-medulla explants during spontaneous activity (same culture as in Fig. VII-4). **A–F:** Rhythmic discharges occurring synchronously between medulla and cerebrum explants (after return from strychnine to control medium). Note that large *positive* cerebral slow waves tend to occur regularly after each prominent spike burst in medulla. This is seen more clearly at a faster sweep rate **(D)**, but at times cerebral discharge may start before onset of medulla burst (**E**; see also Fig. VII-3C$_{2,3,4,6}$). Also note the correlation of silent periods in medulla spike-burst patterns with the occurrence of *negative* cerebral slow waves. **G:** During intervals when spontaneous cerebral activity is absent, spike bursts in medulla appear to be longer lasting and less sharply interrupted by silent periods. (In other cases, however, repetitive sequences of medulla spike bursts alternate with silent periods even in the absence of cerebral activity; see text.) **H–J:** Development of *sustained* oscillatory discharges in cerebrum concomitant with appearance of more rhythmic (ca. 1–2/sec) spike bursts in medulla—in contrast to the more typical occurrence of periodic "damping" of cerebral oscillatory discharges (as in **A–F**; also note transition back to latter state in **J**). **K:** Large positive evoked potentials recorded from two sites in another cerebral explant (CER°) in the same culture but *not* coupled to a medulla explant. No signs of oscillatory afterdischarges or spontaneous activity could be detected in this isolated explant. **L:** After transfer of electrodes back to paired cerebrum-medulla explants, a long-lasting cerebral oscillatory afterdischarge is still evoked by a single stimulus to medulla and the complex discharges also continue to occur spontaneously. (From Crain, Peterson, and Bornstein, 1968*b*.)

periods when the cerebral explant became quiescent (Fig. VII-5G). The latter observation raises the possibility that inhibitory feedback from the cerebral to the medulla explant may play a role under some conditions in quenching medulla spike activity (Fig. VII-5A–F; note the negative cerebral waves concomitant with the silent periods in medulla). In addition, excitatory influences of cerebral neurons on the medulla are probably also involved, since the onset of discharges in the former at times precedes the onset in the latter (Fig. VII-5E; see also Fig. VII-4$C_{2,3,4,6}$). These remarks are of course highly speculative, but they provide a working hypothesis for further experiments on these complex heterogeneous neuronal arrays, incorporating microelectrode recordings at multiple sites within each explant and correlative intracellular measurements (Crain et al., 1968b).

Sustained EEG-like activity has not been generally observed in isolated cerebral neocortex explants (Crain, 1966, 1972a; Calvet, 1974). It is therefore interesting to note the appearance of "undamped" oscillatory (ca. 10/ sec) activity in several medulla-coupled cerebral explants *concomitant* with the occurrence of rhythmic (ca. 1–2/sec) medulla spike bursts (cf. Fig. VII-5H–J versus VII-5A–F). Cerebral excitability may have been sufficiently increased during these periods so that 1/sec bursts of impulses from the medulla explant were now adequate to prevent the cerebral oscillatory discharges from rapidly attenuating within the first second, as they often tend to do (e.g., Figs. VII-4C_2;5A–F; see also Fig. VII-6). The generation of these elaborate activities is in sharp contrast to the absence of spontaneous discharges in an isolated ("control") cerebral explant in the same culture. Responses evoked in the latter explant were also much simpler and briefer in duration (cf. Fig. VII-5K versus VII-5L). Similar differences have been seen in other coupled (as contrasted to isolated) cerebral explants, but wide variations in excitability of isolated cerebral explants (Crain, 1966) indicate that more systematic studies are necessary to clarify the degree to which coupling with medulla (or other CNS) tissues may modify intrinsic cerebral neocortex functions.

2. Possible Significance of Oscillatory Afterdischarges

In a review of the development of "organotypic" bioelectric activities in CNS tissue cultures in 1966, I attempted to interpret the possible physiologic significance of the remarkably complex, yet stereotyped, oscillatory afterdischarges (e.g., Figs. IV-4;5;37) that can be triggered by a single brief stimulus in many mature CNS explants:

The repetitive potential sequences of CNS explants show an interesting resemblance to the secondary cerebral afterdischarges following sensory (or direct) stimulation observed in many animal studies, including even some of the complex patterns characteristic of visual cortex of unanesthetized monkeys (Hughes, 1964) and humans (Barlow, 1960; Brazier, 1960). The records in Fig. [VII-7A,B,C (see also Figs. IV-4;5;37)], for example, display a remarkable similarity to responses reported by Walter (1962) [Fig. VII-7D] from human cortex, which consist of a rhythmic oscillatory (ca. 10/sec) sequence, phase-locked to a brief visual stimulus, appearing with a latency of about 300 msec after the primary evoked potential and lasting several seconds (see also Brazier, 1963) . . . [and more recent review in Shagass, 1972]. Correlation of the physiological aspects of these secondary oscillatory discharges has led Walter (1962) to suggest that they represent "a true reverberatory effect, preserving information about the stimulus as a significant event" (see also Hughes, 1964). Might the repetitive afterdischarges in cultured CNS tissues possibly represent a primitive form of such an information storage process? [Crain, 1966; see also Chap. VIII-A and Fig. VIII-3].

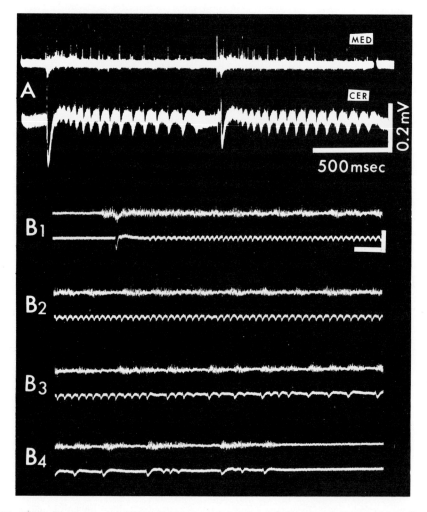

FIG. VII-6. Rhythmic repetitive discharges occurring synchronously between another pair of explants of fetal mouse cerebrum and medulla after formation of interneuronal connections in culture (from 14-day fetus; 3 weeks *in vitro*). **A:** Spontaneous activities of medulla and cerebral explants recorded simultaneously as in Figs. VII-4,5. Note the sudden onset of each medulla spike barrage (**A,** MED) followed closely by a complex

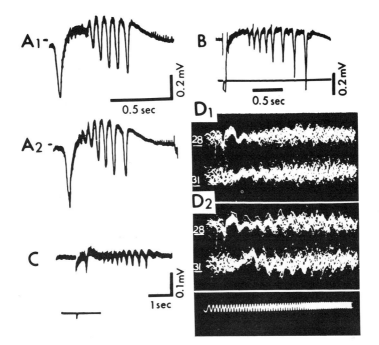

FIG. VII-7. Resemblance of complex oscillatory afterdischarges evoked by a single electric stimulus in mature cerebral and cord explants to rhythmic oscillatory patterns recorded from human visual cortex in response to a single brief visual stimulus. **A**$_{1,2}$, **B**: Repetitive oscillatory afterdischarges evoked in two mouse cerebral neocortex explants (2–6 weeks *in vitro*) by a single stimulus applied several hundred micrometers from the recording site. Note variation in latency of onset of the secondary repetitive discharge following primary, positive evoked potential (**A**$_{1,2}$; same records as in Fig. IV-37D). **C**: Oscillatory afterdischarges evoked by a single stimulus in human spinal cord explant (3–4 months *in vitro*). Note regular, 5–10/sec repetitive sequence including an early evoked potential, followed by a long delay and then a series of diphasic oscillatory potentials of increasing amplitude (same record as in Fig. IV-4A$_3$). **D**: Coherent rhythmic aftereffects of visual stimulation. Twenty responses to single flashes at random intervals of approximately 1 sec. Implanted electrodes were in visual cortex, 2 cm apart. In the upper pair the subject was inattentive (**D**$_1$); in the lower pair the subject was responding with key movement to each flash, indicated by the dotted signal (**D**$_2$). The coherent "ringing" between electrodes 28 and 31 is enhanced during responsive attention. The primary response is localized to electrode 28, but the aftereffect is phase-reversed between 28 and 31 (both of which are referred to the average of 67 other electrodes), indicating electric reciprocation between these regions. After-rhythm frequency: 12.5 cps. Note the transient flattening just before the start of the after-rhythm (cf. records **A, B, C,** and Fig. IV-5A$_4$). Calibration is 50 cps; 100 μV. (The absence of spontaneous EEG activities in the CNS explants permits a clear-cut demonstration of the oscillatory afterdischarge sequence with a single stimulus—in contrast to the large numbers of evoked responses which must be superimposed in cerebral recordings *in situ* in order to average out the spontaneous discharges so that the stimulus-locked repetitive response can be detected.) (**A** and **B** from Crain, 1964a. **C** from Crain and Peterson, 1963. **D** from Walter, 1962.)

---

cerebral oscillatory (ca. 15/sec) discharge sequence (**A**, CER); compare with Fig. VII-4C. **B**$_{1-4}$: Continuous recording of spontaneous discharges at the same electrode loci as in **A**. Note the rhythmic alterations in amplitude of medulla spike-burst patterns and synchronization with some of the cerebral discharges, as in **A**. (From Crain, 1972a.)

Two years later, in an extensive monograph on the physiologic basis of the alpha rhythm, Andersen and Andersson (1968) commented in their concluding chapter:

It is probable that the same basic mechanisms that operate during barbiturate spindles are also active in man when modulated, spindlelike alpha activity occurs. . . . it is tempting to propose that the rhythmic thalamic activity is necessary to produce a sufficiently effective impact by the afferent volleys on the cortical system. A single stimulus to the cortex or to certain thalamic nuclei is not sufficient to produce a perceived reaction. . . . However, even when a single receptor is activated, the ensuing response is perceived. . . . It may be conjectured that a single afferent volley from a receptor is transformed to a train of impulses of about 10/sec by the thalamic recurrent inhibitory mechanism. Such a train may have far greater effect on the cortical synapses than the single excitation by an artificial electrical stimulus. . . . From psychological experiments and electrical stimulation of conscious man, it appears that the cortical system needs a certain number of stimuli in an "activation period" to produce a perceived sensation (Libet et al., 1964). The highly interesting experimental results of Wagman and Battersby (1964) may be related to such an activation period. . . . suggesting that . . . some central process must be left undisturbed for at least 200 msec to have the first, weak visual stimulus perceived. Adopting the idea of Gerard (1955) that reverberation of activity in neural networks is involved in the establishment of learned responses . . . spontaneous spindle activity might be a means by which the brain assures that the information is repeated; in other words, it could be a system by which engrams are formed, taking previous sensory information as the starting point. . . . It could be an essential feature in a reverberating circuits that is necessary to keep the information stored in the right place, ready to be recalled by the cortex.

Wagman and Battersby (1964) noted, moreover:

In recent years, several studies have shown that even a brief stimulus can elicit an electrical response from the cerebral cortex of lightly anesthetized or unanesthetized preparations which persists for some time after the stimulus is terminated. Usually, such sensory responses consist of a transient surface positive ("primary") wave followed by one or more negative-positive sequences ("after-responses"), which may be superimposed upon a long negative wave, the total response lasting as long as 300 msec. [Note the remarkable resemblance of the oscillatory afterdischarge patterns of our CNS explants to this description!] In general, the literature suggests that both "specific" and "unspecific" thalamocortical projections may be involved in the production of after-responses, but the exact mechanism remains unknown. Also unknown is the possible behavioral significance of the phenomenon, although it is clear that the sequence of events in a cortical receiving area only starts with the classic "primary" response. . . . afferent volleys to sensory cortex do not in themselves assure conscious sensation—after all, the [primary evoked] responses remain unaltered in deeply anesthetized animals. . . . The time course of the subjective threshold changes described above could be explained if one postulated that some long-lasting activity in the cerebral visual system was a necessary condition for the perception of a flash of light at threshold [cf. Fig. VII-7D$_2$ versus VII-7D$_1$; see also Shevrin and Fritzler, 1968; Ritter and Vaughan, 1969; Shevrin et al., 1971].

Generation of oscillatory afterdischarges in explants of cerebral neocortex and spinal cord, with such remarkable mimicry of the complex, yet stereotyped, "spindle" activities generated by these radically different networks of neurons *in vitro* and *in situ* provides a valuable model system for further analyses of the basic cellular mechanisms underlying these important rhythmic network discharges in the mammalian CNS.

C. CEREBRAL HYPEREXCITABILITY AND COLLATERAL SPROUTING

On the basis of correlative electrophysiologic and histologic analyses of chronically isolated neonatal cerebral slabs *in situ,* Purpura concluded that extensive axon-collateral sprouting of the regenerating pyramidal neurons may be "the major factor responsible for the increase in excitatory synaptic drives that are reflected in evoked repetitive bursts" (Purpura and Housepian, 1961). Moreover, the "major generators for . . . the surface positive repetitive discharges . . . [appear to be] located at depths corresponding to the cell bodies and proximal portions of apical dendrites of the largest pyramidal neurons" where repetitive focal negativities were recorded concomitantly. However, since these studies have been limited so far to extracellular recordings, the data do not exclude the possibility that generation of IPSPs in superficial cortical regions may play a major role in development of the surface positive discharges (see section D).

It is of course quite reasonable to associate the increased excitability of chronically isolated immature cerebral tissues with growth of larger numbers of excitatory synapses on pyramidal neurons. However, since the evidence rests primarily on histologic analysis of a relatively small fraction of the cells (in Golgi sections), it does not constitute a compelling argument against the alternative concept of "denervation or disuse hypersensitivity," which has been demonstrated in many adult tissues under conditions where substantial growth of additional axon-collaterals and synapses appears to be precluded (Sharpless, 1964, 1969; Rutledge, 1969; Ward, 1969; see also Echlin, 1959; Stavraky, 1961).

Some form of hypersensitivity may also occur in these immature cerebral tissues after neuronal isolation, thereby increasing the potency of existing excitatory synaptic connections. The axon-collaterals which sprout profusely from the regenerating pyramidal cells might actually be making most of their synaptic connections with *inhibitory* interneurons. Growth of new collaterals terminating directly in excitatory synapses on neighboring efferent neurons may be characteristic only of *localized* lesions where, as Ramón y Cajal (1928) suggested, "the nervous impulse that reaches the mutilated neuron is not absolutely lost, since it is now diverted, through the enlarged channel of the collaterals, towards other congenerous neurones . . . thus increasing the energy of the efferent currents."

In *completely* isolated CNS tissues, on the other hand, there are no such normal "congenerous neurons," since not only are *all* efferent neurons surgically severed, they are also partly deafferented. Under these extreme conditions, increased numbers of *inhibitory* collaterals may develop as a major compensatory (homeostatic) reaction, which would neutralize the "super-sensitivity" of the partly denervated (and totally sensory-deprived) efferent neurons and thereby tend to restore the injured CNS tissue toward a more stable state compatible with continued function (Crain, 1966). Such hyper-trophic recurrent innervation of inhibitory interneurons — which ramify pro-fusely and in turn trigger IPSPs in hundreds of neighboring efferent neurons — would greatly enhance the synchronization and regularity of rhythmic waves generated by these cells (in accordance with the inhibitory "phasing" mechanism elaborated by Andersen and Eccles (1962) and others, and would account for the unusually stereotyped character of the oscillatory afterdis-charges in chronically isolated immature cerebral tissues (Crain, 1966, 1969; see also Calvet et al., 1974) (Chap. IV-D,E).

From this point of view, duration of the repetitive oscillatory sequences and amplitude of the periodic sharp-wave components would depend on the strength of the long-lasting excitatory drive impinging on the efferent neu-rons (e.g., summated EPSPs or other graded depolarizing potentials or both; note ca. 1-sec negativities in Figs. IV-29B;31H;37D;39B;42A) relative to the strength of the summated, shorter-duration, recurrent inhibitory dis-charges. If the latter are sufficiently powerful, the discharge sequence may be quenched rapidly following initial triggering of the system. The large positive monophasic evoked potentials observed in many of the older cere-bral explants may be due to such inhibitory dominance (Figs. VI-2A;9A); the latent hyperexcitability and capacity for generation of oscillatory after-discharges can be revealed — by selective enhancement of EPSPs or depres-sion of IPSPs — with drugs such as strychnine, bicuculline, or picrotoxin (Fig. VI-2B,D) or by repetitive electric stimuli (Fig. IV-42). These inter-pretations of extracellularly recorded repetitive discharge patterns in cere-bral explants are of course speculative; correlative intracellular recordings (and more quantitative histologic studies) are required to provide a firmer foundation for analysis of the special excitability properties of isolated im-mature cerebral tissues, both *in situ* and *in vitro*.

D. ROLE OF INHIBITORY SYSTEMS IN MASKING EARLY "BEHAVIORAL REPERTOIRE" OF CNS CULTURES AND EMBRYOS

The potent effects of bicuculline, strychnine, and other antagonists of inhibitory transmitters in enhancing complex evoked and spontaneous discharges in CNS explants shortly after onset of synaptogenesis has been interpreted as evidence that inhibitory synaptic circuits may begin to func-tion rather early in development of the central nervous system (CNS) (Chap. IV-D) (Crain, 1974a; Crain and Bornstein, 1974). In one of the few cases where it has been possible to obtain intracellular recordings of postsynaptic potentials (PSPs) in CNS neurons shortly after synaptogenesis *in situ* — i.e., in neonatal cat cerebral cortex and hippocampus (Purpura et al., 1965, 1968) —"extraordinary" long-duration inhibitory PSPs have been observed along with the expected excitatory PSPs. Purpura (1971) commented, moreover, that:

the immature neocortex and hippocampus are by no means *immature* as regards the differential development of inhibitory synaptic activities. In fact, insofar as *inhibition* is concerned it must be allowed that the cerebral cortex of the neonatal kitten is virtually as "mature" as it will ever be! If, then, there is any problem that requires the immediate attention of neurobiologists interested in the development of behavior, it is the problem of defining the functional significance of the precocious and differential development of inhibition in immature cerebral cortex.

It is of interest in this regard that the earliest potentials recorded from fetal somesthetic cortex in response to tactile stimulation are predominantly surface-*positive,* appearing at 43 days of gestation in the sheep (Molliver, 1967) and at the midfetal stage in the dog (Molliver and Van der Loos, 1970). Large negative evoked potentials do not appear until several days later. Although additional electrophysiologic data are required to clarify the mechanisms underlying these early surface positive potentials, a simple tentative hypothesis would be that they represent extracellular recordings of summated inhibitory (hyperpolarizing) PSPs generated by primitive synaptic networks located relatively close to the cortical surface electrode (see Discussions by Crain and Purpura following paper by Purpura, 1964; see also alternative views by Molliver and Van der Loos, 1970; Meyerson and Persson, 1974).

Cultures of CNS tissues provide a useful model system to study some aspects of this important problem. Extracellular microelectrode recordings at 3–4 days after explantation of late fetal or newborn mouse cerebral cortex may show positive evoked potentials (e.g., Fig. IV-29B, lower sweeps) (Chap. IV-D) with temporal patterns remarkably similar to those of the inhibitory PSPs obtained in the neonatal cat cortex. Furthermore, introduction of low concentrations of strychnine (10^{-6} M) leads to the appearance of prominent spontaneous and evoked slow waves in the explants, which increase in amplitude and decrease in duration during the following week *in vitro* (Crain and Bornstein, 1964) (Chap. IV-D4), clearly resembling the changes in strychnine "sharp waves" seen during ontogenetic development of mammalian cerebral cortex *in situ* (Bishop, 1950; Crain, 1952; Himwich, 1962; Figs. IV-29,30). Strychnine or bicuculline also cause inversion of positive evoked potentials in cerebral explants into characteristic negative slow waves of large amplitude and long duration (Fig. VI-2). These phenomena can be interpreted as evidence of selective strychnine or bicuculline blockade of inhibitory (hyperpolarizing) PSPs, thereby unmasking excitatory (depolarizing) PSP components (Crain, 1969, 1974a) (Chap. VI-A,B).

Direct electrophysiologic data have not yet been obtained regarding the extent to which inhibitory synapses may develop and begin to function during the *early* stages of synaptogenesis in the spinal cord of mammalian or avian embryos *in situ*. Mature inhibitory PSPs have indeed been recorded during late fetal stages in the cat (Naka, 1964), and since polysynaptic circuits apparently form concomitantly with the earliest detectable reflex behavior (Windle, 1934), Naka concluded that "there is no reason to suppose that the inhibitory reaction should appear later than the excitatory one." Strychnine and picrotoxin had produced, moreover, convulsive limb movements in amphibian larvae (Hughes and Prestige, 1967; see also Hughes, 1968); and Weiss's (1941*a,b;* 1950) larval CNS deplantation experiments (Chap. I) also suggested some type of intrinsic tonic "inhibitory" controls in the normal immature, as well as, mature CNS. He noted, for example, that:

deplanted pools of central neurones from a wide variety of sources display rhythmic spontaneous activity. We may assume that the factors generating this activity and determining its pulse are present in all gray matter, but are normally prevented from reaching discharge threshold by *harnessing effects* lying in the organization of the intact nervous system. The appearance of the rhythmic spontaneous discharges in the deplanted fragments may therefore be ascribed to the breakdown (degradation) of the finer central organization. One factor affecting the discharge threshold has definitely been identified as humoral, inasmuch as the threshold fluctuates with the composition of the blood [italics added] [Weiss, 1941*a*].

Furthermore, Székely and Szentágothai (1962) demonstrated that strychnine could greatly enhance the spontaneous activity of similar spinal cord and forelimb deplants, so that the usual 10–20/min muscle contractions increased to more than 100/min and often involved intermittent tetanic bursts at rates too high to be counted by visual observation.[1] On the other hand, preliminary studies in chick embryos failed to detect excitatory effects of strychnine and picrotoxin until relatively *late* stages *in ovo* (Oppenheim et al., 1972; see below).

On the basis of our studies with CNS tissue culture models, correlative experiments were carried out on the development of motility in guppy embryos in an attempt to clarify ambiguities regarding release from *early* CNS inhibition *in situ* (Pollack and Crain, 1972). Neuropharmacologic agents can be more readily introduced into these fish embryos (in contrast to chick embryos *in ovo*) simply by adding the chemicals to the bathing

---

[1] The excitatory effects of strychnine on these deplants of larval cord-innervated limbs did not appear until about a week after the onset of spontaneous muscle contractions (Székely and Szentágothai, 1962). In fact "many preparations with good reflectoric or spontaneous activity never exhibited any characteristic strychnine effect at all." The delayed onset, or frequent absence, of strychnine effects may have been due to the poor development of inhibitory circuits in many of the relatively small cord deplants used in this study, generally containing a "group of scattered [nerve] cells without central organoid structure" (Székely and Szentágothai, 1962). Weiss (1950) also noted that the endogenous discharges of deplanted cord-innervated limbs developed, at times, into convulsive "epileptiform" patterns (possibly related to humoral factors), resembling the acute effects of strychnine obtained by Székely and Szentágothai (1962) (see also Chap. VIII-B4).

fluid as in our tissue culture experiments. Introduction of low concentrations of strychnine (ca. 10^{-6} M) into the fluid bathing 1- to 2-week-old embryos, after removal from the chorionic membrane, led to increased frequency of early spontaneous (nonswimming) movements and/or precocious appearance of more complex movements. At a developmental stage 1–2 days prior to the onset of normal early swimming patterns, strychnine rapidly elicited primitive swimming movements. Furthermore, at the stage when primitive swimming behavior has already developed, strychnine elicited a more complex type of swimming, like that seen in older, "dormant" embryos that are able to swim immediately after release from the normally restrictive chorionic membrane.

These observations suggest that excitatory and inhibitory synaptic systems underlying patterned motility of fish embryos develop and begin to function concomitantly or nearly so. The predominance of quiet periods in the untreated fish embryo and the marked enhancement of motility under strychnine indicate that tonic inhibitory processes may play a major part in maintaining this early immotility rather than a simple lack of development of excitatory synaptic functions. The behavioral repertoire of the developing embryo may therefore be considerably more complex than can be described by overt motility patterns, since it may also involve active CNS *restraints* on embryonic motility (Crain, 1971b, 1974a).

The behavioral studies of strychnine-enhanced motility during early development of fish embryos *in situ* are consonant with electrophysiologic analyses of 13- to 14-day fetal rodent spinal cord explants during synaptogenesis *in vitro* (Crain and Peterson, 1967; Crain, 1974b). Onset of strychnine and bicuculline sensitivity occurs within 1 day after the first detectable complex synaptically mediated bioelectric discharges at 2–3 days in culture (Chap. IV-A), just about the time when behavioral reflexes appear in 15- to 16-day mouse embryos *in utero* (Vaughn et al., 1975). On the other hand, preliminary pharmacologic studies in chick embryos failed to detect any excitatory effects of strychnine on behavioral motility until 15 days *in ovo* (Oppenheim et al., 1972). Even with direct application of strychnine to the spinal cord during microelectrode recordings *in ovo,* no signs of enhanced polyneuronal burst discharges were detected until the 13-day stage (Stokes and Bignall, 1974), which is more than a week after the onset of cord synaptogenesis and the appearance of behavioral reflexes in the chick embryo *in ovo* (Windle and Orr, 1934; Foelix and Oppenheim, 1973). Stokes and Bignall (1974) asserted, in fact, that their "results also support the hypothesis that vertebrate spinal cord inhibition evolves late in embryonic development. This late emergence of spinal cord inhibition (13 days) is suggested by other studies of the development of reflex responses in vertebrate embryos. Such studies have shown that in most vertebrate nervous systems reflex excitation precedes the development of antagonist inhibition. Pollack and Crain (1972), however, describe very early strychnine-sensitive inhibition in teleost embryos. Such observations of increases in motility after strychnine application are subjective in nature, however, since they do not differentiate subliminal movements which the quantitative analysis of neural electrical activity might have done." It is not clear, however, why these authors were so concerned about "subliminal movements" in view of the dramatic onset of vigorous swimming movements after introduction of strychnine (Pollack and Crain, 1972)! These views indicate the degree of controversy that still exists (at least as of 1974) among some neuroembryologists regarding early onset of inhibitory functions during CNS development. Still more recently, Sedlacek (1975) reported strychnine enhancement of spontaneous motility in the chick embryo *in ovo* "even on day 11" (at 10^{-6} g/g egg weight). Depression of motility by GABA, on the other hand, was not observed until day 15 (at 10^{-4} g/g e.w.).

More systematic studies by Oppenheim and Reitzel (1975; see also Oppenheim, 1975; Oppenheim et al., 1975) demonstrated, however, that significant excitatory effects of strychnine on limb motility occur as early as 8 days *in ovo* (at 2×10^{-6} g/g e.w.). Preliminary tests indicate that bicuculline and picrotoxin are effective several days earlier than the onset of strychnine sensitivity (similar to observations in fetal mouse cord explants (Crain, 1975a) (Fig. IV-2). These experiments by Oppenheim and Reitzel (1975; see also Bekoff et al., 1975 and below) provide a dramatic illustration of the value of CNS tissue culture models as a stimulus to correlative studies *in situ*. Demonstration of strychnine-enchanced bioelectric discharges in early fetal rat cord explants (Crain, 1966; Crain, Peterson, 1967) had been a major factor leading to an initially controversial hypothesis regarding early onset of inhibitory functions in the embryonic spinal cord *in situ*, presented at the 1971 AAAS Symposium "Prenatal Ontogeny of Behavior and the Nervous System" (Crain, 1971c). [This Symposium manuscript was unfortunately delayed for several years due to publication problems (Crain, 1974a; see also Crain, 1971b; Pollack and Crain, 1972)]. Discussions on the significance of the CNS tissue culture models with leading neuroembryologists (e.g., Hamburger, Oppenheim, Gottlieb, Corner, and others) at the 1971 Symposium and during the following years appear to have played a significant role in stimulating more serious attempts to utilize pharmacologic agents and electrophysiologic techniques for analyses of inhibitory synaptic functions during early behavioral development *in situ* (see below).

Previous neuroembryologic studies have often focused on overt motility as a major manifestation of behavior in the early embryo (see below). This approach, however, may tend to distract attention away from the forest because of the rustling of the leaves on the trees. Integrated behavior of crucial survival value to the chick embryo growing in a tightly packed shell may also involve *active* restraints on the mobility of a major portion of its body musculature (Crain, 1971b, 1974a). The early overt motility which incessantly and periodically breaks through these postulated restraints as "convulsive . . . jerky uncontrolled movements of . . . individual parts, such as head, trunk, limbs, beak, eyelids" (Hamburger, 1973) may indeed be predominantly uncoordinated, as emphasized by Hamburger (1963, 1968, 1971), but if its major functional significance is merely related to maintenance of joint movements (to preclude ankylosis: Drachman and Sokoloff, 1966), unpatterned muscle contractions may adequately fulfill this requirement. The rhythmic *temporal* patterns of these overt movements, on the other hand, certainly provide significant clues to the primitive synaptic network properties of the embryonic CNS (Hamburger, 1968, 1971, 1973; Provine, 1971, 1972, 1973; Corner and Crain, 1972; Ripley and Provine, 1972). However, Hamburger's interpretation of the *spatially* uncoordinated patterns of overt muscle contractions as evidence which contradicts Coghill's (1929) generalization that "behavior . . . [in all vertebrates] develops from the beginning through the progressive expansion of a perfectly integrated total pattern" detracts from recognition of the possible existence of integrated, active CNS restraints that set limits to the mobility of the body musculature and which could be the major *behavioral* expression of these embryos during certain stages of development. These "restraints" are masked, of course, by the ubiquitous, uncoordinated overt motility of the embryo, but as Kuo (1967) noted "behavior is far more than the visible muscular movements. Besides such movements, the morphological aspect, the physiological (biophysical and biochemical) changes, the developmental history of the animals, and the ever-changing environmental context are interwoven events which are essential and integral parts of behavior."

Integrated CNS restraints on embryonic motility may be based on organized inhibitory synaptic circuits built into the internuncial networks of the early chick spinal cord (Crain, 1971b, 1974a). These diffusely distributed, endogenous negative feedback systems would serve to minimize excessive activation of the body musculature during the long period of organization and sculpturing of the CNS *in ovo* or *in utero*. In such a dynamic growth period when many neurons are selectively degenerating (Hughes, 1968) and many synaptic connections are retracting and others forming, unrestrained excitation of motor neurons could be disastrous, not only in terms of mechanical movements dangerous to the survival of the embryo in a confined though fragile environment, but also in terms of metabolic deficits produced by such excessive muscular contractions. Although large convulsive-like movements of individual parts do indeed occur frequently during normal embryonic development (see above), this degree of motility may still be quite subdued relative to the capacity of the body musculature to undergo violent contractions in response to a *totally* uninhibited CNS. Organized CNS inhibitory systems may include not only those mediated by the well-established post- and presynaptic junctions (Eccles, 1964), but also any other mechanisms by which CNS neurons may *systematically* depress one another. The latter could involve, for example,

diffusion of inhibitory transmitters from terminals of some types of interneurons to widely distributed chemosensitive regions on neighboring
neurons (e.g., glycine- or GABA-receptor sites) (see also Chap. IV-D3).

Provine's (1971) microelectrode recordings, showing widespread, synchronized "burst discharges occurring throughout the rostrocaudal axis
of the ventral portion of spinal cords of embryos between 6 and 20 days of
age," indeed provide a clear-cut bioelectric correlate of the sinusoid "waves
of contraction which pass through the [entire] bodies of young 4- to 6-day
embryos" (Provine, 1973). This type of total body coordinated, patterned
movements, which is the "direct precursor of swimming movements . . . in
fishes and amphibians . . . breaks down soon after its inception at 4 days
. . . in the chick. [After] 5 days, the S-waves disappear altogether" (Hamburger, 1973). Provine's data indicate, nevertheless, maintenance of widespread burst discharges in the ventral cord throughout the *entire* period after
the S-waves disappear, leaving only uncoordinated jerky movements which
may involve highly variable components of the body musculature at any one
moment. This "type I" motility, as described by Hamburger and Oppenheim
(1967), consists of "irregular, *low amplitude* movements . . . [which] may
involve all parts of the embryo simultaneously, or at the other extreme,
one part, such as a single toe or the beak *may move, while all other parts are
momentarily at rest"* [italics added]. Why does a significant and variable
fraction of the skeletal muscles remain immobile in 5-day and older embryos during each stereotyped burst discharge that spreads throughout the
entire rostrocaudal axis of the spinal cord? Widespread modulation or
suppression of motoneuron activity by inhibitory interneurons during these
cord discharges may indeed be the critical factor that accounts for this
apparent discrepancy between spatial patterns of bioelectric CNS activity
and overt body motility, as well as for the more general restraints on motility, e.g., relatively "low amplitudes" (see above) and long interburst
intervals (Provine, 1972). (It should be kept in mind, of course, that Provine's extracellular microelectrode recordings of burst discharges probably
included intermingled arrays of spike potentials generated in the *inhibitory*
as well as the excitatory interneurons of these complex spinal cord networks—cf. more selective recordings by Bekoff et al. (1975) (see below).

Coghill's discussions of inhibition in relation to development of behavior
indicate that his concept of "progressive expansion of a perfectly integrated
total pattern" (Coghill, 1929) clearly assumed a critical role for inhibitory
processes (Coghill, 1940, 1943):

> The progressive individuation of a partial pattern within the total pattern obviously hangs
> on . . . organized . . . inhibition. . . . The major division of the total pattern must be under
> inhibition when a part acquires independence of action, and the same part can be inhibited
> while the major segment of the total pattern acts. So that the whole individual probably acts
> in every response, either in an excitatory or inhibitory way. Therefore, while overtly the in-
> dividuated part acts apparently independently of the total pattern, the latter participates in
> its performance by inhibition.

Early onset of widespread, inhibitory synaptic circuits may also be the means by which stereotyped, specified neuronal cell assemblies become organized during development in "forward reference" (Coghill, 1929) to later functions but without benefit of prior activity of these assemblies— in contrast to the more "plastic" cell assemblies associated with learning in Hebb's (1949) formulation (see also Chap. VIII-A). Perhaps each of these newly formed groups of nerve cells with patterned synaptic interconnections could be kept depressed by innervation from arborizing collaterals of a special type of inhibitory interneuron, similar to the cerebral basket cell whose "axon . . . ramifies profusely and distributes itself to 200–500 pyramidal cells, making a dense plexus enclosing the cell bodies of the pyramidal cells in a basket-like structure ending in terminal synapses" (Andersen et al., 1963). These inhibitory interneurons have been postulated to provide a critical component in the "inhibitory phasing" mechanism underlying synchronized rhythmic, repetitive discharges of various aggregates of adult CNS neurons (Andersen and Eccles, 1962; Andersen et al., 1963), and during embryonic stages they may produce much more potent and sustained depression of the immature postsynaptic neurons in each cell assembly. Regulator inhibitory interneurons might then function as selective "switches," which would keep the complex cell assembly modules— or "mnemons" (Cherkin, 1966; Young, 1966)—"turned off" until critical endogenous or exogenous stimuli *disinhibit* them by direct interference with the synaptic actions of the regulator neurons at later stages of development —providing a cellular basis for "innate releasing mechanisms" (Tinbergen, 1950; see also Lehrman, 1953).

Similar selective disinhibition mechanisms may also underlie generation of stereotyped "fixed action patterns" of behavior (Chap. VIII-A) in adult organisms (Roberts, 1972, 1974, 1975; Maynard, 1972; cf. alternative hypothesis by Kandel et al., 1976a). On the basis of extensive neurochemical and pharmacologic studies of inhibitory systems in adult CNS, Roberts (1972) suggested that "in behavioral sequences, innate or learned, genetically preprogrammed circuits are released to function at varying rates and in various combinations by inhibition of neurons that are tonically holding command neurons in check. The activity of such circuits would be regulated by neurons exerting tonic inhibitory effects on the command neurons. . . . The successful operation of [such] a nervous system . . . requires a coordination of neural activity that can determine from birth, *or even before,* the ability of an individual to prevent the too-frequent firing of preprogrammed circuits of behavioral options spontaneously or maladaptively" (italics added). The similarities are indeed remarkable between Roberts' (1972, 1974) disinhibition hypothesis based primarily on neuropharmacologic analyses in adult CNS and my own, which developed independently during studies of fetal CNS tissue culture models (Crain, 1971b,c; 1974a). These events illustrate once again the potentialities and relevance of the culture models for analyses of rather complex neural functions.

Integrated inhibitory circuits in the CNS may develop with widely different patterns, depending on the specific survival requirements of each species of embryo, as emphasized in Anokhin's (1964) concept of "systemogenesis." Generalized hormonal and other determinants of the physicochemical environment of the embryonic CNS tissues provide, of course, a "range of permissive conditions" (Hamburger, 1971) under which these postulated early inhibitory systems can produce homeostatic *intra*-CNS controls which ensure "from the beginning . . . [a] progressive expansion of a perfectly integrated total pattern [Coghill, 1929]." The hypothesis is also consonant with Young's (1964) views regarding synaptic mechanisms underlying learning which suggest that "in the untrained condition [alternative neural] . . . pathways are held inhibited . . . by the action of small cells [with] inhibitory collaterals. . . . Learning would then consist in removal of inhibition from one path. Such a mechanism recalls the suggestion that enzymes exist in an inhibited form and that demand brings them into action by disinhibition." This similarity between selective derepression of genes and disinhibition of neuronal mnemonic cell assemblies may indeed be not only an interesting analogy but also a clue to mechanisms underlying long-term CNS activities during ontogenetic development as well as in relation to memory and learning (see also Bonner, 1966).

Validation of these postulated integrated inhibitory networks in the early embryo requires systematic microelectrode studies of the CNS during embryologic development *in situ,* using selective pharmacologic agents applied acutely as well as chronically in conjunction with focal electric stimuli. Until the role of such inhibitory systems is directly analyzed, we should continue to entertain the possibility that Coghill's generalizations regarding behavioral development may apply, not only to amphibian embryos but also to mammalian and avian species. These comments on development of early behavior in embryos, formulated on the basis of studies with CNS tissue culture models (Crain, 1971*b,c;* see above), have provided a fruitful stimulus for further experimental studies *in situ* as well as *in vitro*. Recent electromyographic recordings from 7-day chick embryos in Hamburger's laboratory (Bekoff et al., 1975) did in fact demonstrate the existence of coordinated motor output in the hindlimb involving selective neural activation of agonist and antagonist muscles. The results "suggest that functional inhibitory synapses may be present in the lumbosacral central nervous system at this [7-day] stage of development" (Bekoff et al., 1975). Oppenheim was even more emphatic following his recent pharmacologic studies with chick embryos (see above) and concluded that "it is clear that at least some inhibitory processes make their appearance at a remarkably early stage in most vertebrate forms, and that therefore inhibition must be taken into account in any attempt to understand the functional ontogeny of the embryonic and fetal nervous system. . . . The related problem of whether inhibition serves some unique function during neurogenesis — as suggested by Crain (1974a) — or if the embryonic demonstration of inhibition merely represents another manifestation of the functional state of the developing nervous system . . . must also await the accumulation of more basic data on the behavioral, electrophysiologic, anatomical, and biochemical aspects of inhibition" (Oppenheim and Reitzel, 1975).

An analogous homeostatic inhibitory mechanism was previously proposed in connection with the regenerative response of immature (and possibly adult) CNS tissues to severe trauma (Crain, 1966). As suggested above (see section C), the large numbers of collaterals which sprout and ramify profusely from damaged CNS neurons (Purpura and Housepian, 1961; Björklund and Stenevi, 1971; Björklund et al., 1971) may make synaptic connections primarily with neighboring *inhibitory* interneurons (Crain, 1966). This "compensatory (homeostatic) reaction . . . would neutralize the 'supersensitivity' of the partly denervated . . . efferent neurons, and thereby tend to restore the injured CNS tissue toward a more stable state compatible with continued function" (Crain, 1969). The postulated development of inhibitory circuits early in synaptogenesis of the embryonic CNS would of course provide an analogous homeostatic function by minimizing unnecessary activation and motility of the organism during the normal sculpturing of the CNS.

VIII

Tissue Culture Models for Studies of CNS Plasticity, Trophic Factors, and Regeneration

A. CNS PLASTICITY

The studies of cultured CNS tissues have emphasized that development of many organotypic structures and functions appear to be so tightly coupled to genetic factors that the explants continue to organize in rather stereotyped fashion in spite of wide variations in environmental conditions, even after chronic exposure to agents which block all nerve impulses (see below) as well as after random dispersion of immature central nervous system (CNS) neurons in a relatively homogeneous, unpatterned culture environment (Chap. V-B,C). The complex rhythmic oscillatory afterdischarges which develop in these mammalian CNS explants during maturation in culture therefore provide strong support to the concepts of "motor tapes" (Hoyle, 1964, 1970) and "central pattern generators" (Wilson, 1964, 1967), which have been proposed an endogenous CNS mechanisms underlying many complex, yet stereotyped, "instinctive" behavioral patterns ("fixed-action patterns") (Burrows, 1975; Huber, 1975; see also Chap. VII-D). This does not preclude, however, development of still more complex properties in these neuronal networks that are contingent on specific environmental factors. As Dobzhansky (1968) elegantly points out:

what is inherited is . . . a genotypic potentiality for an organism's developmental response to its environment. Given a certain genotype and a certain sequence of environmental situations, the development follows a certain path. The carriers of other genetic endowments in the same environmental sequence might well develop differently. But, also, a given genotype might well develop phenotypically along different paths in different environments. In most abbreviated terms, the observed, phenotypic variance has both a genetic and an environmental component [see also Birch, 1971].

Brain culture models may therefore be useful preparations to investigate mechanisms underlying phenotypic variance of specific components of a given genotype as a function of parametric environmental alterations. It will be of interest to introduce systematically various types of extrinsic stimuli during development of these stereotyped "self-organizing" CNS explants. Electric stimuli can be applied to specific afferent inputs such as neurites of sensory ganglion cells in contrast to inputs from other CNS regions. These stimuli could be random or highly patterned, temporally as well as spatially. The explants can also be directly exposed to chemical agents such as hormones, enzymes, metabolic inhibitors, dispersed uniformly throughout the culture medium or applied locally via micropipettes. Critical experimental alterations may reveal some aspects of the "genotypic potentiality" that are more tightly coupled to environmental factors, by producing selective maturation of particular neuronal circuits or cell assemblies, involving qualitative as well as quantitative changes in the network structure and functions.

Although it is probable that "the patterning of most of the long fiber systems of the CNS . . . is primarily a problem of developmental mechanics" (Sperry and Hibbard, 1968), the "old speculation . . . continues to seem reasonable that the plastic changes imposed by function are located not in these long-axon systems but in Ramón y Cajal's type II neurons" (Sperry, 1971; see also Young, 1964). Many of these small interneurons with short processes are still undergoing cell division late in development and do not differentiate until a major portion of the CNS is already functioning during the postnatal period (Altman and Das, 1965; Altman, 1967). Perhaps these "microneurons" are much more plastic than the long-axon "macroneurons," which differentiate at an earlier stage when relatively little function is occurring in neighboring neurons (Altman, 1967, 1970; see also Jacobson, 1969, 1974). Furthermore, even if the *specificity* of connections of many types of neurons is tightly coupled to genetic factors, the *efficacy* of these synapses may be quite plastic and significantly dependent on environmental factors. Quantitative data must be obtained to determine the critical developmental stage which each type of neuronal network assembly must reach through endogenous mechanisms before these systems become capable of undergoing plastic alterations in response to patterned environmental stimuli, i.e., "functional shaping" (Sperry, 1965, 1971).

Preliminary attempts have been made to detect such signs of plasticity as a result of experimental alteration of the culture environment during development of embryonic CNS tissues, e.g., sustained changes in excitability, in bioelectric discharge patterns, and in synaptic ultrastructure. The possible role of spontaneous bioelectric discharges on early CNS development has been studied in this model system by chronic exposure of fetal rodent spinal cord and cerebral explants to media containing Xylocaine at a concentration (50 μg/ml) sufficient to block all nerve impulses during the entire period *in vitro* (Crain et al., 1968a) (Chap. VI-E). The neurons in these drugged cultures continued, nevertheless, to develop organized synaptic networks as in normal media, and no morphologic deficits could be detected in the explants after weeks of exposure, even at the electron microscopic level (Model et al., 1971). Furthermore, within *minutes* after removing the blocking agent from the bathing fluid, the first electric stimulus applied to such a "virginal" explant often evoked an organotypic cerebral evoked potential of large amplitude and long duration, similar to those seen in mature control explants (Figs. VIII-1A;2B; cf. Fig. IV-37). These experiments suggest that ontogenetic development of some types of complex interneuronal CNS functions may be programmed to occur independent of prior bioelectric excitation of the cellular elements composing the system. Furthermore, after endogenous formation of such a neuronal cell assembly in culture, it can be maintained in a quiescent state for at least several

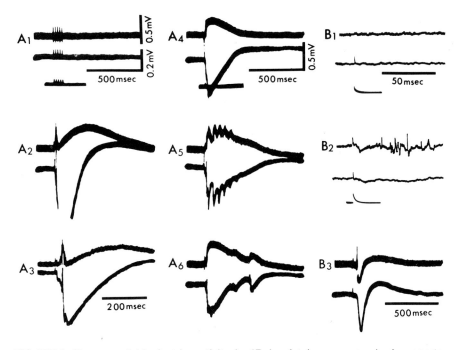

FIG. VIII-1. Absence of bioelectric activity in 17-day fetal mouse cerebral neocortex explants during chronic (1 month) exposure to Xylocaine (50 μg/ml) and rapid recovery in normal medium. **A₁**: No responses are evoked while explant is still in culture medium containing Xylocaine, even with repetitive stimuli at high intensity (as in procaine: Fig. VI-9). **A₂**: After transfer to regular BSS still containing Xylocaine at 50 μg/ml, thereby removing "serum depressants" (Chap. VI-F), the *first* stimulus triggers a characteristic cerebral evoked potential. Note the long duration, large amplitude, and polarity differences; i.e., negative near the original cortical surface (upper sweep) and initially positive at the "deeper" cortical site (lower sweep) (cf. Fig. IV-37). **A₃,₄**: Similar responses after second and later stimuli. **A₅,₆**: After transfer to normal medium, responses are still more complex and longer in duration. **B₁**: Absence of responses in another cerebral explant under same conditions as in **A₁**. **B₂**: Bursts of spikes evoked by single stimulus approximately 2 min after transfer to regular BSS following acute exposure to Xylocaine at 200 μg/ml. **B₃**: Characteristic "slow wave" evoked potentials appear approximately 1 min later. (From Crain, Bornstein, and Peterson, 1968a.)

weeks and yet remain organized with characteristic bioelectric excitability, in mimicry of many CNS networks which appear to form in "forward reference" to their ultimate function (Coghill, 1929). It should be pointed out, however, that generation of miniature postsynaptic potentials (PSPs) by spontaneous quantal release of transmitter at presynaptic terminals may not have been blocked during chronic exposure of the CNS explants to Xylocaine (or high Mg^{++}), since these potentials persist in adult frog spinal cord *in situ* after selective block of synaptically mediated action potentials (Katz and Miledi, 1963). Spontaneous transmitter release at inhibitory presynaptic terminals may be particularly important during early stages of synaptogenesis when extrajunctional sensitivity to inhibitory mediators may be high (Chaps. IV-A,D, VII-D).

The *in vitro* results are in agreement with and extend the classic *in situ* studies of Harrison (1904), Carmichael (1926), and Matthew and Detwiler (1926) on behavioral development in amphibian embryos during chronic anesthesia (see also Gottlieb, 1973). The experiments in whole animals, however, did not rule out the possible role of internuncial neuronal network discharges *within* the CNS during the period of neuromuscular quiescence. The experiments by Fromme (1941), on the other hand, raise the possibility that quantitative deficits in swimming behavior which appear after release from chronic anesthesia may involve sensitive synaptic circuits that are not present in our CNS explants. Alternatively, more quantitative measurements of the bioelectric properties of CNS tissues after return from chronic drug exposure to normal culture medium may yet reveal functional deficits related to Fromme's data *in situ* (cf. Hamburger, 1973).

Although no significant changes in response pattern were detected in some of these virginal explants with subsequent stimuli (Fig. VIII-1A$_{3,4}$), more complex oscillatory (5–20/sec) afterdischarges did indeed appear in a few cases during the first half-hour of intermittent stimulation (Fig. VIII-2C,D$_{3-5}$; see also Fig. VIII-1A$_{5,6}$; in the latter culture, however, the increased complexity of the response may have been due to more complete removal of the blocking agent prior to records A$_{5,6}$). Sustained increase in afterdischarges and in spontaneous activity has also been observed in some CNS explants cultured in normal media, especially following brief periods of repetitive stimulation at the beginning of the electrophysiologic experiment (Crain, 1966; Crain et al., 1968b) (see also recent data in hippocampal explants in Chap. IV-D$_4$). Facilitating effects of suitably spaced, paired stimuli may last many seconds, so that single stimuli which were previously ineffective now evoke long-lasting repetitive sequences (Fig. VIII-3B$_{3-5}$,C$_4$). Appearance of this phenomenon following application of only a few pairs of brief stimuli demonstrates a degree of plasticity in cultured CNS tissues which may be useful for studies of long-lasting alterations of neural activity basic to problems of memory and learning (see below). Sporadic increases in excitability often occurred, however, during the first hour after transfer

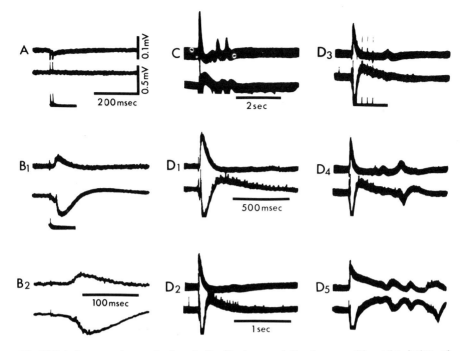

FIG. VIII-2. Increased complexity of afterdischarges following repetitive stimulation of cerebral explant during recovery from chronic exposure to Xylocaine (2-day neonatal mouse; 5 days *in vitro*). **A:** Complete block in original culture medium containing Xylocaine (50 µg/ml). **B₁:** Within a few minutes after transfer to normal medium, the *first* stimulus triggers characteristic cerebral evoked potentials (as in Fig. VIII-1A₂). Note the absence of any secondary oscillatory afterdischarges; the same response is seen after the second stimulus (**B₂**). **C:** After approximately 10 min of intermittent test stimuli, the discharges are much more complex and longer-lasting (and now appear spontaneously as well as after stimulation). **D₁,₂:** Recording electrodes are moved to new sites in the explant, where no secondary oscillatory afterdischarges are evoked; note the repetitive spike barrages which occur concomitantly with the primary slow-wave response. Following a brief application of repetitive (10/sec) stimuli (**D₃**), oscillatory afterdischarges can now be triggered by single stimuli (**D₄**). After further repetitive stimulation, the response to a single stimulus becomes still more complex (**D₅**). (Response durations are longer in record **D₅** because excessive high-pass filtration was used in records **A–D₄**.) (From Crain, Bornstein and Peterson, 1968*a*.)

of an explant from the long-term Maximow culture chamber to open micrurgical recording chambers, *apparently* independent of evoked activity. These studies therefore need to be repeated systematically under more rigorous control of the physicochemical environment than was feasible in the earlier acute recordings in open chambers (see discussion by Crain in Bullock, 1967) by introducing patterned stimuli during longitudinal electrophysiologic experiments on CNS explants maturing for days or weeks in sterile sealed micrurgical chambers (Chap. II-B1; Figs. II-3;4). Preliminary studies were carried out more recently using the sealed chamber arrange-

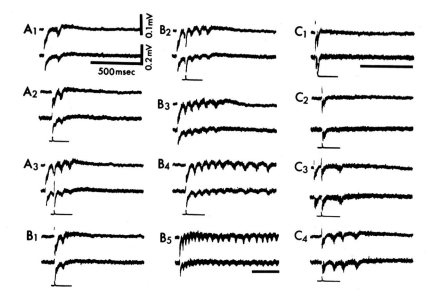

FIG. VIII-3. Development of repetitive oscillatory discharges following successive single and paired stimuli in fetal rat spinal cord explant (1 month *in vitro*). $A_{1,2}$: Simultaneous records of simple diphasic potential evoked in two regions of the explant, 200 μm apart, by single stimulus applied 500 μm from both recording sites. A_3: Paired stimuli, at a nearly 100-msec test interval, evoke a longer (ca. 200 msec) response consisting of two diphasic potentials (each with a pattern similar to those in $A_{1,2}$). B_1: Several minutes later. Single stimulus evokes responses similar to those in **A**, but with shorter latency. B_2: Paired stimuli now elicit a three-cycle repetitive sequence (note synchronization of activity between the two recording sites). B_3: A *single* stimulus, applied several seconds later, now evokes a five-cycle afterdischarge. $B_{4,5}$: Further development of the duration of this repetitive response following application of single stimuli at intervals of several seconds. $C_{1,2}$: Twenty minutes later. A single stimulus elicits an even simpler response than in **A**. C_3: Paired stimuli evoke a one-cycle response similar to that in A_1. C_4: *Single* stimulus applied several seconds later elicits a three-cycle repetitive sequence (cf. B_3 and B_2). (From Crain, 1966.)

ment to characterize various types of response decrement which occur in CNS explants during repetitive stimulation at 5- to 10-sec intervals for periods of several hours (S. C. Baer, *in preparation*). Classic conditioning paradigms with paired stimuli to CNS explants in these closed chambers have also been initiated, and preliminary favorable results must be verified with more critical controls during long-term recordings under sterile conditions (Crain, 1973*a*) (see also Fig. VIII-3).

The culture models may of course be relevant to only some of the rather primitive functional properties of the intact CNS; but in view of the remarkable organotypic bioelectric activities displayed by these isolated bits of tissue, it will certainly be worthwhile to investigate the degree to which they can develop a still more sophisticated "behavioral repertoire" relevant to studies of plasticity, learning, and memory (John, 1967; Kandel and

Spencer, 1968; Horn and Hinde, 1970). Moreover, in contrast to many of the simpler neural systems derived from invertebrates and lower vertebrates, our mammalian brain explant model is based on quantitative and geometric (rather than phylogenetic) simplification which can hopefully be graded so as to permit significant function *in vitro* of the specialized "plastic" tissues associated with memory and learning in higher organisms.

B. CNS NEUROTROPHIC FACTORS

Trophic effects have been defined as "long-term . . . interactions between nerves and other cells which initiate or control molecular modification in the other cell (Guth, 1969) and which may thereby be "responsible for the structural, chemical, and functional integrity of the target tissues (Lentz, 1971). From this point of view, formation and long-term maintenance of synaptic junctions, involving membrane specializations in the postsynaptic cells, are clearly neurotrophic effects; their occurrence *in vitro* in the absence of neural impulse activity (see section A) suggests mediation by neurotrophic chemical agents. The studies in Chaps. IV–VII, then, demonstrate the capacity of embryonic CNS neurons to provide trophic stimulation to neighboring neurons, leading to formation of stable synaptic junctions with characteristic postsynaptic specializations. Maturation and long-term maintenance of organotypic, triggerable synaptic networks in a typical CNS explant therefore involves a complex *set* of neurotrophic interactions between large numbers (e.g., hundreds) of component neurons (Crain and Peterson, 1974*a;* see also Guth and Windle, 1970). Glial cells may also produce trophic effects on synaptic networks, and it may soon be possible to evaluate their role by similar studies in culture of dissociated CNS neurons reaggregating after selective removal of all glial cells by cell fractionation procedures prior to explantation (Barkley et al., 1973; see also Okun et al., 1972; Chap. II-A2).

In view of the complexity and technical problems involved in experimental analysis of trophic interactions between neurons within CNS tissues, attempts have been made to obtain insights into neurotrophic mechanisms by using simpler neuromuscular model systems. We have utilized fetal as well as adult muscle explants to investigate possible trophic actions of spinal cord neurons in our culture systems.

1. Trophic Effects of Fetal Spinal Cord Neurons on Maturation of Fetal Skeletal Muscle Fibers in Culture

When isolated fragments of 18-day fetal rodent skeletal muscle are explanted in culture media and substrate oriented toward optimal maturation of spinal cord tissue, myotube formation occurs, leading to the appearance of cross striations in some of the thicker fibers during the second week (Peterson and Crain, 1970). Fibrillatory contractions occur more frequently during this period. The cross striations may become prominent, but they seem to be quite labile, fading and reappearing unpredictably during the third week. Soon after this period *in vitro* the muscle begins to atrophy. Cross striations disappear completely, fat droplets may form, fusiform swellings develop in the long muscle fibers (Fig. VIII-4A), and muscle contractions are less consistent. Despite gradually increasing areas of fibrosis, these muscle explants can be maintained for months, during which time spontaneous fibrillatory contractions may still be observed at times.

Muscle atrophy in culture is completely prevented when fetal muscle is explanted into a spinal cord-ganglion culture, provided the orientation is favorable to the infiltration of organotypic peripheral motor nerve fascicles (Fig. IV-10A,B). Under these circumstances development is not interrupted, and mature innervated muscle fibers can be maintained for many months. The trophic effects of the nerve complex on muscle, however, are more dramatically demonstrated when a cord-ganglion fragment is added to a muscle culture that has been allowed to atrophy after many weeks of maintenance in isolation. Fetal rodent spinal cord cross sections (0.5–1 mm in thickness) with attached dorsal root ganglia (DRGs) (14–15 days *in utero*) have been added to such cultures up to 9 weeks after muscle explantation (Peterson and Crain, 1970). For optimal development the *ventral* surface of the cord is oriented toward the main mass of muscle, at the edge of the muscle outgrowth zone (as in Figs. II-1 and IV-10A). This ensures that the muscle fibers will be located near the normal growth zone of the emerging ventral cord motor axons. Dorsal and ventral roots grow out from the cord explant onto the muscle tissue and after a short distance break into arborizations that spread over the muscle surface (Fig. VIII-4B). Under optimal conditions significant cytologic changes can be observed in the atrophied muscle fibers within 4 days after presentation of the cord explant. Fatty and granular cytoplasmic inclusions disappear. Cross striations and fibrillations reappear first in muscle fibers close to the cord. By the second week swellings associated with atrophic fibers generally disappear. Most muscle fibers are now cross striated, and they may show increased diameter and peripheral alignment of nuclei (Fig. VIII-4B). Synchronous contractions of large groups of muscle fibers are now seen more frequently. In striking contrast to these neurotrophic effects of peripheral nerve fibers on suitably located muscle tissue, those portions of muscle that become covered by the spinal cord explant and remain in direct contact with CNS tissue generally degenerate completely. In all other regions the muscle differentiation is stable and has been maintained without regression for at least several months. Functional neuromuscular connections have been demonstrated by electrophysiologic studies (Crain, 1970*a*) in cultures carried for 3–8 weeks after presenting a cord explant to an atrophied muscle explant (with the same techniques as used in Fig. IV-13; Chap. IV-A). The

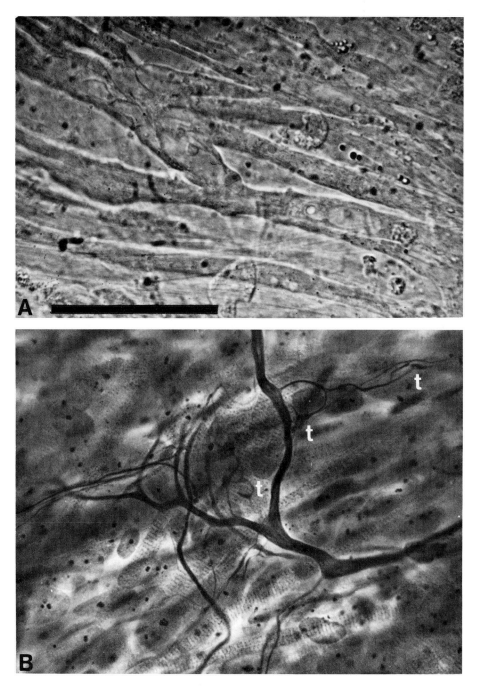

FIG. VIII-4. Atrophy of fetal rat skeletal muscle explant grown in isolation, and recovery after coupling with spinal cord. **A:** Atrophied rat muscle, 8 weeks in culture. Myotubes show abnormal swellings, and myonuclei are centrally located and vary greatly in size. Note the longitudinal striations but absence of cross striations; also note the abundant cytoplasmic fat granules. **B:** Month-old atrophied rat muscle, 5 weeks after addition of mouse spinal cord explant (cord-muscle array similar to that in Fig. II-1). The muscle now shows well-developed cross striations. Note arborization of broad nerve fiber which spreads over muscle tissue; several simple terminals (t) can be seen. Scale: 50 μm. (From Peterson and Crain, 1970.)

cord-evoked muscle responses are comparable to those observed in cultures where the muscle tissue matures from the outset under the more favorable conditions associated with explantation directly into the vicinity of a cord explant. Cholinesterase staining indicates the presence of abundant neuro-muscular junctions in those cultures that show bioelectric evidence of neuromuscular transmission.

The sensitivity of this model system for detection of neurotrophic effects on muscle is greatly enhanced by selectively depressing muscle develop-ment with cortisone. Cord-ganglion explants are not adversely affected by cortisone, and in fact earlier studies by Murray and Peterson (1965) sug-gested that this steroid may "augment the ability of both central and pe-ripheral nervous tissues to cope with toxic environmental conditions." It is only following ventral root invasion that the severe cortisone-induced muscle depression is neutralized and that myoblastic fusion, fibrillations, cross striations, and finally synchronous contractions develop. This result is in striking contrast to the noninnervated muscle grown under these culture conditions where atrophy and even degeneration occur rapidly (as in Fig. VIII-4A) (Peterson and Crain, 1970). The *in vitro* data are conso-nant with studies of muscle atrophy produced by long-term administration of large doses of cortisone in adult rats *in situ* (Faludi et al., 1966), where denervation led to marked increase in sensitivity of the muscle to cortisone-induced atrophy (Goldberg and Goodman, 1969).

It should be noted that isolated muscle fibers from mammalian and espe-cially avian embryos have developed and been maintained for months under some types of culture conditions, with cross striations and other cytologic features of maturity (e.g., Engel, 1961; Shimada et al., 1967; for reviews see Fischman, 1972; Murray, 1965a, 1972), although significant deficits may still exist in these uninnervated fibers, e.g., size, cytochemical proper-ties (Askanas, 1972). In the culture environment used for our studies, however, the muscle fibers were evidently unable to utilize endogenous mechanisms to maintain a fully mature state for more than a few weeks *in vitro*. This culture system therefore provided a more sensitive prepara-tion to detect neurotrophic effects on maintenance of muscle maturation, and addition of cortisone led to a further enhancement in sensitivity, as noted above. A similar strategy was used by Levi-Montalcini and Angeletti (1963) to demonstrate the essentiality of the nerve growth factor (NGF) for maintenance of the integrity of sympathetic neurons. Other laboratories had shown that chick sympathetic neurons could develop and be main-tained for months in culture in a serum and embryo-extract medium without addition of NGF (Crain et al., 1964a; see also Vandervael, 1945). By ex-planting chick embryo sympathetic ganglion cells in a suboptimal nutrient medium, however, they demonstrated that the neurons degenerated within a few days, whereas addition of exogenous NGF to this medium permitted maintenance for more than a month. In addition to differences in chemical composition of the culture medium, the physical substrate or framework may play a significant role in determining the long-term integrity of isolated muscle fibers in culture, e.g., embedment of the muscle within the three-dimensional fibrin meshwork of a plasma clot (Engel, 1961) as opposed to maintenance of the muscle attached to the surface of a collagen-gel film in a fluid medium (Peterson and Crain, 1970, 1972). The degree to which the culture framework provides longitudinal stretch to the muscle fibers also appears to be an important factor in maturation (Nakai, 1965). Another major variable is the frequency with which spontaneous contractions occur in a particular culture medium (for review see Murray, 1965a, 1972), especially in view of the evidence associating overt muscle activity and trophic regulations (Jones and Vrbova, 1970, 1971; Drachman and Witzke, 1972; Lømo and Rosenthal, 1972).

On the other hand, Robbins and Yonezawa (1971) used a culture medium similar to ours, oriented on optimizing development of CNS tissues, and reported that no cross striations could be detected in their fetal rat skeletal muscle fibers until innervation by spinal cord neurites occurred. Furthermore, rapid loss of cross striations occurred within 2–3 days after surgical denervation of these cord-innervated muscle fibers. Perhaps the culture environment used by these investigators contained some factor that depressed isolated muscle development, as in our cultures under cortisone. The immature state of the muscle fibers at the time of denervation (2 weeks *in vitro*) may also have been an important factor in this rapid onset of atrophy.

2. Trophic Effects of Fetal Cord Neurons on Maturation of Adult Skeletal Muscle Regenerates in Culture

In a collagen-substrate culture, 3- to 6-mm lengths of teased adult skeletal muscle fibers oriented toward ventral root nerve fibers of a fetal rodent spinal cord explant regenerate rapidly as the neural outgrowth makes contact with the muscle (Fig. II-1). Trophic enhancement of the *early* regenerative capacity of muscle is relatively nonspecific and can also be produced by contacts with a variety of non-neural fetal cells, e.g., lung, liver, meninges, and with peripheral ganglia. This early regenerative process consists of a complex organotypic sequence of: (1) budding or "satellite cell" activation from the rapidly degenerating parent muscle fibers; (2) myoblast multiplication and fusion into myotubes; (3) formation of a new group of young fibers oriented parallel to the old ones, concomitant with gradual phagocytosis of the remnants of the original parent muscle fibers (see details in Peterson and Crain, 1972; Konigsberg et al., 1975). After undergoing the early regeneration sequence, the young fibers of neurally deprived muscle show fibrillatory contractions and develop transient cross striations at their peak of development (ca. 2–3 weeks) *in vitro,* but soon afterward, as *in situ,* they atrophy (as also occurs in isolated explants of fetal muscle; see above). Further differentiation, maturation, and long-term maintenance requires innervation, *in vitro* as well as *in situ.* In our cultures this is dependent on the organotypic development of both the central and peripheral nerve network of the spinal cord complex. These conclusions are consistent with observations of denervated muscle studied during embryologic development (e.g., Muchmore, 1968; Tweedle et al., 1974), as well as in "minced muscle" preparations implanted into adult hosts (e.g., Studitsky, 1963; see review in Carlson, 1972, and recent supporting data from Carlson's laboratory: Mong, 1975; see also amphibian limb deplant studies by Weiss, 1950).

By 2–3 weeks *in vitro* regenerated muscle may appear well differentiated, with prominent cross striations and peripherally positioned subsarcolemmal nuclei (Fig. VIII-5; see also Fig. IV-12). During the following weeks in culture, gradual maturation of the motor endplate structure occurs, including increased complexity of nerve terminals and postsynaptic specializations, as illustrated by silver impregnation (Fig. IV-10) and cholinesterase staining (Fig. VIII-5B) (Peterson and Crain, 1972), and by electron microscopy. The latter studies, by Pappas et al. (1971*a,b*), show that after 4 weeks of coupling the postsynaptic endplate structure has developed simple infoldings, and a normal terminal Schwann cell relationship to the presynaptic terminal is present. Further differentiation of the postsynaptic membrane develops gradually, and at 10 weeks *in vitro* complex infoldings characteristic of mature motor endplates have formed (Fig. IV-11). The muscle fibers maintain highly ordered cross striations, elaborate networks of sarcoplasmic reticulum, triads, and subsarcolemmal nuclei for many months (Fig. IV-12).

Maintenance of healthy, mature, innervated skeletal muscle fibers for periods as long as a year of isolation *in vitro* sets limits to interpretations of "disuse atrophy" based on neuronally isolated cord techniques *in situ* (Tower, 1937*b*; Klinkerfuss and Haugh, 1970). Since the atrophy observed by Tower (1937*b*) and the autolytic changes reported by Klinkerfuss and Haugh (1970) do not occur in these long-term ganglion-cord-muscle cultures, factors other than "disuse" may underlie the muscle alterations *in situ,* e.g., deficits in the trophic effects provided by the isolated motoneurons. These deficits might arise either directly following surgical trauma (Drachman, 1971) or as a sequel to loss of synaptic connections with sensory ganglion cells. Muscle activity in some of these long-term cultures becomes highly irregular, so that there are many periods of complete absence of contractions during routine microscopic examinations (which may last for periods of approximately 15 min/day). Electrophysiologic studies indicate, moreover, that spontaneous discharges in older spinal cord explants occur infrequently (on the basis of random samples in acute experiments lasting several hours). This phenomenon may be due to de-

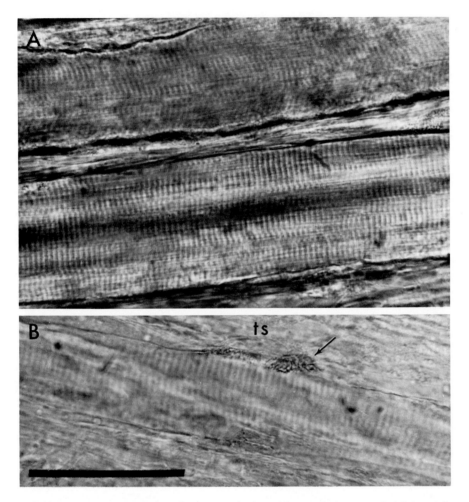

FIG. VIII-5. Photomicrographs of mature, spinal cord-innervated mouse skeletal muscle fibers (2 months *in vitro;* after regeneration from adult muscle explant—see text; see also low-power view in Fig. II-1). **A:** Typical appearance in living culture. Note the well-developed cross striations extending uniformly across the girth of each fiber (see electron microscopic view in Fig. IV-12); subsarcolemmal nuclei are not visible in this field (Figs. IV-10;12). **B:** Mature motor endplate after staining the culture for cholinesterase. Note selective staining of the endplate structure (*arrow*) and the well-defined terminal Schwann cell (ts); see electron microscopic view in Fig. IV-11. Scale: 50 μm. (From Peterson and Crain, 1972; Crain and Peterson, 1974a.)

velopment of inhibitory synaptic mechanisms which suppress discharges of the older CNS explants (Chaps. VI-A, VII-D). The long-term integrity of innervated muscle *in vitro* is therefore difficult to attribute to a greater degree of overt muscle activity than the "sporadic" contractions that occur in the cord-isolation model *in situ* (Tower, 1937*a,b*). Quantitative determina-

tions must be made, however, to evaluate the extent of spontaneous contractions that occur in these cultured muscle fibers during the months *in vitro* (see also section 4).

3. Surgical Denervation

Sustained maintenance of differentiated cross-striated muscle fibers after regeneration in culture is dependent on innervation by organotypic spinal cord tissue. Thus improperly oriented muscle explants that are not in the path of ventral root fibers generally atrophy. Sensory (dorsal root) and sympathetic ganglia can indeed provide a stimulus to early regeneration of isolated muscle, but they do not lead to sustained maintenance of the differentiated state in the absence of cord innervation (Peterson and Crain, 1972). (The presence of DRGs and associated meningeal tissue may, however, play an additional role by facilitating development of well-organized arrays of myelinated peripheral motor axons.) On the other hand, surgical extirpation of the spinal cord portion of the neural complex results in degeneration of the motor nerve fascicles and atrophy of the muscle (Fig. VIII-6A). The DRGs and their sensory nerve fibers remain unchanged and continue to spread over the muscle regenerate and the regions beyond. Denervation atrophy generally occurs within 2–4 weeks after removal of the cord neurons and consists of disruption of characteristic cross striations, fusiform swellings, reduced fiber diameters, and translocation of muscle nuclei from subsarcolemmal to more central loci (Fig. VIII-6B,C). Limited regions of abnormal cross striations may persist in some muscle fibers for extended periods (ca. 2 months) after denervation, but they are always associated with gross pathologic alterations (Fig. VIII-6C). The strength of muscle contractions appeared to diminish as atrophic cytologic alterations developed after surgical denervation, but quantitative measurements of twitch tension have not yet been feasible in these cultures.

Attempts have also been made to interfere with the trophic effects of spinal cord on muscle by chronic exposure of the cultures to selective blocking agents, e.g., Xylocaine and *d*-tubocurarine (Crain and Peterson,

---

FIG. VIII-6. Atrophy of mature mouse skeletal muscle fibers after denervation *in vitro* by extirpation of spinal cord explant. **A:** Low-power view of 5-month-old culture, 6 weeks after extirpation of spinal cord tissue, as shown by the clear zone (c); silver impregnation. DRGs (g) are undisturbed, and sensory nerve fibers are still present in the muscle strip (m) and beyond. Scale: 1 mm. **B:** High-power view of living muscle fibers in another 5-month-old culture similar to that in **A,** 3 weeks after denervation. Note disruption of cross striations, translocation of myonuclei to central loci, and moderate irregularities in the fiber diameter, in contrast to the highly ordered array prior to denervation (e.g., Fig. VIII-5). **C:** Silver impregnation of a similar long-term culture 3.5 weeks after denervation shows progressive stages in disruption of cross striations in several muscle fibers (center) and complete disappearance in others (top). Many of the myonuclei have shifted to more central positions. In contrast, note the typical silver-impregnated array of innervated muscle fibers in Fig. IV-10. Scale (**B** and **C**): 50 μm. (From Crain and Peterson, 1974a.)

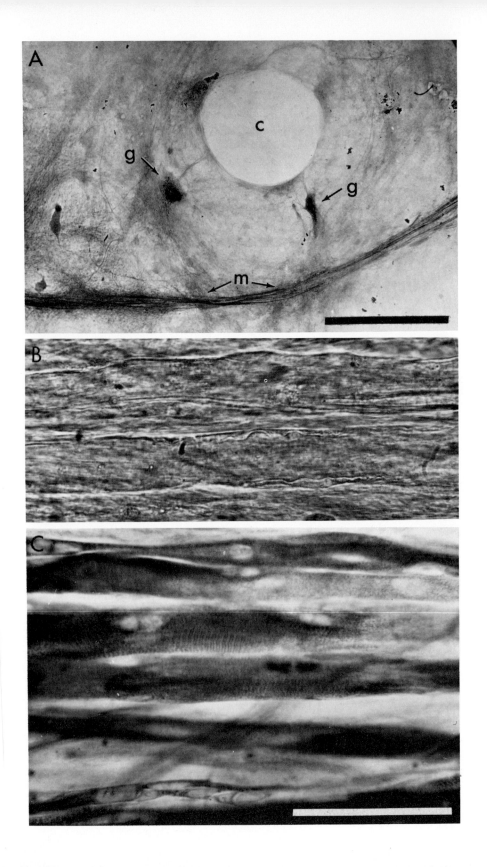

1974*a*), but the muscle atrophy that occurred after their addition to the cultures, at 50–100 μg/ml, may also involve direct toxic effects on the cultured muscle fibers. Further control experiments are needed to clarify this ambiguity. During the course of these studies, we also demonstrated that in the presence of high concentrations of *d*-tubocurarine (up to 100 μg/ml) during the entire 4- to 6-week period in culture many muscle fibers still regenerated and formed functional neuromuscular connections (Crain and Peterson, 1971) as well as characteristic motor endplates (Pappas et al., 1971*b*). Similar evidence for formation of functional neuromuscular junctions was obtained by Cohen (1972) after chronic exposure (9 days) of early frog embryo cord-muscle explants to *d*-tubocurarine at 100–300 μg/ml. The data suggest, therefore, that neuromuscular connections may form and mature even when the acetylcholine receptor sites on the muscle fibers are rendered ineffective to acetylcholine by the action of *d*-tubocurarine. Drug tolerance effects may, however, complicate interpretation of these experiments since muscle contractions could still be evoked by brief tetanic (50/sec) or even single cord stimuli in some of our cultures maintained for weeks in curare at 100 μg/ml (see also Drachman, 1965), although neuromuscular block did appear to be effective in other cases (Crain and Peterson, 1974*a*) and was indeed observed in the experiments with cultured frog tissues (Cohen, 1972).

4. Trophic Effects of Fetal Sympathetic Ganglia on Adult Muscle Regenerates after Cord Denervation *In Vitro*

Attempts to counteract the atrophy produced in mature cultures of adult muscle regenerates following surgical denervation should provide valuable clues to neurotrophic mechanisms. These cultures may provide a useful model system to supplement *in situ* studies of the effects of exogenous spinal cord or other neural extracts (Lentz, 1971, 1972; Oh et al., 1972; Oh, 1975; Kuromi and Hasegawa, 1975) or specific chemicals that may mimic neurotrophic effects (Drachman, 1971; Lentz, 1972, 1974). Chronic electric stimulation of the cultured muscle fibers should clarify the degree to which overt muscle contractions may substitute for normal innervation in maintenance of the structural integrity of muscle fibers (e.g., cross striations, subsarcolemmal myonuclei, etc.), as has been demonstrated in regard to restriction of ACh sensitivity to motor endplate regions (Jones and Vrbova, 1970,1971; Drachman and Witzke, 1972; Lømo and Rosenthal, 1972; Cohen and Fischbach, 1973; Fischbach et al., 1974*a*). Alternatively, the role of overt muscle activity may be clarified by chronic exposure of mature cord-innervated muscle cultures to low concentrations of tetrodotoxin (Chaps. IV-A and V-B) which may selectively prevent spontaneous muscle contractions without interfering with normal neurotrophic effects on the muscle fibers.

Another experimental approach along these lines involves "presentation"

of different types of neurons to cultures of cord-denervated muscle fibers. A start has been made by explantation of sympathetic ganglion chains, from 17-day fetal mice (Crain et al., 1964a) (Chap. III-B) approximately 1 mm from cord-innervated adult mouse skeletal muscle regenerates 3-4 weeks after cord-muscle coupling (Fig. VIII-7A). The culture medium was supplemented with salivary NGF (2 units/ml) during the first 2 weeks to enhance neuritic outgrowth from the sympathetic neurons (Levi-Montalcini and Cohen, 1960; Crain et al., 1964a). Three to four weeks later, after an abundant neuritic arborization had grown into the muscle explant (Fig. VIII-7B), the spinal cord tissue was surgically removed, leaving the DRGs intact, as in cultures without added sympathetic ganglia (Fig. VIII-7A). In contrast to the denervation atrophy which generally occurs within 2-4 weeks after removal of the cord neurons (Fig. VIII-6B), some of the cord-denervated muscle coupled to sympathetic ganglia showed large numbers of healthy cross-striated fibers and no major cytologic signs of atrophy for as long as 6-9 weeks (Fig. VIII-7B,C).[1] Although, as noted above (Chaps. III-B, IV-A, V-A) selective stimulation of sympathetic neurons could evoke contractions in some of the cord-denervated muscle explants, no signs of innervation could be detected in many muscle fibers even though their cytologic integrity suggested that they were under trophic sympathetic influence (Crain and Peterson, 1974a).

These data provide an interesting extension of studies by Mendez et al. (1970) in the adult cat, in which postganglionic fibers of the superior cervical ganglion were sutured to skeletal muscle prior to denervation of the somatic nerve supply. This procedure markedly decreased the frequency of fibrillation potentials that characteristically appeared after the denervation method used by Mendez et al. (1970) on this muscle *in situ*, although no contractions could be evoked by stimulation of the postganglionic fibers. Since "more than 99% of these fibers are adrenergic," the authors concluded that the normal antifibrillation effect is not mediated by acetylcholine but instead by a "hypothetical trophic factor." Attempts are being made to determine whether the sympathetic neurites that provide trophic influence on cord-denervated muscle in our cultures are actually adrenergic or if they derive from the small fraction of cholinergic neurons that may be present in the sympathetic ganglia used in this study (see also Chaps. III-B, V-A). The

---

[1] Analogous experiments have recently been carried out on cultures of smooth muscle cells (from neonatal guinea pig) which begin to dedifferentiate after 5 days *in vitro*. Introduction of an *extract* of sympathetic ganglia, or dibutyryl cyclic AMP (5×10^{-4}g/ml), into the culture medium leads to maintenance of differentiated muscle cells for an additional 3-7 days (Chamley and Campbell, 1975), as also occurs when sympathetic nerve fibers arborize close to cultured smooth muscle cells (Chamley et al., 1974). Similar studies of the effects of spinal cord extracts on the maintenance of denervated skeletal muscle fibers in culture may provide valuable insights into these neurotrophic mechanisms (see Oh et al., 1972; Oh, 1975; Kuromi and Hasegawa, 1975).

tissue culture results are also consistent with evidence by Landmesser (1971) that cholinergic parasympathetic and possibly sympathetic nerves under some conditions not only make functional synaptic connections with skeletal muscle in the adult frog *in situ,* but they can also trophically maintain various structural and functional properties of these fibers for more than a year.

Weiss' (1950) studies of deplants of larval amphibian spinal cord-innervated limbs (Chaps. I-A, VII-D) have also provided valuable data on neurotrophic effects. He showed that a wide variety of internuncial CNS neurons from dorsal spinal cord and medulla could establish stable neuromuscular connections with limb deplants, as evidenced by the characteristic reflexive and "epileptiform" muscle contractions (Chap. VII-D) observed during months of longitudinal study. "Primary sensory neurons were lacking in all cord and most medulla deplants, and primary motoneurons were either absent or when present, were mostly not involved in the innervation of the limb deplants. Significantly, therefore, intracentral neurons can, under proper conditions, form adequate substitutes morphologically and functionally for peripheral motor and sensory nerve fibers" (Weiss, 1950). On the other hand, in cases where nerves grew from deplants of midbrain, cerebellum, thalamus, forebrain, and spinal or cranial ganglia, to limb deplants characteristic reflexive or epileptiform activity was never observed. Furthermore, the muscles of these limbs showed progressive atrophy and generally degenerated. It will be of interest to determine if mammalian CNS internuncial neurons can show similar degrees of plasticity in regard to innervation and long-term maintenance of muscle. Observations of trophic effects of sympathetic ganglion cells on skeletal muscle *in vitro* and *in situ* (see above) and their formation of functional neuromuscular connections under some conditions in culture (Chap. III-B, IV-A) need to be extended more systematically to other types of CNS neurons, presented to muscle fibers alone as well as in competition with spinal cord motoneurons.

FIG. VIII-7. Long-term maintenance of the integrity of mature mouse skeletal muscle fibers in proximity to fetal mouse sympathetic ganglia after denervation *in vitro* by extirpation of the spinal cord explant. **A:** Low-power view of muscle strip (m) with two sympathetic ganglion chains (sy) and a dorsal root ganglion (drg) in close proximity. Sympathetic ganglia had been added at 3 weeks *in vitro;* spinal cord was removed 3 weeks later (note the clear zone, c); and muscle was cultured for an additional 4.5 weeks (silver impregnation). Scale: 1 mm. **B:** High-power view (at m₁ in **A**) shows that these cord-denervated muscle fibers have retained the characteristic cross-striated appearance in the presence of the sympathetic ganglia (note the delicate neurites intertwining muscle), in contrast to the usual denervation atrophy as in Fig. VIII-6. (The muscle fibers are small in diameter in this peripheral end of muscle strip; larger fibers in the central zone were too densely stained to photograph the whole-mount preparation.) **C:** Similar type of culture showing fully matured muscle denervated after 2 months *in vitro* that remained healthy for an additional 9 weeks in the presence of invading sympathetic nerve fibers (living culture). Note the well-organized cross striations similar to the structure of mature innervated muscle in the controls (e.g., Fig. VIII-5). Scale (**B** and **C**): 50 μm. (From Crain and Peterson, 1974a.)

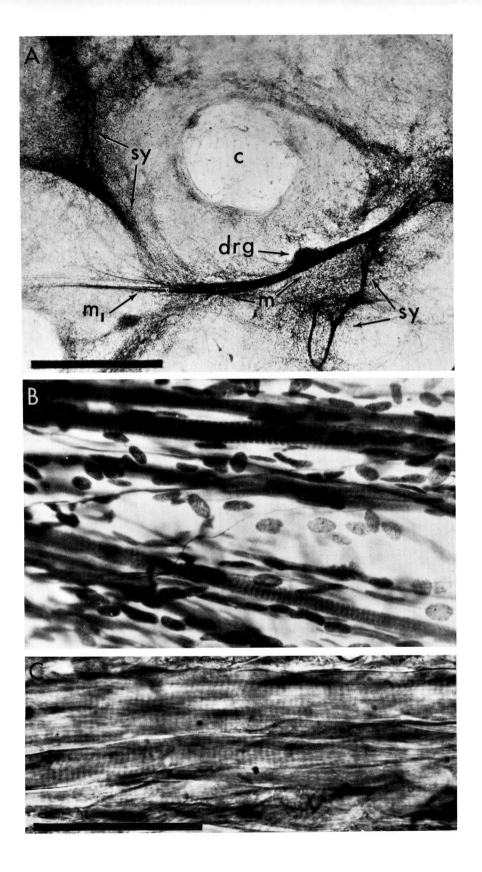

5. Long-term Effects of Direct Electric Currents on Neurons in Culture

In 1964 I prepared a brief review of early studies attempting to detect signs of trophic or tropic effects of electric currents on neurons in culture (Murray, 1965*b*):

Studies of the effects of sustained electric current applied to cultures of growing nerve cells have yielded conflicting reports. Ingvar (1920) claimed that current densities of 0.001–0.002 $\mu A/mm^2$ produced orientation of outgrowing nerve fibers along the "lines of force," but later attempts to confirm this phenomenon (Weiss, 1934) were unsuccessful. More recently, Marsh and Beams (1946) repeated these experiments, using much higher currents. They demonstrated clear-cut deflection of the outgrowing neurites towards the cathode with current densities of 100–500 $\mu A/mm^2$ applied for 3–28 h after explanation (and in some cases for 3–12 h after an initial neuritic outgrowth had developed without current). Perhaps Ingvar had really meant to report current densities of 0.001–0.002 $\mu A/\mu^2$. This would bring his results quite close to those of Marsh and Beams. Although the orienting influences of the plasma clot in which the neural tissue was embedded may have complicated these experiments the data suggest that electric current *may* play a significant role in controlling the growth of nerve fibers. Since the potential gradient produced by the current applied to these cultures was only of the order of 100 mV/mm it "may be considered physiologically attainable" (Marsh and Beams, 1946; see, however, Weiss, 1955). Better controlled experiments along these lines, *in vitro* as well as *in situ,* are clearly needed.

No dramatic developments occurred during the following decade (see also the more recent review by Gottlieb, 1973). Claims have been made (Sisken and Smith, 1975) that application of extremely low currents, ranging up to 0.01 $\mu A/mm^2$ (via platinum wires dipping into the culture fluid), to explants of chick embryo trigeminal ganglia enhanced neuritic outgrowth and neuronal survival, and stimulated growth toward the cathode. The experimental data provided by Sisken and Smith (1975), however, are quite crude, and they do not include adequate controls to eliminate ambiguities and possible artifacts, e.g., chemical effects due to the use of metallic electrodes. "Better controlled experiments . . . are [still] clearly needed"!

C. CNS REGENERATION

Until recently most studies of synaptogenesis *in vitro* were limited to embryonic or neonatal neurons since reliable methods for culture of neural tissues from adult mammals have not yet been available (see Chap. II-A$_1$). An alternative approach was recently developed in conjunction with our muscle denervation experiments (see section B) involving surgical removal of spinal cord tissue from mature, organotypic cord-ganglion-muscle cultures at 1–4 months *in vitro* (Figs. VIII-6;7) and transfer to fresh collagen-coated coverglasses (Peterson and Crain, 1973). Neuritic and meningeal outgrowth developed around all of the transplants in these "subcultures" and peripheral nerve developed, showing characteristic Schwann-type myelination. Where meninges were absent, occasional CNS-type myelination occurred. Silver-impregnation studies of these transplants, and electron microscopy (by E. B. Masurovsky), showed normal neuronal, glial, and synaptic relationships. Complex synaptically mediated bioelectric discharges were recorded after 3–4 weeks of regeneration *in vitro,* comparable to those in cord explants after maturation without transfer (Chap. IV-A). Electrophysiologic analyses of transferred cord paired with fetal cord explants (Crain and Peterson, 1973) demonstrated that the "mature" neurons could form characteristic functional interneuronal connections with newly explanted fetal neurons, and vice versa, via neuritic bridges of 0.5–1 mm as occurs between regular CNS explants (Crain et al., 1968*b*) (Chap. IV-C). Similar tests on pairs of transferred cord explants showed functional connections in only two of six cultures, even though characteristic network discharges could be generated within each explant. Furthermore, in one of the successful pairs where subcultures were made after nearly 3 months *in vitro,* electrophysiologic tests (2 months after pairing) indicated extremely labile connections with long latencies between the discharges initiated in one explant and responses in the other. These experiments demonstrate that "mature" rodent spinal cord neurons can indeed regenerate a second time *in vitro,* and they retain the capacity to establish synaptic relations with other cord neurons. Although functional contacts with fetal nerve cells were more effective, the fact that at least some mature CNS neurons could form new connections with other mature CNS neurons in culture indicates the potentialities of this model system for further studies of the role of trophic factors in CNS regeneration in the adult mammal (Guth and Windle, 1970; Guth, 1974).[2]

Presentation of adult skeletal muscle strips near subcultured cord explants showed, moreover, that the new peripheral axons which grow out from mature cord neurons can also establish characteristic functional neuromuscular junctions after providing the initial stimulus to early phases of muscle regeneration, as occurs with fetal cord neurons (see section B$_2$; see also Chap. IV-A).

Our tissue culture models led me to suggest, at a conference on "The Enigma of Central Nervous Regeneration", that "since fetal rodent spinal

---

[2] An alternative tissue culture model for studies of CNS regeneration has recently been developed by positioning fresh explants of fetal mouse spinal cord and DRGs near mature explants of spinal cord or medulla. This technique permits analyses of the degree to which CNS neurons may retain their receptivity as targets for synaptic connections even after long periods of deafferentation. Preliminary experiments demonstrate that fetal mouse DRG neurons can make characteristic functional synaptic connections with sensory target regions in deafferented spinal cord and medulla explants even when the latter have been initially isolated for periods up to 3 weeks in culture (Crain and Peterson, 1976). Since the sensory-evoked network discharges, which develop in the target regions after DRG innervation, may include potentials generated by CNS interneuronal axons synapsing on DRG terminals (Chap. IV-B,C), our staggered-explant experiments suggest that neurons in the deafferented cord and medulla tissues may also retain the capacity to sprout new collaterals after the long-delayed arrival of DRG neurites (e.g., Fig. IV-26).

cord neurons produce such powerful growth-stimulating trophic effects on dormant adult human skeletal muscle fibers in culture, perhaps similar trophic interactions can be produced by apposition of fetal CNS tissues to explants of adult human brain and spinal cord tissues. This type of culture has not been tried heretofore, and it may prove to be a valuable new approach to the problem of growth stimulation of adult CNS neurons. Crain also proposed that fetal rodent spinal cord cross sections be *transplanted* into gaps prepared in adult rodent spinal cord *in situ* to determine whether *fetal* CNS tissue might provide a more plastic array of cells which could facilitate regeneration and reorganization of damaged adult CNS" (Guth and Windle, 1970). In fact, attempts have been made recently to implant strips of 15-day cultured fetal rat spinal cord (10–15 mm in length) so as to bridge a transected region in adult rat spinal cord (Olson and Bunge, 1974; see also Bunge and Wood, 1973).[3] Serious tissue reactions to the trauma of cord transection appeared to prevent survival of the fetal cord implant, and no functional recovery occurred in the host animal during these preliminary trials. Tests have apparently not yet been carried out with freshly isolated fetal spinal cord transplanted directly into the transected region of adult spinal cord (similar to fetal rat cerebellar and cerebral transplants into neo-natal rat cerebellum—Das and Altman, 1972; Das, 1975). In view of our experiments demonstrating that neurons in fetal spinal cord explants can make functional synaptic connections with *in vitro*-matured cord explants (see above), further attempts to apply this tissue culture model to regeneration in the adult CNS *in situ* may still be fruitful (see also recent reviews by Sidman and Wessells, 1975; Varon, 1975).

---

[3] See also Aihara, 1970; Kao et al., 1970; Kao, 1974.

IX

Overview

A. LIMITATIONS OF CNS CULTURE MODELS

Tissue culture techniques are still not sufficiently standardized, especially with regard to development of complex CNS networks with characteristic synaptic activities, and criteria based on microscopic observations of the living cultures are not yet adequate to estimate the probable functional integrity of these interneuronal relationships. Potent "biochemical lesions" may occur which involve no detectable morphologic alterations, even at the electron microscopic level. This is especially important to keep in mind in evaluating the functional significance of biochemical and cytologic properties of cultured CNS tissues studied without correlative bioelectric tests on the same specimens. There are often serious variations between CNS cultures prepared under "standard" conditions even in a well-established laboratory, so that inferences about the functional integrity of *particular* explants based on bioelectric studies of this *type* of culture in another laboratory may be unwarranted extrapolations. No morphologic deficits have been detected, for example, during weeks of exposure of fetal cerebral cortex and spinal cord explants to Xylocaine at concentrations which block (reversibly) generation of all nerve impulses and characteristic synaptically mediated network discharges (Crain et al., 1968a; Model et al., 1971) (Chap. VIII-A). Selective, yet serious, molecular or ultrastructural deficits could easily occur in groups of central nervous system (CNS) explants, and elaborate biochemical analyses of such tissues would be of limited value without functional "validation." Electrophysiologic analyses currently provide the only clear-cut means of determining if a neural assembly is operating normally in a given set of cultures — morphologic or chemical tests demonstrate only that essential, but not necessarily *sufficient,* components are present. On the other hand, significant cytologic or molecular deficits may occur in cultured CNS tissues which can still generate synaptic network activities. This dichotomy is of course useful since it helps to define the cytologic and molecular components essential for specific types of physiologic functions of the nervous system. Interest can then be focused on the possible functional significance of the apparently "unessential" cytologic or molecular features. Characteristic cholinergic neuromuscular transmission occurs, for example, in cultures of dissociated neurons and skeletal muscle cells after formation of relatively simple synaptic junctions (Fischbach, 1974). Further analyses are therefore needed to determine the functional significance of the elaborate primary and secondary infoldings that form at the motor endplates in more organized cultures of spinal cord and muscle explants (Chap. IV-A; Figs. IV-11;12). Similar questions can be raised regarding the role of the terminal Schwann cells at these endplates (Fig. IV-10), and the cholinesterase localizations (Fig. VIII-5B), which are also apparently absent at the junctions between dissociated nerve and muscle cells. Limits are also set to the functional role of myelin sheaths in CNS tissues in view of our observations that organized synaptic network activities still develop and are maintained for months in spinal cord explants where myelin formation is completely blocked during chronic exposure to low concentrations (1–3%) of serum from animals with experimental allergic encephalomyelitis (Chap. VI-F; see also discussions by Crain, Bornstein, and Lehrer in Purpura and Reaser, 1974).

Even under optimal culture conditions CNS explants generally develop some structural and functional deficits or abnormalities relative to their *in situ* counterparts. Separation of these small fragments of CNS tissue from their normal connections with other neurons undoubtedly leads to alterations, at least in neuronal excitability (Crain, 1969) and often in synaptic network properties (e.g., Chap. IV-C,D). Moreover, isolation in culture may selectively damage or eliminate those types of neurons in a CNS explant that are more sensitive to mechanical trauma or to chemical deficiencies in the nutrient medium. Furthermore, even if synapses do form under a particular set of conditions *in vitro,* the resulting network may be significantly unbalanced in regard to normal excitatory and inhibitory components, e.g., abnormal shifts toward inhibitory synaptic dominance may develop in older CNS explants (Chaps. VI-A, VII-D) (Crain, 1969). Altered chemosensitivity of some types of neuronal membranes may also be produced by chronic exposure during maturation to certain metabolites which may be present at relatively high (and currently uncontrolled) concentrations in routine serum-based tissue culture media, e.g., glycine and other amino acids involved in synaptic mediation (Chaps. V-B, VI-A). (Diffusion barriers comparable to the blood-brain barrier are probably not generally present between our CNS explants and the overlying culture media.) It is of interest in this regard that tolerance to *d*-tubocurarine may develop during chronic exposure of *in vitro*-coupled cord-muscle explants to this agent throughout the period when neuromuscular junctions are forming in culture (Chap. VIII-B).

Furthermore, current use of Maximow depression-slide culture chambers (Chap. II-A) involves marked alterations in the biochemical milieu during the 3- to 4-day period between feedings. Anabolites may dwindle and catabolites accumulate (including shifts to acidic pH as carbon dioxide levels increase). Although these environmental fluctuations have been compatible with development and maintenance of "normal" CNS morphology in culture, they may be partly responsible for some of the observed variability in bioelectric excitability properties and pharmacologic sensivity. Relatively minor technologic improvements in culture chamber design will probably permit far more rigid regulation of the culture medium (Chap. II-A1). In view of all the variables in the physicochemical environment of CNS cultures, it is indeed fortunate that fetal CNS explants develop the remarkable degree of organotypic synaptic network functions described above, including characteristic sensitivity to a substantial number of specific neuropharmacologic and metabolic agents.

B. POTENTIALITIES

Although these technical problems in standardizing cultures of neural explants are even more difficult in the case of dissociated cells, substantial numbers of fetal CNS neurons do indeed survive injury related to cell separation procedures, regenerate their torn processes, and develop the capacity to form functional synaptic relationships (Chap. V). In low-density dissociated cultures, the entire surface of neuron perikarya and their processes are exquisitely exposed in all their glory for critical microelectrode analyses (Chap. V-B,C). Methods for identification of cell types have not, however, been adequately developed (Ransom and Nelson, 1975) (see also Chap. II-A2). In cultures of dissociated spinal cord cells, for example, it has not yet been possible to determine if any of the large neurons are really ventral-horn motoneurons (Chap. V-B). The fact that dissociated cord cells can innervate skeletal muscle fibers is not sufficient evidence to characterize these neurons since even sympathetic ganglion cells have been shown to form cholinergic synaptic junctions with skeletal muscle fibers in culture (Nurse and O'Lague, 1975) (Chap. V-A). Improved techniques will undoubtedly soon be developed to permit isolation in culture of identified neurons obtained by careful dissection of localized regions of CNS tissue prior to dissociation or by refined cell-fractionation procedures (Chap. II-A2; Fischbach, 1976). On the other hand, although most neurons within CNS explants are far less visible and accessible (e.g. Fig. IV-9B), prior knowledge of the *regional* localization of specific types of neurons within accurately dissected tissue slabs can often provide information to guide valuable electrophysiologic analyses of complex neuronal networks (Chap. IV-B,C; Crain and Peterson, 1974b, 1975a, 1976).

Patterned migration *in vitro* of embryonic DRG perikarya attached to a spinal cord explant — forming organized dorsal roots — and outgrowth of orderly fascicles of ventral root fibers onto a homogeneous collagen substrate in the absence of target tissues (Chap. IV-A,B) may be interpreted as evidence that neurons in organotypic cultures can grow complex 3-dimensional neuritic arborizations with patterns that are determined by genetic programs which develop in relation to the position of the neuron perikaryon in "body-space."[1] The concept of body-space in a culture may be useful in cases of organotypic CNS explants which include sufficient components to provide a coded representation of the original body axes in its geometrical array of neurons and glial cells. Note, for example, the clearcut designation of dorsal and ventral regions in the spinal cord and medulla explants in Figs. IV-25, 26, and the reasonable attempts, in these preliminary model experiments, to specify ipsilateral and contralateral arrays of "dorsal column" nerve fascicles bridging the gap between the cord and medulla explants in Fig. IV-26. The third—rostro-caudal—axis in these particular cultures is specified by prior dissection of selected cross-sectional slabs, e.g., lumbar cord and medulla at the level of the cuneate nucleus. Analyses of these complex types of tissue cultures may provide clues to some of the fundamental aspects of spatial relationships between arrays of CNS neurons that are invariant to drastic environmental transformation.

Organized neural architectonics may be based on existence of a variety of complex, yet stereotyped, intracellular neuronal systems, each consisting of a perikaryon with all of its patterned neuritic arborizations specified in 3 dimensions (analogous to the highly patterned arborizations with characteristic contours as occur in development of trees). Perhaps there are dynamic feedback systems which provide information to the perikaryon regarding the growth and terminal arborization of *all* of the branches of the neuron, so that local disturbances in any particular terminal lead to regulatory (homeostatic) processes in the perikaryon which tend to restore programmed patterns of neuritic arborizations which may be *relatively* independent of local target cues (but critically modulatable by these cues)[1]. *Sets* of neurons in suitably prepared CNS explants *may* retain in culture complex properties which determine, not only the formation of connections between specific types of neurons (i.e., phenotypic specificity), but also the development of an organized spatial framework in which the neurons make synaptic connections at particular positions within the cell population, leading to functional patterns related to the 3-dimensional body axes, i.e., locus specificity (Hunt and Jacobson, 1973; see also Sperry, 1965). If this high degree of order can occur in culture it would permit experimental analyses of some of the basic principles which regulate development of the intricate spatial organization and precise regional localizations in the central nervous system. Our recent studies of patterned neuritic

---

[1] This concept of body-space in relation to nerve territorial fields was recently proposed by Diamond et al. (1976) following systematic studies of patterns of nerve sprouting after local colchicine exposure and surgical manipulation of individual peripheral nerves in the salamander (see also Aguilar et al., 1973). The authors emphasize that trophic factors brought to the periphery by neuronal transport may play an important role in determining and regulating the territory occupied by each nerve fiber in body-space, operating together with the well-established local influences provided by the target tissue (e.g., Ramón y Cajal, 1960; see reviews in Hughes, 1968; Jacobson, 1970; Hunt and Jacobson, 1973).

growth of isolated dorsal root ganglia in relation to target neurons in explants of spinal cord and medulla (Chap. IV-B,C2) (Crain and Peterson, 1975a,b, 1976, Peterson and Crain, 1975) constitute a step in this direction.[2]

It should be emphasized that preparation of organotypic CNS explants requires considerable skill and experience both in dissecting and carefully manipulating the fragile neural tissues of the embryonic CNS as well as in the techniques of long-term maintenance. The remarkable structural and functional integrity of many of the CNS explants described above demonstrate the feasibility of these methods, but the importance of thorough training (preferably by apprenticeship) should be considered by investigators seriously interested in utilizing these types of tissue culture preparations.

Tissue culture models of brain functions have undergone vigorous development during the past decade as a result of the systematic extension of earlier morphologic studies with electrophysiologic and pharmacologic analyses. From esoteric exercises limited to a few isolated laboratories prior to 1960, neural tissue culture techniques are now becoming recognized as a reproducible method for supplementing and extending many neurobiologic studies *in situ*. The power of CNS culture models rests on the accessibility of mammalian neurons for direct experimental manipulation coupled with the capacity of these cells to form organotypic synaptic networks even after dramatic geometric simplification under rigidly controlled physiochemical conditions *in vitro*. Coordinated physiologic, cytologic, and biochemical studies of CNS culture models will undoubtedly lead to increasingly valuable insights into cellular mechanisms underlying significant

---

[2] Bunge (1976) has expressed the view that ". . . in the period from 1955 to 1968 the art of nerve tissue culture entered briefly into what might be termed a baroque interval. The zealots of this period proclaimed the beauty of their preparations; the detractors questioned their scientific usefulness. That a baroque era should follow a classical period is perhaps not surprising, just as it is not surprising that the work of the chief baroque artisans (particularly Bornstein, Hild, Murray, Peterson, and Pomerat) was inevitably to spur a younger generation to reverse the trend and to attempt to take apart the whole into its component cells . . . [thereby leading to] the present 'cubist' era in nerve tissue culture." From this point of view, Bunge (1976) refers to our recent study of organized arrays of DRG, spinal cord and medulla explants (Crain and Peterson, 1975a) as "a masterpiece of baroque culture art"! Although his subsequent comments indicate recognition of the significance of these studies of regionally specific sensory synaptic network functions *in vitro*, the term "baroque" is inappropriate since it could be misconstrued to imply that use of these complex CNS explants may be so needlessly ornate as to impede analysis of the underlying biological principles. The neurophysiologic and correlative studies of CNS explants described in Chaps. IV, VI–VIII provide, on the contrary, ample evidence supporting the usefulness of a wide variety of tissue culture models incorporating sufficient complexity to facilitate significant analyses at each level of neural organization. Furthermore, the true beauty of these CNS cultures derives not merely from an esthetic appreciation of the elegantly patterned structural contours which develop *in vitro* — as described in Chaps. IV and VIII (see also the exquisite photomicrographs of explants of the organ of Corti by Sobkowicz et al., 1975) — but more significantly from recognition that the formation of these organotypic structural arrays in isolation from the organism provides an exciting opportunity to manipulate complex *systems* of mammalian CNS neurons under unusually flexible experimental conditions.

aspects of normal and abnormal functions of the nervous system, especially during critical stages of development, and perhaps even in relation to memory and learning.

The tissue culture "window" to the brain has been opened for all who wish to observe more directly parts of that "enchanted loom," so elegantly depicted by Sherrington (1951), "where millions of flashing shuttles weave a dissolving pattern, always a meaningful pattern though never an abiding one; a shifting harmony of subpatterns." Perhaps some of the "subpatterns" still generated by bits of CNS tissues *in vitro* may provide further clues to understanding this wondrous "shifting harmony" of the cerebral fugues.

References

Aguilar, C. E., Bisby, M. A., Cooper, E., and Diamond, J. (1973): Evidence that axoplasmic transport of trophic factors is involved in the regulation of peripheral nerve fields in salamanders. *J. Physiol. (Lond.)*, 234:449–464.

Aihara, H. (1970): Autotransplantation of the cultured cerebellar cortex for spinal cord reconstruction. *Brain Nerve (Tokyo)*, 22:769–784.

Aladjalova, N. A. (1964): *Slow Electrical Processes in the Brain*. Elsevier, Amsterdam.

Altman, J. (1967): Postnatal growth and differentiation of the mammalian brain with implications for a morphological theory of memory. In: *The Neurosciences: A Study Program*, edited by G. C. Quarton, T. Melnechuk, and F. O. Schmitt, pp. 723–743. Rockefeller University Press, New York.

Altman, J. (1970): Postnatal neurogenesis and the problem of neural plasticity. In: *Developmental Neurobiology*, edited by W. A. Himwich, pp. 197–237. Charles C Thomas, Springfield, Ill.

Altman, J., and Das, G. D. (1965): Post-natal origin of microneurones in the rat brain. *Nature (Lond.)*, 207:953–956.

Andersen, P., and Andersson, S. A. (1968): *Physiological Basis of the Alpha Rhythm*. Appleton-Century-Crofts, New York.

Andersen, P., and Eccles, J. C. (1962): Inhibitory phasing of neuronal discharge. *Nature (Lond.)*, 196:645–647.

Andersen, P., Eccles, J. C., and Løyning, Y. (1963): Recurrent inhibition in the hippocampus with identification of the inhibitory cell and its synapses. *Nature (Lond.)*, 198:540–542.

Andersen, P., Eccles, J. C., Schmidt, R. F., and Yokota, T. (1964): Slow potential waves produced in the cuneate nucleus by cutaneous volleys and by cortical stimulation. *J. Neurophysiol.*, 27:78–91.

Andres, K. H. (1961): Untersuchungen Uber den Feinbau von Spinalganglion. *Z. Zellforsch.*, 55:1–48.

Anokhin, P. K. (1964): Systemogenesis as a general regulator of brain development. In: *The Developing Brain*, edited by W. A. Himwich and H. E. Himwich, pp. 54–86. American Elsevier, New York.

Araki, T., and Otani, T. (1955): Responses of single motoneurones to direct stimulation in toad's spinal cord. *J. Neurophysiol.*, 18:472–485.

Armstrong-James, M. A., and Williams, T. D. (1963): Post-natal development of the direct cortical response in the rat. *J. Physiol. (Lond.)*, 168:19–20.

Armstrong-James, M. A., and Williams, T. D. (1964): Differences in the direct cortical-response to unifocal stimuli during the post-natal development of the rat cerebral cortex. *J. Physiol. (Lond.)*, 170:15P–16P.

Askanas, V. (1972): Histochemistry of cultured aneural chick muscle. Morphological maturation without differentiation of fiber types. *Exp. Neurol.*, 37:218–230.

Auerbach, A. A., and Purpura, D. P. (1972): Effects of dibutyryl cyclic AMP at giant fiber synapses in the hatchetfish. *Fed. Proc.*, 31:403.

Ayala, G. F., Dichter, M., Gumnit, R. J., Matsumoto, H., and Spencer, W. A. (1973): Genesis of epileptic interictal spikes: New knowledge of cortical feedback systems suggest a neurophysiological explanation of brief paroxysms. *Brain Res.*, 52:1–17.

Baer, S. C., and Crain, S. M. (1971): Magnetically coupled micromanipulator for use within a sealed chamber. *J. Appl. Physiol.*, 31:926–929.

Baker, P. F., Hodgkin, A. L., and Ridgway, E. B. (1971): Depolarization and calcium entry in squid giant axon. *J. Physiol. (Lond.)*, 218:709–755.

Barber, R. F., and Saito, K. (1975): Light microscopic visualization of GAD and GABA-T in immunocytochemical preparations of rodent CNS. In: *GABA in Nervous System Function*, edited by E. Roberts, T. N. Chase, and D. B. Tower, pp. 113–132. Raven Press, New York.

Barker, J. L., and Nicoll, R. A. (1973): The pharmacology and ionic dependency of amino acid responses in the frog spinal cord. *J. Physiol. (Lond.)*, 228:259–278.

Barker, J. L., Crayton, J. A., and Nicoll, R. A. (1971): Noradrenaline and acetylcholine responses of supra-optic neurosecretory cells. *J. Physiol. (Lond.),* 218:19–32.

Barkley, D. S., Rakie, L. L., Chaffee, J. K., and Wong, D. L. (1973): Cell separation by velocity sedimentation of postnatal mouse cerebellum. *J. Cell Physiol.,* 81:271–280.

Barlow, J. S. (1960): Rhythmic activity induced by photic stimulation in relation to intrinsic alpha activity of the brain in man. *Electroencephalogr. J.,* 12:317–325.

Beer, B., Chasin, M., Clody, D. E., Vogel, J. R., and Horovitz, Z. P. (1972): Cyclic adenosine monophosphate phosphodiesterase in brain: Effect on anxiety. *Science,* 176:428–430.

Bekoff, A., Stein, P. S., and Hamburger, V. (1975): Coordinated motor output in the hindlimb of the 7-day chick embryo. *Proc. Natl. Acad. Sci. U.S.A.,* 72:1245–1248.

Bell, N. H., Avery, S., Sinha, T., Clark, C. M., Allen, D. O., and Johnston, C. (1972): Effects of dibutyryl cyclic adenosine 3′,5′-monophosphate and parathyroid extract on calcium and phosphorus metabolism in hypoparathyroidism and pseudohypoparathyroidism. *J. Clin. Invest.,* 51:816–823.

Benda, P., DeVitry, F., Picart, R., and Tixier-Vidal, A. (1975): Dissociated cell cultures from fetal mouse hypothalamus: Patterns of organization and ultrastructural features. *Exp. Brain Res.,* 23:29–48.

Benitez, H. H., Masurovsky, E. B., and Murray, M. R. (1974): Interneurons of the sympathetic ganglia, in organotypic culture: A suggestion as to their function, based on three types of study. *J. Neurocytol.,* 3:363–384.

Benitez, H. H., Murray, M. R., and Coté, L. J. (1973): Responses of sympathetic chain-ganglia isolated in organotypic culture to agents affecting adrenergic neurons. *Exp. Neurol.,* 39:424–448.

Benoist, J. M., Besson, J. M., and Boissier, J. R. (1974): Modifications of presynaptic inhibition of various origins by local application of convulsant drugs on cat's spinal cord. *Brain Res.,* 71:172–177.

Bhargava, V. K., and Meldrum, B. S. (1969): The strychnine-like action of curare and related compounds on the somatosensory evoked response of the rat cortex. *Br. J. Pharmacol.,* 37:112–122.

Bhargava, V. K., and Meldrum, B. S. (1971): Blockade by eserine of the cerebral cortical effects of strychnine and curare. *Nature [New Biol.],* 230:152.

Biales, B., Dichter, M., and Tischler, A. (1975): Electrical excitability of cultured adrenal medulla. In: *Society of Neuroscience, 5th Annual Meeting, New York,* p. 460.

Birch, H. G. (1971): Levels, categories and methodological assumptions in the study of behavioral development. In: *Biopsychology of Development,* edited by E. Tobach, R. Aronson, and E. Shaw, pp. 503–513. Academic Press, New York.

Bird, M. M., and James, D. W. (1973): The development of synapses in vitro between previously dissociated chick spinal cord neurons. *Z. Zellforsch.,* 140:203–226.

Bird, M. M., and James, D. W. (1975): The culture of previously dissociated embryonic chick spinal cord cells on feeder layers of liver and kidney, and the development of paraformaldehyde induced fluorescence upon the former. *J. Neurocytol.,* 4:633–645.

Birks, R. I. (1966): The fine structure of motor nerve endings at frog myoneural junction. *Ann. N.Y. Acad. Sci.,* 135:8–19.

Bishop, E. J. (1950): The strychnine spike as a physiological indicator of cortical maturity in the postnatal rabbit. *Electroencephalogr. Clin. Neurophysiol.,* 2:309–315.

Bjerre, B., Björklund, A., and Stenevi, U. (1973): Stimulation of growth of new axonal sprouts from lesioned monoamine neurones in adult rat brain by nerve growth factor. *Brain Res.,* 60:161–176.

Björklund, A., and Stenevi, U. (1971): Growth of central catecholamine neurones into smooth muscle grafts in the rat mesencephalon. *Brain Res.,* 31:1–20.

Björklund, A., Katzman, R., Stenevi, U., and West, K. A. (1971): Development and growth of axonal sprouts from noradrenaline and 5-hydroxytryptamine neurones in the rat spinal cord. *Brain Res.,* 31:21–34.

Blaustein, M. P., and Goldman, D. E. (1966): Action of anionic and cationic nerve-blocking agents: Experiment and interpretation. *Science,* 153:429–432.

Bodian, D., Melby, E. C., and Taylor, N. (1968): Development of fine structure of spinal cord in monkey fetuses. II. Pre-reflex period to period of long intersegmental reflexes. *J. Comp. Neurol.,* 133:113–166.

Bonner, J. (1966): Molecular biological approaches to the study of memory. In: *Macro-molecules and Behavior,* edited by J. Gaito, pp. 158–164. Appleton-Century-Crofts, New York.

Bornstein, M. B. (1958): Reconstituted rat-tail collagen used as substrate for tissue culture on coverslips in Maximow slides and roller tubes. *Lab. Invest.,* 7:134–140.

Bornstein, M. B. (1963): Morphological development of cultured mouse cerebral neocortex. *Trans. Am. Neurol. Assoc.,* 88:22–24.

Bornstein, M. B. (1964): Morphological development of neonatal mouse cerebral cortex in tissue culture. In: *Neurological and Electroencephalographic Correlative Studies in Infancy,* edited by P. Kellaway and I. Petersén, pp. 1–11. Grune & Stratton, New York.

Bornstein, M. B. (1973*a*): Organotypic mammalian central and peripheral nerve tissue. In: *Tissue Culture Methods and Applications,* edited by P. F. Kruse and M. K. Patterson, pp. 86–92. Academic Press, New York.

Bornstein, M. B. (1973*b*): The immunopathology of demyelinative disorders examined in organotypic cultures of mammalian central nerve tissues. In: *Progress in Neuropathology,* Vol. 2, edited by H. M. Zimmerman, pp. 69–90. Grune & Stratton, New York.

Bornstein, M. B. (1973*c*): Patterns of development and response of cultured mammalian nerve tissue. In: *Metabolic Compartmentation in the Brain,* edited by R. Balázs and J. E. Cremer, pp. 267–283. Macmillan, London.

Bornstein, M. B., and Breitbart, L. M. (1964): Anatomical studies of mouse embryo spinal cord-skeletal muscle in long-term tissue culture. *Anat. Rec.,* 148:362.

Bornstein, M. B., and Crain, S. M. (1965): Functional studies of cultured mammalian CNS tissues as related to "demyelinative disorders." *Science,* 148:1242–1244.

Bornstein, M. B., and Crain, S. M. (1971): Lack of correlation between changes in bioelectric functions and myelin in cultured CNS tissues chronically exposed to sera from animals with EAE. *J. Neuropathol. Exp. Neurol.,* 30:129P.

Bornstein, M. B., and Model, P. G. (1971): Development of neurons and synapses in cultures of dissociated spinal cord, brain stem and cerebrum of the embryo mouse. In: *American Society of Cell Biology,* 11th Annual Meeting, New Orleans, p. 35.

Bornstein, M. B., and Model, P. G. (1972): Development of synapses and myelin in cultures of dissociated embryonic mouse spinal cord medulla and cerebrum. *Brain Res.,* 37:287–293.

Bornstein, M. B., and Murray, M. R. (1958): Serial observations on patterns of growth, myelin formation, maintenance and degeneration in cultures of newborn rat and kitten cerebellum. *J. Biophys. Biochem. Cytol.,* 4:499–504.

Bornstein, M. B., Iwanami, H., Lehrer, G. M., and Breitbart, L. (1968): Observations on the appearance of neuromuscular relationships in cultured mouse tissues. *Z. Zellforsch.,* 92:197–206.

Bradley, K., Easton, D. M., and Eccles, J. C. (1953): An investigation of primary or direct inhibition. *J. Physiol. (Lond.),* 122:474–488.

Bray, D. (1970): Surface movements during the growth of single explanted neurons. *Proc. Natl. Acad. Sci. U.S.A.,* 65:906–910.

Brazier, M. A. (1960): Long-persisting electrical traces in the brain of man and their possible relationship to higher nervous activity. *Electroencephalogr. J., (Suppl.),* 13:347–359.

Brazier, M. A. (1963): The problem of periodicity in the electroencephalogram: Studies in the cat. *Electroencephalogr. J.,* 15:287–298.

Breckenridge, B. McL. (1970): Cyclic AMP and drug action. *Ann. Rev. Pharmacol.,* 10:19–34.

Breckenridge, B. McL., and Bray, J. J. (1970): Cyclic AMP and nerve function. In: *Role of Cyclic AMP in Cell Function,* edited by P. Greengard and E. Costa, pp. 325–333. Raven Press, New York.

Bullock, T. H. (1967): Simple systems for the study of learning mechanisms. VI. Related studies on tissue cultures. In: *Neurosciences Research Symposium Summaries,* Vol. 2, edited by F. O. Schmitt, T. Melnechuk, G. C. Quarton, and G. Adelman, pp. 253–257. M.I.T. Press, Cambridge, Mass.

Bunge, M. B., Bunge, R. P., and Peterson, E. R. (1967*a*): The onset of synapse formation in spinal cord culture as studied by electron microscopy. *Brain Res.,* 6:728–749.

Bunge, M. B., Bunge, R. P., Peterson, E. R., and Murray, M. R. (1967*b*): A light and electron microscope study of long-term organized cultures of rat dorsal root ganglia. *J. Cell Biol.,* 32:439–466.

Bunge, R. P. (1976): Changing uses of nerve tissue culture 1950-1975. In: *The Nervous System, Vol. 1: Basic Neurosciences,* edited by R. O. Brady, pp. 31–42. Raven Press, New York.

Bunge, R. P., and Wood, P. (1973): Studies on the transplantation of spinal cord tissue in the rat. I. The development of a culture system for hemisections of embryonic spinal cord. *Brain Res.,* 57:261–276.

Bunge, R. P., Bunge, M. B., and Peterson, E. R. (1965): An electron microscope study of cultured rat spinal cord. *J. Cell Biol.,* 24:163–191.

Bunge, R. P., Rees, R., Wood, P., Burton, H., and Ko, C.-P. (1974): Anatomical and physiological observations on synapses formed on isolated autonomic neurons in tissue culture. *Brain Res.,* 66:401–412.

Burn, J. H., and Rand, M. J. (1965): Acetylcholine in adrenergic transmission. *Ann. Rev. Pharmacol.,* 5:163–182.

Burns, B. D. (1958): *The Mammalian Cerebral Cortex.* Edward Arnold, London.

Burns, B. D. (1968): *The Uncertain Nervous System.* Edward Arnold, London.

Burrows, M. (1975): Integration by motoneurones in the insect cerebral nervous system. In: *'Simple' Nervous Systems,* edited by P. N. R. Usherwood and D. R. Newth, pp. 345–379. Edward Arnold, London.

Burton, H., and Bunge, R. P. (1975): A comparison of the uptake and release of [^{3}H] norepinephrine in rat autonomic and sensory ganglia in tissue culture. *Brain Res.,* 97:157–162.

Burton, H., Ko, C.-P., and Bunge, R. P. (1975): Cholinergic synapses between sympathetic neurons in tissue culture. In: *Society of Neuroscience, 5th Annual Meeting, New York,* p. 816.

Butcher, R. W., and Sutherland, E. W. (1962): Adenosine 3',5'-phosphate in biological materials. I. Purification and properties of cyclic 3',5'-nucleotide phosphodiesterase and use of this enzyme to characterize adenosine 3',5'-phosphate in human urine. *J. Biol. Chem.,* 237:1244–1250.

Caldwell, P. C., and Downing, A. C. (1955): The preparation of capillary microelectrodes. *J. Physiol. (Lond.),* 128:31.

Caley, D. W., and Maxwell, D. S. (1971): Ultrastructure of developing cerebral cortex in the rat. In: *Brain Development and Behavior,* edited by M. B. Sterman, D. J. McGinty, and A. M. Adinolfi, pp. 89–107. Academic Press, New York.

Calvet, M. C. (1974): Patterns of spontaneous electrical activity in tissue cultures of mammalian cerebral cortex vs. cerebellum. *Brain Res.,* 69:281–295.

Calvet, M. C., Drian, M. J., and Privat, A. (1974): Spontaneous electrical patterns in cultured Purkinje cells grown with an antimitotic agent. *Brain Res.,* 79:285–290.

Calvet, M. C., and Lepault, A. M. (1975): In vitro Purkinje cell electrical behavior related to tissular environment. *Exp. Brain Res.,* 23:249–258.

Capps-Covey, P., and McIlwain, D. L. (1975): Bulk isolation of large ventral spinal neurons. *J. Neurochem.,* 25:517–521.

Carlson, B. M. (1972): *The Regeneration of Minced Muscles.* Karger, Basel.

Carmichael, L. (1926): The development of behavior in vertebrates experimentally removed from the influence of external stimulation. *Psychol. Rev.,* 33:51–58.

Carpenter, F. G., and Bergland, R. M. (1957): Excitation and conduction in immature nerve fibers of the developing chick. *Am. J. Physiol.,* 190:371–376.

Ceccarelli, B., Hurlbut, W. P., and Mauro, A. (1972): Depletion of vesicles from frog neuromuscular junctions by prolonged tetanic stimulation. *J. Cell Biol.,* 54:30–38.

Ceccarelli, B., Hurlbut, W. P., and Mauro, A. (1973): Turnover of transmitter and synaptic vesicles at the frog neuromuscular junction. *J. Cell Biol.,* 57:499–524.

Cechner, R. L., Fleming, D. G., and Geller, H. M. (1970): Neurons in vitro: a tool for basic and applied research in neural electrodynamics. In: *Biomedical Engineering Systems,* edited by M. Clynes and J. H. Milsum, pp. 595–653. McGraw-Hill, New York.

Cerf, J. A., and Carels, G. (1966): Multiple sclerosis: Serum factor producing reversible alterations in bioelectric responses. *Science,* 152:1066–1068.

Chalazonitis, A., Greene, L. A., and Nirenberg, M. (1974): Electrophysiological characteristics of chick embryo sympathetic neurons in dissociated cell culture. *Brain Res.,* 68:235–252.

Chambers, R., and Kopac, M. J. (1950): Micrurgical technique for the study of cellular phenomena. In: *McClung's Handbook of Microscopical Technique,* edited by R. M. Jones, pp. 492–543. Hoeber, New York.

Chamley, J. H., and Campbell, G. R. (1975): Trophic influences of sympathetic nerves and cyclic AMP on differentiation and proliferation of isolated smooth muscle cells in culture. *Cell Tiss. Res.,* 161:497–510.

Chamley, J. H., Campbell, G. R., and Burnstock, G. (1973): An analysis of the interactions between sympathetic nerve fibers and smooth muscle cells in tissue culture. *Dev. Biol.,* 33:344–361.

Chamley, J. H., Campbell, G. R., and Burnstock, G. (1974): Dedifferentiation, redifferentiation and bundle formation of smooth muscle cells in tissue culture: The influence of cell number and nerve fibers. *J. Embryol. Exp. Morphol.,* 32:297–323.

Chamley, J. H., Mark, G. E., Campbell, G. R., and Burnstock, G. (1972): Sympathetic ganglia in culture. I. Neurons. *Z. Zellforsch.,* 135:287–314.

Chang, H.-T. (1953): Similarity in action between curare and strychnine on cortical neurons. *J. Neurophysiol.,* 16:221–233.

Chasin, M., Harris, D. N., Phillips, M. B., and Hess, S. M. (1972): 1-Ethyl-4-(isopropyli-denehydrazino)-1 H-pyrazolo (3,4,-β)-pyridine-5-carboxylic acid, ethyl ester, hydrochloride (SQ 20009)—a potent new inhibitor of cyclic 3′,5′-nucleotide phosphodiesterases. *Biochem. Pharmacol.,* 21:2443–2450.

Chen, J. S., and Levi-Montalcini, R. (1969): Axonal outgrowth and cell migration in vitro from nervous system of cockroach embryos. *Science,* 166:631–632.

Cherkin, A. (1966): Toward a quantitative view of the engram. *Proc. Natl. Acad. Sci. U.S.A.,* 55:88–91.

Cheung, W. Y. (1970): Cyclic nucleotide phosphodiesterase. In: *Role of Cyclic AMP in Cell Function,* edited by P. Greengard and E. Costa, pp. 51–65. Raven Press, New York.

Cheung, W. Y., and Salganicoff, L. (1967): Cyclic 3′,5′-nucleotide phosphodiesterase: Localization and latent activity in rat brain. *Nature (Lond.),* 214:90–91.

Chowdhury, T. K. (1969): Techniques of intracellular microinjection. In: *Glass Microelectrodes,* edited by M. Lavellée, O. F. Schanne, and N. C. Hébert, pp. 404–423. Wiley, New York.

Christ, D. D., and Nishi, S. (1971): Site of adrenaline blockade in the superior cervical ganglion of the rabbit. *J. Physiol. (Lond.),* 213:107–117.

Coghill, G. E. (1929): *Anatomy and the Problem of Behavior.* Macmillan, New York.

Coghill, G. E. (1940): Early embryonic somatic movements in birds and in mammals other than man. *Monogr. Soc. Res. Child Dev.,* 5:1–48.

Coghill, G. E. (1943): Flexion spasms and mass reflexes in relation to the ontogenetic development of behavior. *J. Comp. Neurol.,* 79:463–486.

Cohen, M. W. (1972): The development of neuromuscular connexions in the presence of d-tubocurarine. *Brain Res.,* 41:457–463.

Cohen, S. A., and Fischbach, G. D. (1973): Regulation of muscle activity in cell culture. *Science,* 181:76–78.

Comandon, J., and de Fonbrune, P. (1938): La chambre à huile. *Ann. Inst. Pasteur Lille,* 60:113–141.

Cook, R. D., and Peterson, E. R. (1974): The growth of smooth muscle and sympathetic ganglia in organotypic tissue cultures: Light and electron microscopy. *J. Neurol. Sci.,* 22:25–38.

Corner, M. A. (1964a): Localization of capacities for functional development in the neural plate of Xenopus laevis. *J. Comp. Neurol.,* 123:243–256.

Corner, M. A. (1964b): Rhythmicity in the early swimming of anuran larvae. *J. Embryol. Exp. Morphol.,* 12:665–671.

Corner, M. A., and Crain, S. M. (1965): Spontaneous contractions and bioelectric activity after differentiation in culture of presumptive neuromuscular tissues of the early frog. *Experientia,* 21:422–424.

Corner, M. A., and Crain, S. M. (1969): The development of spontaneous bioelectric activities and strychnine sensitivity during maturation in culture of embryonic chick and rodent central nervous tissues. *Arch. Int. Pharmacodyn.,* 182:404–406.

Corner, M. A., and Crain, S. M. (1972): Patterns of spontaneous bioelectric activity during maturation in culture of fetal rodent medulla and spinal cord tissues. *J. Neurobiol.,* 3:25–45.

Corrigall, W. A., Crain, S. M., and Bornstein, M. B. (1975): Electrophysiological studies during synaptogenesis in cultures of fetal mouse olfactory bulb. In: *Society of Neuroscience, 5th Annual Meeting, New York,* p. 771.

Corrigall, W. A., Crain, S. M., and Bornstein, M. B. (1976): Electrophysiological studies of fetal mouse olfactory bulb explants during development of synaptic functions. *J. Neurobiol.* (*in press*).

Coté, L. J., Benitez, H. H., and Murray, M. R. (1975): Biosynthesis of catecholamines in organotypic cultures of the peripheral autonomic nervous system: Modifications by biopterin and other agents. *J. Neurobiol.*, 6:233–243.

Coyle, J. T., Jacobowitz, D., Klein, D., and Axelrod, J. (1973): Dopaminergic neurons in explants of substantia nigra in culture. *J. Neurobiol.*, 4:461–470.

Crain, S. M. (1952): Development of electrical activity in the cerebral cortex of the albino rat. *Proc. Soc. Exp. Biol. Med.*, 81:49–51.

Crain, S. M. (1954a): Electrical activity in tissue cultures of chick embryo spinal ganglia. University Microfilms, Ann Arbor, No. 10,785 (Ph.D. thesis, Columbia University).

Crain, S. M. (1954b): Action potentials in tissue cultures of chick embryo spinal ganglia. *Anat. Rec.*, 118:292.

Crain, S. M. (1956): Resting and action potentials of cultured chick embryo spinal ganglion cells. *J. Comp. Neurol.*, 104:285–330.

Crain, S. M. (1963): Development of complex bioelectric activity during growth and differentiation of cultured mouse cerebral neocortex. *Trans. Am. Neurol. Assoc.*, 88:19–21.

Crain, S. M. (1964a): Development of bioelectric activity during growth of neonatal mouse cerebral cortex in tissue culture. In: *Symposium: Neurological and Electroencephalographic Correlative Studies in Infancy,* edited by P. Kellaway and I. Petersén, pp. 12–26. Grune & Stratton, New York.

Crain, S. M. (1964b): Electrophysiological studies of cord-innervated skeletal muscle in long-term tissue cultures of mouse embryo myotomes. *Anat. Rec.*, 148:273.

Crain, S. M. (1965a): Nervous and muscle tissues in vitro: Electrophysiological properties. In: *Cells and Tissues in Culture,* edited by E. N. Willmer, pp. 335–339, 344–347, 422–431. Academic Press, London.

Crain, S. M. (1965b): Bioelectric activities of cortical and subcortical regions in mouse cerebral tissue cultures. *Neurology (Minneap.)*, 15:291.

Crain, S. M. (1966): Development of "organotypic" bioelectric activities in central nervous tissues during maturation in culture. *Int. Rev. Neurobiol.*, 9:1–43.

Crain, S. M. (1968): Development of functional neuromuscular connections between separate explants of fetal mammalian tissues after maturation in culture. *Anat. Rec.*, 160:466.

Crain, S. M. (1969): Electrical activity of brain tissue developing in culture. In: *Basic Mechanisms of the Epilepsies,* edited by H. H. Jasper, A. A. Ward, and A. Pope, pp. 506–516. Little, Brown, Boston.

Crain, S. M. (1970a): Bioelectric interactions between cultured fetal rodent spinal cord and skeletal muscle after innervation in vitro. *J. Exp. Zool.*, 173:353–370.

Crain, S. M. (1970b): Tissue culture studies of developing brain function. In: *Developmental Neurobiology,* edited by W. A. Himwich, pp. 165–196. Charles C Thomas, Springfield, Ill.

Crain, S. M. (1970c): Long-term recordings from spinal cord explants in closed chamber with sealed-in manipulatable microelectrodes. *J. Cell Biol.*, 47:43a.

Crain, S. M. (1971a): Intracellular recordings suggesting synaptic functions in chick embryo spinal sensory ganglion cells isolated in vitro. *Brain Res.*, 26:188–191.

Crain, S. M. (1971b): Discussion in: *The Biopsychology of Development,* edited by E. Tobach, L. R. Aronson, and E. Shaw, pp. 65–66. Academic Press, New York.

Crain, S. M. (1971c): Tissue culture models of developing brain functions. In: *Amer. Assn. Adv. Sci. Symposium, Prenatal Ontogeny of Behavior and the Nervous System,* New York (see Crain, 1974a).

Crain, S. M. (1972a): Tissue culture models of epileptiform activity. In: *Experimental Models of Epilepsy,* edited by D. P. Purpura, J. K. Penry, D. Tower, D. M. Woodbury, and R. Walter, pp. 291–316. Raven Press, New York.

Crain, S. M. (1972b): Depression of complex bioelectric activity of mouse spinal cord explants by glycine and γ-aminobutyric acid. *In Vitro*, 7:249.

Crain, S. M. (1972c): Selective depression of organotypic bioelectric discharges of CNS explants by glycine and γ-aminobutyric acid. In: *Society of Neuroscience, 2nd Annual Meeting, Houston*, p. 131.

Crain, S. M. (1973a): Microelectrode recording in brain tissue cultures. In: *Methods in Phys-*

iological Psychology, Vol. 1: Bioelectric Recording Techniques: Cellular Processes and Brain Potentials, edited by R. F. Thompson and M. M. Patterson, pp. 39–75. Academic Press, New York.

Crain, S. M. (1973*b*): Tissue culture studies of central nervous system maturation. *Proc. Assoc. Res. Nerv. Ment. Dis.,* 51:113–131.

Crain, S. M. (1973*c*): Book review: *Nerve Growth Factor and its Antiserum,* edited by E. Zaimis and J. Knight. *Science,* 179:1316–1317.

Crain, S. M. (1974*a*): Tissue culture models of developing brain functions. In: *Studies on the Development of Behavior and the Nervous System, Vol. 2: Aspects of Neurogenesis,* edited by G. Gottlieb, pp. 69–114. Academic Press, New York.

Crain, S. M. (1974*b*): Selective depression of organotypic bioelectric activities of CNS tissue cultures by pharmacologic and metabolic agents. In: *Drugs and the Developing Brain,* edited by A. Vernadakis and N. Weiner, pp. 29–57. Plenum Press, New York.

Crain, S. M. (1974*c*): Paroxysmal discharges after release from tonic inhibition in mouse CNS tissue cultures during acute exposure to chloride-free medium. *Fed. Proc.,* 33:285.

Crain, S. M. (1974*d*): Progress Reports to National Multiple Sclerosis Society and National Institute of Neurological Diseases and Stroke.

Crain, S. M. (1975*a*): Onset of inhibitory functions during synaptogenesis in fetal mouse brain cultures. In: *Golgi Centennial Symposium,* edited by M. Santini, pp. 625–634. Raven Press, New York.

Crain, S. M. (1975*b*): Tissue culture models of brain functions. In: *Methods in Brain Research,* edited by P. B. Bradley, pp. 379–411. Wiley, New York.

Crain, S. M. (1975*c*): Development of complex synaptic functions in 'simple' neuronal arrays in culture. In: *'Simple' Nervous Systems,* edited by P. N. R. Usherwood and D. R. Newth, pp. 67–117. Edward Arnold, London.

Crain, S. M. (1975*d*): Physiology of CNS tissues in culture. In: *Metabolic Compartmentation and Neurotransmission. Relation to Brain Structure and Function,* edited by S. Berl, D. D. Clarke, and D. J. Schneider, pp. 273–303. Plenum Press, New York.

Crain, S. M. (1976): Development of specific sensory-evoked synaptic networks in CNS tissue cultures. In: *Electrobiology of Nerve, Synapses, and Muscle (Grundfest Festschrift),* edited by J. Reuben. Raven Press, New York (*in press*).

Crain, S. M., and Baer, S. C. (1969): A new tissue culture chamber for long-term studies with sealed-in manipulatable microelectrodes. *J. Cell Biol.,* 43:27a.

Crain, S. M., and Bornstein, M. B. (1964): Bioelectric activity of neonatal mouse cerebral cortex during growth and differentiation in tissue culture. *Exp. Neurol.,* 10:425–450.

Crain, S. M., and Bornstein, M. B. (1971): Development of organotypic bioelectric activities in cultured reaggregates of rodent CNS cells after complete dissociation. In: *Society of Neuroscience, 1st Annual Meeting, Washington, D.C.,* p. 181.

Crain, S. M., and Bornstein, M. B. (1972): Organotypic bioelectric activity in cultured reaggregates of dissociated rodent brain cells. *Science,* 176:182–184.

Crain, S. M., and Bornstein, M. B. (1974): Early onset in inhibitory functions during synaptogenesis in fetal mouse brain cultures. *Brain Res.,* 68:351–357.

Crain, S. M., and Peterson, E. R. (1963): Bioelectric activity in long-term cultures of spinal cord tissues. *Science,* 141:427–429.

Crain, S. M., and Peterson, E. R. (1964): Complex bioelectric activity in organized tissue cultures of spinal cord (human, rat and chick). *J. Cell. Comp. Physiol.,* 64:1–15.

Crain, S. M., and Peterson, E. R. (1966): Formation of functional interneuronal connections between explants of rat brainstem and spinal cord during development in culture. *Fed. Proc.,* 25:701.

Crain, S. M., and Peterson, E. R. (1967): Onset and development of functional interneuronal connections in explants of rat spinal cord-ganglia during maturation in culture. *Brain Res.,* 6:750–762.

Crain, S. M., and Peterson, E. R. (1971): Development of paired explants of fetal spinal cord and adult skeletal muscle during chronic exposure to curare and hemicholinium. *In Vitro,* 6:373.

Crain, S. M., and Peterson, E. R. (1973): A tissue culture model for studies of regeneration and formation of new functional connections in adult CNS. In: *Society of Neuroscience, 3rd Annual Meeting, San Diego,* p. 402.

Crain, S. M., and Peterson, E. R. (1974*a*): Development of neural connections in culture. *Ann. N.Y. Acad. Sci.,* 228:6–34.

Crain, S. M., and Peterson, E. R. (1974*b*): Enhanced afferent synaptic functions in fetal mouse spinal cord-sensory ganglion explants following NGF-induced ganglion hypertrophy. *Brain Res.,* 79:145–152.

Crain, S. M., and Peterson, E. R. (1975*a*): Development of specific sensory-evoked synaptic networks in fetal mouse cord-brainstem cultures. *Science,* 188:275–278.

Crain, S. M., and Peterson, E. R. (1975*b*): Enhanced sensory-evoked synaptic discharges in fetal mouse spinal cord and brainstem explants following nerve growth factor-induced hypertrophy of attached dorsal root ganglia. In: *Golgi Centennial Symposium,* edited by M. Santini, pp. 635–642. Raven Press, New York.

Crain, S. M., and Peterson, E. R. (1975*c*): Selective innervation of target tissues in spinal cord and medulla explants by isolated dorsal root ganglia. In: *Society of Neuroscience, 5th Annual Meeting, New York,* p. 751.

Crain, S. M., and Peterson, E. R. (1976): Development of specific synaptic networks in cultures of CNS tissues. In: *Reviews of Neuroscience,* edited by S. Ehrenpreis and I. Kopin. Raven Press, New York (*in preparation*).

Crain, S. M., and Pollack, E. D. (1972): Restorative effects of cyclic AMP on complex bioelectric activities after acute Ca^{++} deprivation in cultured CNS tissues. *J. Cell Biol.,* 55:52a.

Crain, S. M., and Pollack, E. D. (1973): Restorative effects of cyclic AMP on complex bioelectric activities of cultured fetal rodent CNS tissues after acute CA^{++}-deprivation. *J. Neurobiol.,* 4:321–342.

Crain, S. M., and Wiegand, R. G. (1961): Catecholamine levels of mouse sympathetic ganglia following hypertrophy produced by salivary nerve-growth factor. *Soc. Exp. Biol. Med. Proc.,* 107:663–665.

Crain, S. M., Alfei, L., and Peterson, E. R. (1970): Neuromuscular transmission in cultures of adult human and rodent skeletal muscle after innervation *in vitro* by fetal rodent spinal cord. *J. Neurobiol.,* 1:471–489.

Crain, S. M., Benitez, H., and Vatter, A. E. (1964*a*): Some cytologic effects of salivary nerve-growth factor on tissue cultures of peripheral ganglia. *Ann. N.Y. Acad. Sci.,* 118:206–231.

Crain, S. M., Bornstein, M. B., and Lennon, V. A. (1975*a*): Depression of complex bioelectric discharges in cerebral tissue cultures by thermolabile complement-dependent serum factors. *Exp. Neurol.,* 49:330–335.

Crain, S. M., Bornstein, M. B., and Peterson, E. R. (1968*a*): Maturation of cultured embryonic CNS tissues during chronic exposure to agents which prevent bioelectric activity. *Brain Res.,* 8:363–372.

Crain, S. M., Peterson, E. R., and Bornstein, M. B. (1968*b*): Formation of functional interneuronal connections between explants of various mammalian central nervous tissues during development in vitro. In: *Ciba Foundation Symposium, Growth of the Nervous System,* edited by G. E. W. Wolstenholme and M. O'Connor, pp. 13–31. Churchill, London.

Crain, S. M., Raine, C. S., and Bornstein, M. B. (1975*b*): Early formation of synaptic networks in cultures of fetal mouse cerebral neocortex and hippocampus. *J. Neurobiol.,* 6:329–336.

Crain, S. M., Bunge, R. P., Bunge, M. B., and Peterson, E. R. (1964*b*): Bioelectric and electron microscopic evidence for development of synapses in spinal cord cultures. *J. Cell Biol.,* 23:114–115A.

Crain, S. M., Grundfest, H., Mettler, F. A., and Flint, T. (1953): Electrical activity from tissue cultures of chick embryo spinal ganglia. *Trans. Am. Neurol. Assoc.,* 78:236–239.

Crain, S. M., Peterson, E. R., Masurovsky, E. B., and Pappas, G. D. (1976): Early formation and development of functional synaptic networks in organotypic cultures of fetal mouse spinal cord with attached dorsal root ganglia. *In preparation.*

Cunningham, A. W. B. (1961): Spontaneous potentials from explants of chick embryo spinal cord in tissue culture. *Naturwissenschaften,* 48:719–720.

Cunningham, A. W. B. (1962): Qualitative behavior of spontaneous potentials from explants of 15 day chick embryo telencephalon in vitro. *J. Gen. Physiol.,* 45:1065–1076.

Cunningham, A. W. B., and Stephens, S. G. (1961): Qualitative effects of strychnine and brucine on spontaneous potentials from explants of telencephalon. *Experientia,* 17:569–571.

Cunningham, A. W. B., Hamilton, A. E., King, M. F., Rojas-Corona, R. R., and Songster, G. F. (1970): Slow spontaneous signals from brain tissue culture. *Experientia,* 26:13–16.

Cunningham, A. W. B., O'Lague, P., Rojas-Corona, R. R., and Freeman, J. A. (1966): Microelectrode studies of spontaneous potentials from chick embryo telencephalon in vitro. *Experientia,* 22:439–441.

Curtis, D. R. (1975): Gamma-aminobutyric and glutamic acids as mammalian central transmitters. In: *Metabolic Compartmentation and Neurotransmission. Relation to Brain Structure and Function,* edited by S. Berl, D. D. Clarke, and D. J. Schneider, pp. 11–36. Plenum Press, New York.

Curtis, D. R., and Johnston, G. A. R. (1974): Amino acid transmitters in the mammalian central nervous system. *Ergeb. Physiol.,* 69:97–188.

Curtis, D. R., and Watkins, J. C. (1965): The pharmacology of amino acids related to γ-aminobutyric acid. *Pharmacol. Rev.,* 17:347–391.

Curtis, D. R., Duggan, A. W., and Johnston, G. A. R. (1971a): The specificity of strychnine as a glycine antagonist in the mammalian spinal cord. *Exp. Brain Res.,* 12:547–565.

Curtis, D. R., Duggan, A. W., Felix, D., and Johnston, G. A. R. (1971b): Bicuculline, an antagonist of GABA and synaptic inhibition in the spinal cord of the cat. *Brain Res.,* 32: 69–96.

Curtis, D. R., Duggan, A. W., Felix, D., Johnston, G. A. R., and McLennan, H. (1971c): Antagonism between bicuculline and GABA in the cat brain. *Brain Res.,* 33:57–73.

Curtis, D. R., Game, C. J. A., Johnston, G. A. R., McCulloch, R. M., and Maclachlan, R. M. (1972): Convulsive action of penicillin. *Brain Res.,* 43:242–245.

Curtis, D. R., Hösli, L., and Johnston, G. A. R. (1967): Inhibition of spinal neurones by glycine. *Nature (Lond.),* 215:1502–1503.

Curtis, D. R., Hösli, L., Johnston, G. A. R., and Johnston, I. H. (1968): The hyperpolarization of spinal motoneurones by glycine and related amino acids. *Exp. Brain Res.,* 5:235–258.

Dambach, G. E., and Erulkar, S. D. (1973): The action of calcium at spinal neurones of the frog. *J. Physiol. (Lond.),* 228:799–817.

Daniels, J. C., and Spehlmann, R. (1973): The convulsant effect of topically applied atropine. *Electroencephalogr. Clin. Neurophysiol.,* 34:83–87.

Das, G. D. (1975): Differentiation of dendrites in the transplanted neuroblasts in the mammalian brain. In: *Advances in Neurology,* Vol. 12, edited by G. W. Kreutzberg, pp. 181–199. Raven Press, New York.

Das, G. D., and Altman, J. (1972): Studies on the transplantation of developing neural tissue in the mammalian brain. I. Transplantation of cerebellar slabs into the cerebellum of neonate rats. *Brain Res.,* 38:233–249.

Davidoff, R. A. (1972a): Gamma-aminobutyric acid antagonism and presynaptic inhibition in the frog spinal cord. *Science,* 175:331–333.

Davidoff, R. A. (1972b): The effects of bicuculline on the isolated spinal cord of the frog. *Exp. Neurol.,* 35:179–193.

Davidoff, R. A. (1972c): Penicillin and presynaptic inhibition in the amphibian spinal cord. *Brain Res.,* 36:218–222.

Davidson, N., and Southwick, C. A. P. (1971): Amino acids and presynaptic inhibition in the rat cuneate nucleus. *J. Physiol. (Lond.),* 219:689–708.

Davison, A. N., and Kaczmarek, L. K. (1971): Taurine – a possible neurotransmitter? *Nature (Lond.),* 234:107–108.

Deadwyler, S. A., Dudek, F. E., Cotman, C. W., and Lynch, G. (1975): Intracellular responses of rat dentate granule cells in vitro: Posttetanic potentiation to perforant path stimulation. *Brain Res.,* 88:80–85.

DeBoni, U., Scott, J. W., and Crapper, D. R. (1975): Neuron culture from adult goldfish. In: *Society of Neuroscience, 5th Annual Meeting, New York,* p. 812.

DeBoni, U., Scott, J. W., and Crapper, D. R. (1976): Neuron culture from adult goldfish. *J. Neurobiol. (in press).*

deFonbrune, P. (1949): *Technique de Micromanipulation.* Masson, Paris.

DeGroat, W. C. (1970): The action of γ-aminobutyric acid and related amino acids on mammalian autonomic ganglia. *J. Pharmacol. Exp. Ther.,* 176:384–396.

DeGroat, W. C. (1972): GABA-depolarization of a sensory ganglion: Antagonism by picrotoxin and bicuculline. *Brain Res.,* 38:429–432.

DeGroat, W. C., Lalley, P. M., and Saum, W. R. (1972): Depolarization of dorsal root ganglia in the cat by GABA and related amino acids: Antagonism by picrotoxin and bicuculline. *Brain Res.,* 44:273–277.

DeLong, G. R. (1970): Histogenesis of fetal mouse isocortex and hippocampus in reaggregating cell cultures. *Dev. Biol.* 22:563–583.

Dettbarn, W. D. (1971): Local anesthetics. In: *Handbook of Neurochemistry*, Vol. 6, edited by A. Lajtha, pp. 423–439. Plenum Press, New York.

Deza, L., and Eidelberg, E. (1967): Development of cortical electrical activity in the rat. *Exp. Neurol.*, 17:425–438.

Dhawan, B. N., Sharma, J. N., and Srimal, R. C. (1972): Selective inhibition by glycine of some somatic reflexes in the cat. *Br. J. Pharmacol.*, 44:404–412.

Diamond, J., Cooper, E., Turner, C., and Macintyre, L. (1976): Trophic regulation of nerve sprouting. (*submitted for publication*).

Diamond, J., and Miledi, R. (1962): A study of foetal and new-born rat muscle fibres. *J. Physiol. (Lond.)*, 162:393–408.

Dichter, M. A. (1973): Intracellular single unit recording. In: *Methods in Physiology Psychology, Vol. 1, Bioelectric Recording Techniques: Cellular Processes and Brain Potentials*, edited by R. F. Thompson and M. M. Patterson, pp. 3–21. Academic Press, New York.

Dichter, M. A. (1975): Physiological properties of vertebrate nerve cells in tissue culture. In: *Brain Mechanisms in Mental Retardation*, edited by N. A. Buchwald and M. A. B. Brazier, pp. 101–114. Academic Press, New York.

Dickinson, J. C., and Hamilton, P. B. (1966): The free amino acids of human spinal fluid determined by ion exchange chromatography. *J. Neurochem.*, 13:1179–1187.

Dobzhansky, T. (1968): On genetics, sociology, and politics. *Perspect. Biol. Med.*, 11:544–554.

Drachman, D. B. (1965): The developing motor end-plate: Curare tolerance in the chick embryo. *J. Physiol. (Lond.)*, 180:735–740.

Drachman, D. B. (1971): Neuromuscular transmission of trophic effects. *Ann. N.Y. Acad. Sci.*, 183:158–170.

Drachman, D. B., and Sokoloff, L. (1966): The role of movement in embryonic joint development. *Dev. Biol.*, 14:401–420.

Drachman, D. B., and Witzke, F. (1972): Trophic regulation of acetylcholine sensitivity of muscle: Effect of electrical stimulation. *Science*, 176:514–516.

Drayton, M. R., and Kiernan, J. A. (1973): Effects of aprotinin on organ cultures of the cerebellum of the adult rat. *Exp. Neurol.*, 39:381–388.

Dreifuss, J. J., and Kelly, J. S. (1972): The activity of identified supraoptic neurons and their response to acetylcholine applied by iontophoresis. *J. Physiol. (Lond.)*, 220:105–118.

Eccles, J. C. (1964): *The Physiology of Synapses*. Springer-Verlag, Berlin.

Echlin, F. A. (1959): The supersensitivity of chronically "isolated" cerebral cortex as a mechanism in focal epilepsy. *Electroencephalogr. Clin. Neurophysiol.*, 11:697–722.

El-Badry, H. M. (1963): *Micromanipulators and Micromanipulation*. Academic Press, New York.

Ellingson, R. J., and Rose, G. H. (1970): Ontogenesis of the electroencephalogram. In: *Developmental Neurobiology*, edited by W. A. Himwich, pp. 441–474. Charles C Thomas, Springfield, Ill.

Elmqvist, D., and Feldman, D. S. (1965): Calcium dependence of spontaneous acetylcholine release at mammalian motor nerve terminals. *J. Physiol. (Lond.)*, 181:487–497.

Engel, W. K. (1961): Cytological localization of cholinesterase in cultured skeletal muscle cells. *J. Histochem. Cytochem.*, 9:66–72.

Evans, M. H. (1972): Tetrodotoxin, saxitoxin, and related substances: Their application in neurobiology. *Int. Rev. Neurobiol.*, 15:83–166.

Faludi, G., Gotlieb, J., and Meyers, J. (1966): Factors influencing the development of steroid-induced myopathies. *Ann. N.Y. Acad. Sci.*, 138:61–72.

Farbman, A. I., and Gesteland, R. C. (1974): Developmental and electrophysiological studies of olfactory mucosa in organ culture. *1st ECRO Congress, Université Paris-Sud, Orsay*, p. 20.

Farese, R. V. (1971): Calcium as a mediator of adrenocorticotrophic hormone action on adrenal protein synthesis. *Science*, 173:447–450.

Farley, B. G. (1962): Some similarities between the behavior of a neural network model and electrophysiological experiments. In: *Self-organizing Systems*, edited by M. C. Yovits, G. T. Jacobi, and G. D. Goldstein, pp. 535–550. Spartan Press, Washington, D.C.

Feldberg, W., and Fleischhauer, K. (1962): The site of origin of the seizure discharge produced by tubocurarine acting from the cerebral ventricles. *J. Physiol. (Lond.)*, 160:258–283.

Feldberg, W., and Fleischauer, K. (1963): The hippocampus as the site of origin of the seizure discharge produced by tubocurarine acting from the cerebral ventricles. *J. Physiol. (Lond.)*, 168:435–442.

Feldman, S., and Dafny, N. (1970): Effects of cortisol on unit activity in the hypothalamus of the rat. *Exp. Neurol.*, 27:375–387.

Felix, D., and McLennan, H. (1971): The effect of bicuculline on the inhibition of mitral cells of the olfactory bulb. *Brain Res.*, 25:661–664.

Fell, H. B. (1951): Histogenesis in tissue culture. In: *Cytology and Cell Physiology*, 2nd ed., edited by G. Bourne, pp. 419–444. Clarendon Press, Oxford.

Feltz, P., and Rasminsky, M. (1974): A model for the mode of action of GABA on primary afferent terminals: Depolarizing effects of GABA applied iontophoretically to neurones of mammalian dorsal root ganglia. *Neuropharmacology*, 13:553–564.

Fischbach, G. D. (1970): Synaptic potentials recorded in cell cultures of nerve and muscle. *Science*, 169:1331–1333.

Fischbach, G. D. (1972): Synapse formation between dissociated nerve and muscle cells in low density cell cultures. *Dev. Biol.*, 28:407–429.

Fischbach, G. D. (1974): Some aspects of neuromuscular junction formation. In: *Cell Communication*, edited by R. P. Cox, pp. 43–66. Wiley, New York.

Fischbach, G. D. (1976): Nerve-muscle junction formation in vitro. *Cold Spring Harbor Symp. Quant. Biol. (in press)*.

Fischbach, G. D., and Dichter, M. A. (1974): Electrophysiologic and morphologic properties of neurons in dissociated chick spinal cord cell cultures. *Dev. Biol.*, 37:100–116.

Fischbach, G. D., Cohen, S. A., and Henkart, M. P. (1974a): Some observations on trophic interaction between neurons and muscle fibers in cell culture. *Ann. N.Y. Acad. Sci.*, 228:35–46.

Fischbach, G. D., Fambrough, D., and Nelson, P. G. (1973): A discussion of neuron and muscle cell cultures. *Fed. Proc.*, 32:1636–1642.

Fischbach, G. D., Henkart, M. P., Cohen, S. A., Breuer, A. C., Whysner, J., and Neal, F. M. (1974b): Studies on the development of neuromuscular junctions in cell culture. *Soc. Gen. Physiol.*, 26th Symp., pp. 259–283. Raven Press, New York.

Fischman, D. A. (1972): Development of striated muscle. In: *The Structure and Function of Muscle*, Vol. 1, 2nd ed., edited by G. Bourne, pp. 75–148. Academic Press, New York.

Florendo, N. T., Barrnett, R. J., and Greengard, P. (1971): Cyclic 3′,5′-nucleotide phosphodiesterase: Cytochemical localization in cerebral cortex. *Science*, 173:745–747.

Foelix, R. F., and Oppenheim, R. W. (1973): Synaptogenesis in the avian embryo: ultrastructure and possible behavioral correlates. In: *Developmental Studies of Behavior and the Nervous System, Vol. 1: Behavioral Embryology*, edited by G. Gottlieb, pp. 104–139. Academic Press, New York.

Forn, J., Tagliamonte, A., Tagliamonte, P., and Gessa, G. L. (1972): Stimulation by dibutyryl cyclic AMP of serotonin synthesis and tryptophan transport in brain slices. *Nature [New Biol.]*, 237:245–247.

Frank, K., and Becker, M. C. (1964): Microelectrodes for recording and stimulation. In: *Physical Techniques in Biological Research, Vol. V: Electrophysiological Methods, Part A*, edited by W. L. Nastuk, pp. 22–87. Academic Press, New York.

Fromme, A. (1941): An experimental study of the factors of maturation and practice in the behavioral development of the embryo of the frog, Rana pipiens. *Genet. Psychol. Monogr.*, 24:219–256.

Furshpan, E. J., and Potter, D. D. (1968): Low resistance junctions between cells in embryos and tissue culture. In: *Current Topics in Developmental Biology*, Vol. 3, edited by A. Moscona and A. Monroy, pp. 95–127. Academic Press, New York.

Gähwiler, B. H. (1975): The effects of GABA, picrotoxin and bicuculline on the spontaneous bioelectric activity of cultured cerebellar Purkinje cells. *Brain Res.*, 99:85–96.

Gähwiler, B. H. (1976a): Spontaneous bioelectric activity of cultured Purkinje cells during exposure to glutamate, glycine and strychnine. *J. Neurobiol.*, 7:97–107.

Gähwiler, B. H. (1976b): Inhibitory action of noradrenaline and cyclic adenosine monophosphate in explants of rat cerebellum. *Nature (Lond.)*, 259:483–484.

Gähwiler, B., and Stähelin, H. (1975): Response of cultured cerebellar Purkinje cells to GABA and GABA-antagonists. *Experientia*, 31:728.

Gähwiler, B. H., Mamoon, A. M., and Tobias, C. A. (1973): Spontaneous bioelectric activity of cultured cerebellar Purkinje cells during exposure to agents which prevent synaptic transmission. *Brain Res.*, 53:71–79.

Gähwiler, B. H., Mamoon, A. M., Schlapfer, W. T., and Tobias, C. A. (1972): Effects of temperature on spontaneous bioelectric activity of cultured nerve cells. *Brain Res.*, 40: 527–533.

Gaillard, P. J. (1955): Parathyroid gland tissue and bone in vitro. *Exp. Cell Res. (Suppl.)*, 3:154–169.

Gaillard, P. J., and Schaberg, A. (1965): Endocrine glands. In: *Cells and Tissue in Culture*, Vol. 2, edited by E. N. Willmer, pp. 631–695. Academic Press, New York.

Garber, B. B., and Moscona, A. A. (1972): Reconstruction of brain tissue from cell suspensions. I. Aggregation patterns of cells dissociated from different regions of the developing brain. *Dev. Biol.*, 27:217–234.

Geller, H. M. (1975): Phasic discharge of neurons in long-term cultures of tuberal hypothalamus. *Brain Res.*, 93:511–515.

Geller, H. M., and Woodward, D. J. (1974): Responses of cultured cerebellar neurons to iontophoretically applied amino acids. *Brain Res.*, 74:67–80.

Gerard, R. W. (1955): The biological roots of psychiatry. *Am. J. Psychiatry*, 112:81–90.

Gessa, G. L., Krishna, G., Forn, J., Tagliamonte, A., and Brodie, B. B. (1970): Behavioral and vegetative effects produced by dibutyryl cyclic AMP injected into different areas of the brain. In: *Role of Cyclic AMP in Cell Function*, edited by P. Greengard and E. Costa, pp. 371–381. Raven Press, New York.

Giller, E. L., Schrier, B. K., Shainberg, A., Fisk, H. R., and Nelson, P. G. (1973): Increased choline acetyltransferase activity in combined cultures of spinal cord and muscle cells from the mouse. *Science*, 182:588–589.

Giller, E. L., Breakefield, X. O., Christian, C. N., Neale, E. A., and Nelson, P. G. (1975): Expression of neuronal characteristics in culture: some pros and cons of primary cultures and continuous cell lines. In: *Golgi Centennial Symposium*, edited by M. Santini, pp. 603–623. Raven Press, New York.

Godfrey, E. W., Nelson, P. G., Schrier, B. K., Breuer, A. C., and Ransom, B. R. (1975): Neurons from fetal rat brain in a new cell culture system: A multidisciplinary analysis. *Brain Res.*, 90:1–21.

Goldberg, A. L., and Goodman, H. M. (1969): Relationship between cortisone and muscle work in determining muscle size. *J. Physiol. (Lond.)*, 200:667–675.

Goldberg, A. L., and Singer, J. J. (1969): Evidence for a role of cyclic AMP in neuromuscular transmission. *Proc. Natl. Acad. Sci. U.S.A.*, 64:134–144.

Goldberg, N. D., O'Dea, R. F., and Haddox, M. K. (1973): Cyclic GMP. In: *Advances in Cyclic Nucleotide Research*, Vol. 3, edited by P. Greengard and G. A. Robison, pp. 155–213. Raven Press, New York.

Gottlieb, G. (1973): Introduction to behavioral embryology. In: *Studies on the Development of Behavior and the Nervous System, Vol. 1: Behavioral Embryology*, edited by G. Gottlieb, pp. 3–45. Academic Press, New York.

Grafstein, B. (1963): Postnatal development of the transcallosal response in the cerebral cortex of the cat. *J. Neurophysiol.*, 26:79–99.

Grafstein, B., and Sastry, P. B. (1957): Some preliminary electrophysiological studies on chronic neuronally isolated cerebral cortex. *Electroencephalogr. Clin. Neurophysiol.*, 9:723–725.

Granit, R., and Phillips, C. G. (1956): Excitatory and inhibitory processes acting upon individual Purkinje cells of the cerebellum in cats. *J. Physiol.*, 133:520–547.

Green, J. D., Mancia, M., and von Baumgarten, R. (1962): Recurrent inhibition in the olfactory bulb. I. Effects of antidromic stimulation of the lateral olfactory tract. *J. Neurophysiol.*, 25:467–488.

Greengard, P., and Kuo, J. F. (1970): On the mechanism of action of cyclic AMP. In: *Role of Cyclic AMP in Cell Function*, edited by P. Greengard and E. Costa, pp. 287–306. Raven Press, New York.

Grosse, G., and Lindner, G. (1968): Untersuchungen zur Morphologie des Zentralnervasen Gewebes von Ambystoma mexicanum in vitro. *Z. Mikr. Anat. Forsch.*, 79:343–362.

Guillery, R., Sobkowicz, H. M., and Scott, G. L. (1968): Light and electron microscopical observation of the ventral horn and ventral root in long-term cultures of the spinal cord of the fetal mouse. *J. Comp. Neurol.,* 134:433–476.

Guth, L. (1969): "Trophic" effects of vertebrate neurons. *Neurosci. Res. Prog. Bull.,* 7:1–73.

Guth, L. (1974): Axonal regeneration and functional plasticity in the central nervous system. *Exp. Neurol.,* 45:606–654.

Guth, L., and Windle, W. F. (1970): The enigma of central nervous regeneration. *Exp. Neurol. (Suppl. 5),* 28:1–43.

Hackett, J. T. (1972): Electrophysiological properties of neuronal circuits in the frog cerebellum in vitro. *Brain Res.,* 48:385–389.

Hackett, J. T. (1975): Calcium is essential for chemical synaptic transmission in the frog cerebellum in vitro. In: *Society of Neuroscience, 5th Annual Meeting, New York,* p. 642.

Halgren, E., and Varon, S. (1972): Serotonin turnover in cultured raphé nuclei from newborn rat: In vitro development and drug effects. *Brain Res.,* 48:438–442.

Hamburger, V. (1963): Some aspects of the embryology of behavior. *Q. Rev. Biol.,* 38:342–365.

Hamburger, V. (1968): Emergence of nervous coordination. IV. Origins of integrated behavior. *Dev. Biol.* 2:251–271.

Hamburger, V. (1971): Development of embryonic motility. In: *The Biopsychology of Development,* edited by E. Tobach, L. R. Aronson, and E. Shaw, pp. 45–66. Academic Press, New York.

Hamburger, V. (1973): Anatomical and physiological basis of embryonic motility in birds and mammals. In: *Development Studies of Behavior and the Nervous System, Vol. 1: Behavioral Embryology,* edited by G. Gottlieb, pp. 51–76. Academic Press, New York.

Hamburger, V., and Balaban, M. (1963): Observations and experiments on spontaneous rhythmical behavior in the chick embryo. *Dev. Biol.,* 7:533–545.

Hamburger, V., and Oppenheim, R. W. (1967): Prehatching motility and hatching behavior in the chick. *J. Exp. Zool.,* 166:171–194.

Hardman, J. G., Robison, G. A., and Sutherland, E. W. (1971): Cyclic nucleotides. *Ann. Rev. Physiol.,* 33:311–336.

Harris, A. J. (1974a): Inductive functions of the nervous system. *Ann. Rev. Physiol.,* 36:251–305.

Harris, A. J. (1974b): Role of acetylcholine receptors in synapse formation. *Soc. Gen. Physiol.,* 26th Symp., pp. 315–337. Raven Press, New York.

Harrison, R. G. (1904): An experimental study of the relation of the nervous system to the developing musculature in the embryo of the frog. *Am. J. Anat.,* 3:197–219.

Harrison, R. G. (1907): Observations on the living developing nerve fiber. *Proc. Soc. Exp. Biol. Med.,* 4:140–143; *Anat. Rec.,* 1:116–118.

Harrison, R. G. (1910): The outgrowth of the nerve fiber as a mode of protoplasmic movement. *J. Exp. Zool.,* 9:787–846.

Harrison, R. G. (1969): *Organization and Development of the Embryo,* edited by S. Wilens, Yale University Press, New Haven.

Hayes, B. P., and Roberts, A. (1973): Synaptic junction development in the spinal cord of an amphibian embryo: An electron microscope study. *Z. Zellforsch.,* 137:251–269.

Hebb, D. O. (1949): *The Organization of Behavior.* Wiley, New York.

Henkart, M. (1972): Structure and function of the endoplasmic reticulum in the squid giant axon. *Society of Neuroscience, 2nd Annual Meeting, Houston,* p. 103.

Herschman, H. R. (1974): Culture of neural tissue and cells. In: *Research Methods in Neurochemistry,* Vol. 2, edited by N. Marks and R. Rodnight, pp. 101–160. Plenum Press, New York.

Heuser, J. E., and Reese, T. S. (1973): Evidence of recycling of synaptic vesicle membrane during transmitter release at the frog neuromuscular junction. *J. Cell Biol.,* 57:315–344.

Hild, W. (1957): Myelinogenesis in cultures of mammalian central nervous tissue. *Z. Zellforsch.,* 46:71–95.

Hild, W., and Tasaki, I. (1962): Morphological and physiological properties of neurons and glial cells in tissue culture. *J. Neurophysiol.,* 25:277–304.

Hild, W., and Tasaki, I. (1964): Neurophysiology. *Methods Med. Res.,* 10:327–334.

Hill, C. E., and Burnstock, G. (1975): Amphibian sympathetic ganglia in tissue culture. *Cell Tiss. Res.,* 162:209–234.

Hill, R. G., Simmonds, M. A., and Straughan, D. W. (1972): Convulsive properties of d-tubocurarine and cortical inhibition. *Nature (Lond.)*, 240:51–52.

Himwich, W. A. (1962): Biochemical and neurophysiological development of the brain in the neonatal period. *Int. Rev. Neurobiol.*, 4:117–158.

Hintzsche, E. (1954): Uber die Wirkung von Succinodinitril auf kulturen isolierter Spinal-ganglienzellen. *Z. Mikr. Anat. Forsch.*, 60:75–80.

Hirst, G. D. S., and Spence, I. (1973): Calcium action potentials in mammalian peripheral neurons. *Nature [New Biol.]*, 243:54–56.

Hoffer, B. J. (1971): Symposium on cyclic AMP and cell function: Discussion. *Ann. N.Y. Acad. Sci.*, 185:555.

Hoffer, B., Freedman, R., Olson, L., and Seiger, A. (1975b): Pharmacological properties of neonatal rat hippocampus transplanted to the anterior chamber of the eye. In: *Sixth International Congress of Pharmacology, Helsinki, Finland,* p. 428.

Hoffer, B., Olson, L., Seiger, A., and Bloom, F. (1975a): Formation of a functional adrenergic input to intraocular cerebellar grafts: Ingrowth of inhibitory sympathetic fibers. *J. Neurobiol.*, 6:565–585.

Hoffer, B., Seiger, A., Ljungberg, T., and Olson, L. (1974): Electrophysiological and cytological studies of brain homografts in the anterior chamber of the eye: Maturation of cerebellar cortex *in oculo. Brain Res.*, 79:165-184.

Hoffer, B., Seiger, A., Freedman, R., Olson, L., and Taylor, D. (1976): Electrophysiology and cytology of hippocampal formation transplants in the anterior chamber of the eye. II. Cholinergic mechanisms. *Brain Res. (in press)*.

Holtzman, E., Crain, S. M., and Peterson, E. R. (1973): Endocytosis at nerve endings in spinal cord cultures. *J. Gen. Physiol.*, 61:253.

Holtzman, E., Freeman, A. F., and Kashner, L. (1971): Stimulation dependent alterations in peroxidase uptake at lobster neuromuscular junctions. *Science*, 175:733–736.

Horn, G., and Hinde, R. A., editors (1970): *Short Term Changes in Neural Activity and Behaviour.* University Press, Cambridge.

Hösli, E., Bucher, U. M., and Hösli, I. (1975b): Uptake of ^{3}H-noradrenaline and ^{3}H-5-hydroxytryptamine in cultured rat brainstem. *Experientia*, 31:354–356.

Hösli, L., Andres, P. F., and Hösli, E. (1971): Effects of glycine on spinal neurones grown in tissue culture. *Brain Res.*, 34:399–402.

Hösli, L., Hösli, E., and Andres, P. F. (1973): Nervous tissue cultures—a model to study action and uptake of putative neurotransmitters such as amino acids. *Brain Res.*, 62:597–602.

Hösli, L., Hösli, E., Andres, P. F., and Wolff, J. R. (1975a): Amino acid transmitters—action and uptake in neurons and glial cells of human and rat CNS tissue culture. In: *Golgi Centennial Symposium*, edited by M. Santini, pp. 473–488. Raven Press, New York.

Hoyle, G. (1964): Exploration of neuronal mechanisms underlying behavior. In: *Neuronal Theory and Modeling*, edited by R. F. Reiss, pp. 346–376. Stanford University Press, Stanford, Calif.

Hoyle, G. (1970): Cellular mechanisms underlying behavior-neuroethology. In: *Advances in Insect Physiology*, edited by J. E. Freheme and J. W. L. Beament, pp. 349–444. Academic Press, New York.

Hoyle, G. (1974): Neural machinery underlying behavior in insects. In: *The Neurosciences, Third Study Program*, edited by F. O. Schmitt and F. G. Worden, pp. 397–410. M.I.T. Press, Cambridge.

Huber, F. (1975): Principles of motor co-ordination in rhythmical behaviour in insects. In: *'Simple' Nervous Systems*, edited by P. N. R. Usherwood and D. R. Newth, pp. 381–413. Edward Arnold, London.

Hughes, A. F. W. (1968): *Aspects of Neural Ontogeny.* Academic Press, New York.

Hughes, A. F. W., and Prestige, M. C. (1967): Development of behaviour in the hindlimb of Xenopus laevis. *J. Zool.*, 152:347–359.

Hughes, J. R. (1964): Responses from the visual cortex of unanesthetized monkeys. *Int. Rev. Neurobiol.*, 7:99–153.

Hunt, R. K., and Jacobson, M. (1973): Neuronal specificity revisited. In: *Current Topics in Developmental Biology*, edited by A. Moscona and A. Monroy, pp. 203–258. Academic Press, New York.

Ikeda, K., and Kaplan, W. D. (1970): Patterned neural activity of a mutant Drosophila melano-gaster. *Proc. Natl. Acad. Sci. U.S.A.*, 66:765–772.

Ingvar, D. H. (1955): Electrical activity of isolated cortex in the unanesthetized cat with intact brain stem. *Acta Physiol. Scand.*, 33:151–168.

Ingvar, S. (1920): Reactions of cells to the galvanic current in tissue cultures. *Proc. Soc. Exp. Biol.*, 17:198–199.

Ito, M., Kostyuk, P. G., and Oshima, T. (1962): Further study on anion permeability in cat spinal motoneurones. *J. Physiol. (Lond.)*, 164:150–156.

Ito, Y., Miledi, R., and Vincent, A. (1974): Transmitter release induced by a 'factor' in rabbit serum. *Proc. R. Soc. Lond.*, 187:235–241.

Iversen, L. L., Dick, F., Kelly, J. S., and Schon, F. (1975): Uptake and localization of transmitter amino acids in the nervous system. In: *Metabolic Compartmentation and Neurotransmission. Relation to Brain Structure and Function,* edited by S. Berl, D. D. Clarke, and D. J. Schneider, pp. 65–89. Plenum Press, New York.

Iversen, L. L., Kelly, J. S., Minchin, M., Schon, F., and Snodgrass, S. R. (1973): Role of amino acids and peptides in synaptic transmission. *Brain Res.*, 62:567–576.

Jacobson, M. (1969): Development of specific neuronal connections. *Science,* 163:543–547.

Jacobson, M. (1970): *Developmental Neurobiology.* Holt, Rinehart and Winston, New York.

Jacobson, M. (1974): A plentitude of neurons. In: *Studies on the Development of Behavior and the Nervous System, Vol. 2: Aspects of Neurogenesis,* edited by G. Gottlieb, pp. 151–166. Academic Press, New York.

Jansen, J. K. S., and Nicholls, J. G. (1972): Regeneration and changes in synaptic connections between individual nerve cells in the central nervous system of the leech. *Proc. Natl. Acad. Sci. U.S.A.*, 69:636–639.

Jenkinson, D. H., Stamenovi, B. A., and Whitaker, B. D. L. (1968): The effect of noradrenaline on the end-plate potential in twitch fibers of the frog. *J. Physiol. (Lond.)*, 195:743–754.

John, E. R. (1967): *Mechanisms of Memory.* Academic Press, New York.

Johnson, D. G., Silberstein, S. D., Hanbauer, I., and Kopin, I. J. (1972a): The role of nerve growth factor in the ramification of sympathetic nerve fibres into the rat iris in organ culture. *J. Neurochem.*, 19:2025–2029.

Johnson, G. A., Boukma, S. J., Lahti, R. A., and Mathews, J. (1972b): Cyclic AMP and cyclic nucleotide phosphodiesterase activity in synaptic vesicles. *Fed. Proc.*, 31:513.

Johnson, R., and Armstrong-James, M. (1970): Morphology of superficial postnatal cerebral cortex with special reference to synapses. *Z. Zellforsch.*, 110:540–558.

Jones, R., and Vrbova, G. (1970): Effect of muscle activity on denervation hypersensitivity. *J. Physiol. (Lond.)*, 210:144P–145P.

Jones, R., and Vrbova, G. (1971): Can denervation hypersensitivity be prevented? *J. Physiol. (Lond.)*, 217:67P.

Kakiuchi, S., Rall, T. W., and McIlwain, H. (1969): The effect of electrical stimulation upon the accumulation of adenosine 3',5'-phosphate in isolated cerebral tissue. *J. Neurochem.*, 16:485–491.

Kandel, E. R., and Spencer, W. A. (1968): Cellular neurophysiological approaches in the study of learning. *Physiol. Rev.*, 48:65–134.

Kandel, E. R., Carew, T., and Koester, J. (1976a): Some rules relating the biophysical properties of neurons and their pattern of interconnections to behavior. In: *Electrobiology of Nerve, Synapses, and Muscle (Grundfest Festschrift),* edited by J. Reuben. Raven Press, New York (*in press*).

Kandel, E. R., Castellucci, V., and Brunelli, M. (1976b): A common presynaptic locus for the synaptic mechanisms underlying short-term habituation and sensitization of the gill-withdrawal reflex in Aplysia. *Cold Spring Harbor Symp. Quant. Biol. (in press).*

Kao, C. C. (1974): Comparison of healing process in transected spinal cords grafted with autogenous brain tissue, sciatic nerve, and nodose ganglion. *Exp. Neurol.*, 44:424–439.

Kao, C. C., Shimizu, Y., Perkins, L. C., and Freeman, L. W. (1970): Experimental use of cultured cerebellar cortical tissue to inhibit the collagenous scar following spinal cord transection. *J. Neurosurg.*, 33:127–139.

Kao, C. Y. (1966): Tetrodotoxin, saxitoxin and their significance in the study of excitation phenomena. *Pharmacol. Rev.*, 18:997–1049.

Katz, B. (1969): *The Release of Neural Transmitter Substances,* pp. 1–60. Charles C Thomas, Springfield, Ill.

Katz, B., and Miledi, R. (1963): A study of spontaneous miniature potentials in spinal moto-neurones. *J. Physiol. (Lond.),* 168:389–422.

Katz, B., and Miledi, R. (1965a): The measurement of synaptic delay, and the time course of acetylcholine release at the neuromuscular junction. *Proc. R. Soc. Lond. [Biol.],* 161:483–495.

Katz, B., and Miledi, R. (1965b): The effect of calcium on acetylcholine release from motor nerve terminals. *Proc. Soc. Lond. [Biol.],* 161:496–503.

Katz, B., and Miledi, R. (1968): The role of calcium in neuromuscular facilitation. *J. Physiol. (Lond.),* 195:481–492.

Kawai, N., and Yamamoto, C. (1967): Effects of γ-amino-butyric acid on the potentials evoked in vitro in the superior colliculus. *Experientia,* 23:1–4.

Kelly, A. M., and Zacks, S. I. (1969): The fine structure of motor endplate morphogenesis. *J. Cell Biol.,* 42:154–169.

Kennard, D. W. (1958): Glass microcapillary electrodes used for measuring potential in living tissues. In: *Electronic Apparatus for Biological Research,* edited by P. E. K. Donaldson, pp. 534–567. Butterworths, London.

Kiernan, J. A., and Pettit, D. R. (1971): Organ culture of the central nervous system of the adult rat. *Exp. Neurol.,* 32:111–120.

Kim, S. U. (1972a): Light and electron microscope study of mouse cerebral neocortex in tissue culture. *Exp. Neurol.,* 35:305–321.

Kim, S. U. (1972b): Light and electron microscope study of neurons and synapses in neonatal mouse olfactory bulb cultured *in vitro. Exp. Neurol.,* 36:336–349.

Kim, S. U., Oh, T. H., and Johnson, D. D. (1972): Developmental changes of acetylcho-linesterase and pseudocholinesterase in organotypic cultures of spinal cord. *Exp. Neurol.,* 35:274–281.

Kim, S. U., Oh, T. H., and Wenger, E. L. (1974): Biochemical and cytochemical studies of the development of choline acetyltransferase and acetylcholinesterase in organotypic cultures of chick neural tube. *J. Neurobiol.,* 5:305–315.

Klinkerfuss, G. H., and Haugh, M. J. (1970): Disuse atrophy of muscle. *Arch. Neurol.,* 22:309–320.

Ko, C.-P., Burton, H., and Bunge, R. P. (1975): Cholinergic synapses between spinal cord and sympathetic neurons in tissue culture. In: *Society of Neuroscience, 5th Annual Meeting, New York,* p. 816.

Ko, C.-P., Burton, H., and Bunge, R. P. (1976a): Synaptic transmission between rat spinal cord explants and dissociated superior cervical ganglion neurons in tissue culture. *Brain Res. (in press).*

Ko, C.-P., Burton, H., Johnson, M. I., and Bunge, R. P. (1976b): Synaptic transmission be-tween rat superior cervical ganglion neurons in dissociated cell cultures. *Brain Res. (in press).*

Kobayashi, T., Inman, O., Buno, W., and Himwich, H. E. (1963): A multidisciplinary study of changes in mouse brain with age. *Recent Adv. Biol. Psychiatry,* 5:293–308.

Koketsu, K. (1969): Cholinergic synaptic potentials and the underlying ionic mechanisms. *Fed. Proc.,* 28:101–112.

Koketsu, K., and Nishi, S. (1969): Calcium and action potentials of bullfrog sympathetic ganglion cells. *J. Gen. Physiol.,* 53:608–623.

König, N., Roch, G., and Marty, R. (1975): The onset of synaptogenesis in rat temporal cortex. *Anat. Embryol.,* 148:73–87

Konigsberg, U. R., Lipton, B. H., and Konigsberg, I. R. (1975): The regenerative response of single mature muscle fibers isolated in vitro. *Dev. Biol.,* 45:260–275.

Kopac, M. J. (1959): Micrurgical studies on living cells. In: *The Cell,* Vol. 1, edited by J. Brachet and A. E. Mirsky, pp. 161–192. Academic Press, New York.

Kopac, M. J. (1964): Micromanipulators: principles of design, operation, and application. In: *Physical Techniques in Biological Research,* Vol. V, Part A, edited by W. L. Nastuk, pp. 193–233. Academic Press, New York.

Korneliussen, H. (1972): Ultrastructure of normal and stimulated motor endplates. *Z. Zell-forsch.,* 130:28–57.

Kravitz, E. A., Talamo, B. R., Grossfeld, R. M., and Epstein, K. (1973): Demonstration of lobster CNS tissue in monolayer cell culture. *Biol. Bull.,* 145:444.

Kristiansen, K., and Courtois, G. (1949): Rhythmic electrical activity from isolated cerebral cortex. *Electroencephalogr. Clin. Neurophysiol.,* 1:265–272.

Krnjevic, K., and Miledi, R. (1958): Some effects produced by adrenaline upon neuromuscular propagation in rats. *J. Physiol. (Lond.),* 141:291–304.

Kudo, Y., Abe, N., Goto, S., and Fukuda, H. (1975): The chloride-dependent depression by GABA in the frog spinal cord. *Eur. J. Pharmacol.,* 32:251–259.

Kuffler, S. W., Dennis, M. J., and Harris, A. J. (1971): The development of chemosensitivity in extra-synaptic areas of the neuronal surface after denervation of parasympathetic ganglion cells in the heart of the frog. *Proc. R. Soc. Lond. [Biol.],* 177:555–563.

Kuo, Z.-Y. (1967): *The Dynamics of Behavior Development,* p. 25. Random House, New York.

Kuperman, A. S., Altura, B. T., and Chezar, J. A. (1968): Action of procaine on calcium efflux from frog nerve and muscle. *Nature (Lond.),* 217:673–675.

Kuromi, H., and Hasagawa, S. (1975): Neurotrophic effect of spinal cord extract on membrane potentials of organ-cultured mouse skeletal muscle. *Brain Res.,* 100:178–181.

Lahdesmaki, P., and Oja, S. S. (1972): Effect of electrical stimulation in the influx and efflux of taurine in brain slices of newborn and adult rats. *Exp. Brain Res.,* 15:430–438.

Lambert, E. H., and Elmqvist, D. (1971): Quantal components of end-plate potentials in the myasthenic syndrome. *Ann. N.Y. Acad. Sci.,* 183:183–199.

Landmesser, L. (1971): Contractile and electrical responses of vagus-innervated frog sartorius muscles. *J. Physiol. (Lond.),* 213:707–725.

LaVail, J. H., and Wolf, M. K. (1973): Postnatal development of the mouse dentate gyrus in organotypic cultures of the hippocampal formation. *Am. J. Anat.,* 137:47–66.

Lehrer, G. M., Bornstein, M. B., Weiss, C., and Silides, D. J. (1970): Enzymatic maturation of mouse cerebral neocortex in vitro and in situ. *Exp. Neurol.,* 26:595–606.

Lehrman, D. S. (1953): A critique of Konrad Lorenz's theory of instinctive behavior. *Q. Rev. Biol.,* 28:337–363.

Leiman, A. L., and Seil, F. J. (1973): Spontaneous and evoked bioelectric activity in organized cerebellar tissue cultures. *Exp. Neurol.,* 40:748–758.

Leiman, A. L., Seil, F. J., and Kelly, J. M. (1975): Maturation of electrical activity of cerebral neocortex in tissue culture. *Exp. Neurol.,* 48:275–291.

Lentz, T. L. (1971): Nerve trophic function: In vitro assay of effects of nerve tissue on muscle cholinesterase activity. *Science,* 171:187–189.

Lentz, T. L. (1972): A role of cyclic AMP in a neurotrophic process. *Nature [New Biol.],* 238:154–155.

Lentz, T. L. (1974): Neurotrophic regulation at the neuromuscular junction. *Ann. N.Y. Acad. Sci.,* 228:323–337.

Levi, G. (1915–1916): La constitusione del protoplasma studiata su cellule viventi coltivati in vitro. *Arch. Fisiol.,* 14:101–112.

Levi, G., and Meyer, H. (1937): Die Struktur der lebenden Neuronen: Die Frage der Pra-existenz der Neurofibrillen. *Anat. Anz.,* 83:401.

Levi, G., and Meyer, H. (1938): Présentation de cultures d'un nombre restreint d-éléments nerveux avec quelques considerations sur les rapports d'interdepéndence entre les neurones. *C. R. Assoc. Anat.,* 33:321–328.

Levi, G., and Meyer, H. (1945): Reactive, regressive and regenerative processes of neurons, cultivated in vitro and injured with micromanipulator. *J. Exp. Zool.,* 99:141–182.

Levi-Montalcini, R. (1958): Chemical stimulation of nerve growth. In: *Symposium on the Chemical Basis of Development,* edited by W. D. McElroy and B. Glass, pp. 646–664. Johns Hopkins Press, Baltimore.

Levi-Montalcini, R., and Angeletti, P. U. (1963): Essential role of the nerve growth factor in the survival and maintenance of dissociated sensory and sympathetic embryonic nerve cells in vitro. *Dev. Biol.,* 7:653–659.

Levi-Montalcini, R., and Angeletti, P. U. (1968a): Biological aspects of the nerve growth factor. In: *Ciba Foundation Symposium, Growth of the Nervous System,* edited by G. E. W. Wolstenholme and M. O'Connor, pp. 126–147. Churchill, London.

Levi-Montalcini, R., and Angeletti, P. U. (1968*b*): Nerve growth factor. *Physiol. Rev.,* 48:534–569.

Levi-Montalcini, R., and Booker, B. (1960): Excessive growth of the sympathetic ganglia evoked by a protein isolated from mouse salivary glands. *Proc. Natl. Acad. Sci. U.S.A.,* 46:373–384.

Levi-Montalcini, R., and Cohen, S. (1960): Effects of the extract of the mouse submaxillary salivary glands on the sympathetic system of mammals. *Ann. N.Y. Acad. Sci.,* 85:324–341.

Levi-Montalcini, R., and Seshan, K. R. (1973): Long-term cultures of embryonic and mature insect nervous and neuroendocrine systems. In: *Tissue Culture of the Nervous System,* edited by G. Sato, pp. 1–33. Plenum Press, New York.

Levitt, P., Moore, R. Y., and Garber, B. B. (1975): Brain histogenesis in vitro: Reconstruction of substantia nigra structures in midbrain cell aggregates. In: *Society of Neuroscience, 5th Annual Meeting, New York,* p. 743.

Li, C.-L., Cullen, C., and Jasper, H. H. (1956): Laminar microelectrode analysis of cortical unspecific recruiting responses and spontaneous rhythms. *J. Neurophysiol.,* 19:131–143.

Li, C. L., Engel, K., and Klatzo, I. (1959): Some properties of cultured chick skeletal muscle with particular reference to fibrillation potential. *J. Cell. Comp. Physiol.,* 53:421–444.

Liberman, E. A., Minina, S. V., and Golubstov, K. V. (1975): The study of metabolic synapse. I. Effect of intracellular microinjection of 3'-5'-AMP. *Biofizika,* 20:451–456.

Libet, B., and Gerard, R. W. (1939): Control of the potential rhythm of the isolated frog brain. *J. Neurophysiol.,* 2:153–169.

Libet, B., Alberts, W. W., Wright, E. W., Delattre, L. D., Levin, G., and Feinstein, B. (1964): Production of threshold levels of conscious sensation by electrical stimulation of human somatosensory cortex. *J. Neurophysiol.,* 27:546–578.

Lieberman, M. (1967): Effects of cell density and low K on action potentials of cultured chick hearts. *Circ. Res.,* 21:879–888.

Llinás, R. (1975): Electroresponsive properties of dendrites in central neurons. In: *Advances in Neurology,* Vol. 12, edited by G. W. Kreutzberg, pp. 1–13. Raven Press, New York.

Llinás, R., Blinks, J. R., and Nicholson, C. (1972): Calcium transient in presynaptic terminal of squid giant synapse: Detection with aequorin. *Science,* 176:1127–1129.

Lodin, Z., Faltin, J., Booher, J., Hartman, J., and Sensenbrenner, M. (1973): Formation of intercellular contacts in cultures of dissociated neurons from embryonic chicken dorsal root ganglia. *Neurobiology,* 3:376–390.

Lømo, T., and Rosenthal, J. (1972): Control of ACh sensitivity of muscle activity in the rat. *J. Physiol. (Lond.),* 221:493–513.

Lumsden, C. E. (1951): Aspects of neurite outgrowth in tissue culture. *Anat. Rec.,* 110:145–179.

Lumsden, C. E. (1968): Nervous tissue in culture. In: *The Structure and Function of Nervous Tissue,* edited by G. H. Bourne, pp. 67–140. Academic Press, New York.

Lumsden, C. E. (1972): The clinical immunology of multiple sclerosis. In: *Multiple Sclerosis,* edited by D. McAlpine, C. E. Lumsden, and E. D. Acheson, pp. 512–621. Churchill Livingstone, London.

Lumsden, C. E., Howard, L., Aparicio, S. R., and Bradbury, M. (1975): Antisynaptic antibody in allergic encephalomyelitis. II. The synapse-blocking effects in tissue culture of demyelinating sera from experimental allergic encephalomyelitis. *Brain Res.,* 93:283–299.

Mains, R. E., and Patterson, P. H. (1973): Primary cultures of dissociated sympathetic neurons. I. Establishment of long-term growth in culture and studies of differentiated properties. *J. Cell Biol.,* 59:329–345.

Mark, V. H., and Gasteiger, E. L. (1953): Observations on the role of afferent and descending impulses on the spontaneous potentials of the spinal cord. *Electroencephalogr. Clin. Neurophysiol.,* 5:251–258.

Marks, B. H., Sakai, K. K., George, J. M., and Koestner, A. (1973): Effects of catecholamines on supra-optic nucleus neurones in organ cultures. In: *Frontiers in Catecholamine Research,* edited by E. Usdin and S. Snyder, pp. 811–813. Pergamon Press, London.

Marsh, G., and Beams, H. W. (1946): In vitro control of growing chick nerve fibers by applied electric currents. *J. Cell. Comp. Physiol.,* 27:139–157.

Marshall, K. C., Wojtowicz, J. M., and Hendelman, W. J. (1975): Depression by magnesium ion of neuronal excitability in tissue cultures of cerebellum. *Society of Neuroscience, 5th Annual Meeting, New York,* p. 814.

Masurovsky, E. B., and Benitez, H. H. (1967): Apparent innervation of chick cardiac muscle by sympathetic neurons in organized culture. *Anat. Rec.*, 157:285.

Masurovsky, E. B., and Bunge, R. P. (1968): Fluoroplastic coverslips for long-term nerve tissue culture. *Stain Technol.*, 43:161–165.

Masurovsky, E. B., and Peterson, E. R. (1973): Photo-reconstituted collagen gel for tissue culture substrates. *Exp. Cell Res.*, 76:447–448.

Masurovsky, E. B., Benitez, H. H., and Murray, M. R. (1972): Synaptic development in long-term organized cultures of murine hypothalamus. *J. Comp. Neurol.*, 143:263–278.

Masurovsky, E. B., Peterson, E. R., and Crain, S. M. (1971): ACLAR film reticles for precise cell localization in nerve tissue cultures. *In Vitro*, 6:379.

Matsumoto, H., and Ajmone Marsan, C. (1964): Cortical cellular phenomena in experimental epilepsy: Interictal manifestations. *Exp. Neurol.*, 9:286–304.

Matthew, S. A., and Detwiler, S. R. (1926): The reaction of Amblystoma embryos following prolonged treatment with chloretone. *J. Exp. Zool.*, 45:279–292.

Maximow, A. (1925): Tissue cultures of young mammalian embryos. *Contr. Embryol. Carnegie Inst.*, 16:47–114.

May, M. K., and Biscoe, T. J. (1975): An investigation of the foetal rat spinal cord. II. An ultrastructural study on the development of synapses with the aid of observations on some electrophysiological properties. *Cell Tissue Res.*, 158:251–268.

Maynard, D. M. (1972): Simpler networks. *Ann. N.Y. Acad. Sci.*, 193:59–72.

McAfee, D. A., and Greengard, P. (1972): Adenosine 3′,5′-monophosphate: Electrophysiological evidence for a role in synaptic transmission. *Science*, 178:310–312.

McDonald, W. I. (1974): Pathophysiology in multiple sclerosis. *Brain*, 97:179–196.

McIlwain, H. (1963): *Chemical Exploration of the Brain, A Study of Cerebral Excitability and Ion Movement.* Elsevier, Amsterdam.

McLaughlin, B. J., Barber, R., Saito, K., Roberts, E., and Wu, J. Y. (1975): Immunocytochemical localization of glutamate decarboxylase in rat spinal cord. *J. Comp. Neurol.*, 164:305–322.

McLennan, H. (1971): The pharmacology of inhibition of mitral cells in the olfactory bulb. *Brain Res.*, 29:177–184.

Meller, K., Breipohl, W., Wagner, H. H., and Knuth, A. (1969): Die Differenzierung isolierter Nerven-und Gliazellen aus trypsiniertem Ruckenmark von Huhnerembryonen in Gewebekulturen. *Z. Zellforsch.*, 101:135–151.

Mendez, J., Aranda, L. C., and Luco, J. V. (1970): Antifibrillary effect of adrenergic fibers on denervated striated muscles. *J. Neurophysiol.*, 33:882–890.

Mettler, F. A., Grundfest, H., Crain, S. M., and Murray, M. R. (1952): Spontaneous electrical activity from tissue cultures. *Trans. Am. Neurol. Assoc.*, 77:52–53.

Meyerson, B. A., and Persson, H. E. (1974): Early epigenesis of recipient functions in the neocortex. In: *Aspects of Neurogenesis, Vol. 2: Studies on the Development of Behavior and the Nervous System,* edited by G. Gottlieb, pp. 171–204. Academic Press, New York.

Miledi, R., and Thies, R. E. (1967): Post-tetanic increase in frequency of miniature end-plate potentials in calcium-free solutions. *J. Physiol. (Lond.)*, 192:54–55.

Miller, R., Varon, S., Kruger, L., Coates, P. W., and Orkand, P. M. (1970): Formation of synaptic contacts on dissociated chick embryo sensory ganglion cells in vitro. *Brain Res.*, 24:356–358.

Miller, W. H., Gorman, R. E., and Bitensky, M. W. (1971): Cyclic adenosine monophosphate: Function in photoreceptors. *Science*, 174:295–297.

Miyata, Y., and Otsuka, M. (1972): Distribution of γ-aminobutyric acid in cat spinal cord and the alteration produced by local ischaemia. *J. Neurochem.*, 19:1833–1834.

Model, P. G., Bornstein, M. B., Crain, S. M., and Pappas, G. D. (1971): An electron microscopic study of the development of synapses in cultured fetal mouse cerebrum continuously exposed to Xylocaine. *J. Cell Biol.*, 49:362–371.

Molliver, M. E. (1967): An ontogenetic study of evoked somesthetic cortical responses in the sheep. *Prog. Brain Res.*, 26:78–91.

Molliver, M. E., and Van der Loos, H. (1970): The ontogenesis of cortical circuitry: The spatial distribution of synapses in somesthetic cortex of newborn dog. *Adv. Anat. Embryol. Cell Biol.*, 42:1–53.

Mong, F. S. F. (1975): Nervous influences on minced muscle regeneration in rats. *Anat. Rec.*, 181:429.

Morrell, F. (1961): Electrophysiological contributions to neural basis of learning. *Physiol. Rev.*, 41:443–494.

Morrell, F. (1963): Effect of transcortical polarizing currents. In: *Brain Function*, Vol. 1, pp. 125–176. University of California Press, Berkeley.

Moscona, A. A. (1965): Recombination of dissociated cells and the development of cell aggregates. In: *Cells and Tissues in Culture*, edited by E. N. Willmer, pp. 489–529. Academic Press, New York.

Moscona, A. A., Trowell, O. A., and Willmer, E. N. (1965): Methods. In: *Cells and Tissues in Culture*, Vol. 1, edited by E. N. Willmer, pp. 19–98. Academic Press, New York.

Muchmore, W. B. (1968): The influence of neural tissue on the early development of somatic muscle in ventrolateral implants in Ambystoma. *J. Exp. Zool.*, 169:251–257.

Murray, M. R. (1959): Factors bearing on myelin formation in vitro. In: *The Biology of Myelin*, edited by S. R. Korey, pp. 201–229. Harper & Row, New York.

Murray, M. R. (1965a): Muscle tissues in vitro. In: *Cells and Tissues in Culture*, Vol. 2, edited by E. N. Willmer, pp. 311–372. Academic Press, New York.

Murray, M. R. (1965b): Nervous tissues in vitro. In: *Cells and Tissues in Culture*, Vol. 2, edited by E. N. Willmer, pp. 373–455. Academic Press, New York.

Murray, M. R. (1971): Nervous tissues isolated in culture. In: *Handbook of Neurochemistry*, Vol. 5A, edited by A. Lajtha, pp. 373–438. Plenum Press, New York.

Murray, M. R. (1972): Skeletal muscle in culture. In: *Structure and Function*, Vol. 1, 2nd ed., edited by G. H. Bourne, pp. 237–299. Academic Press, New York.

Murray, M. R., and Kopech, G. (1953): *A Bibliography of the Research in Tissue Culture*, Vols. I and II. Academic Press, New York.

Murray, M. R., and Peterson, E. R. (1965): Action of cortisone in myelinated cultures of nervous tissues, pp. E221–222. Excerpta Medica Foundation Congress Series 94. Excerpta Medica Foundation, Amsterdam.

Murray, M. R., and Stout, A. P. (1947): Adult human sympathetic ganglion cells cultivated in vitro. *Am. J. Anat.*, 80:225–273.

Myslivecek, J. (1970): Electrophysiology of the developing brain. In: *Developmental Neurobiology*, edited by W. A. Himwich, pp. 475–527. Charles C Thomas, Springfield, Ill.

Naka, K.-I. (1964): Electrophysiology of the fetal spinal cord. II. Interaction among peripheral inputs and recurrent inhibition. *J. Gen. Physiol.*, 47:1023–1038.

Nakai, J. (1956): Dissociated dorsal root ganglia in tissue culture. *Am. J. Anat.*, 99:81–130.

Nakai, J. (1965): Skeletal muscle in organ culture. *Exp. Cell Res.*, 40:307–315.

Nandy, K. (1972): Brain-reactive antibodies in serum of germ-free mice. *Mech. Ageing Dev.*, 1:133–138.

Nandy, K. (1973): Brain-reactive antibodies in serum of aged mice. *Prog. Brain Res.*, 40:437–454.

Narayanan, C. H., Fox, M. W., and Hamburger, V. (1971): Prenatal development of spontaneous and evoked activity in the rat (Rattus norvegicus albinus). *Behaviour*, 40:100–134.

Nelson, P. G. (1967): Brain mechanisms and memory. In: *The Neurosciences: A Study Program*, edited by G. C. Quarton, T. Melnechuk, and F. O. Schmitt, pp. 772–775. Rockefeller University Press, New York.

Nelson, P. G. (1973): Electrophysiological studies of normal and neoplastic cells in tissue culture. In: *Tissue Culture of the Nervous System*, edited by G. Sato, pp. 135–160. Plenum Press, New York.

Nelson, P. G. (1975): Nerve and muscle cells in culture. *Physiol. Rev.*, 55:1–61.

Nelson, P. G., Christian, C. N., and Nirenberg, M. W. (1976): Synapse formation between clonal neuroblastoma × glioma hybrid cells and striated muscle cells. *Proc. Natl. Acad. Sci. U.S.A.*, 73:123–127.

Nelson, P. G., and Peacock, J. H. (1973): Electrical activity in dissociated cell cultures from fetal mouse cerebellum. *Brain Res.*, 61:163–174.

Nicholls, J. G., and Baylor, D. A. (1968): Specific modalities and receptive fields of sensory neurons in the CNS of the leech. *J. Neurophysiol.*, 31:740–756.

Nicholls, J. G., and Van Essen, D. (1974): The nervous system of the leech. *Sci. Am.*, 230:38–48.

Nicholls, J. G., Miyazaki, S., and Wallace, B. (1976): Modification and regeneration of synaptic connections in cultured leech ganglia. *Cold Spring Harbor Symp. Quant. Biol.*, (in press).

Nicoll, R. A. (1971): Pharmacological evidence for GABA as the transmitter in granule cell inhibition in the olfactory bulb. *Brain Res.,* 35:137–149.

Nishi, S., Minota, S., and Karczmar, A. G. (1974): Primary afferent neurones: The ionic mechanism of GABA-mediated depolarization. *Neuropharmacol.,* 13:215–219.

Nurse, C. A., and O'Lague, P. H. (1975): Formation of cholinergic synapses between dissociated sympathetic neurons and skeletal myotubes of the rat in cell culture. *Proc. Natl. Acad. Sci. U.S.A.,* 72:1955–1959.

Obata, K. (1974): Transmitter sensitivities of some nerve and muscle cells in culture. *Brain Res.,* 73:71–88.

Oh, T. H. (1975): Neurotrophic effects: Characterization of the nerve extract that stimulates muscle development in culture. *Exp. Neurol.,* 46:432–438.

Oh, T. H., Johnson, D. D., and Kim, S. U. (1972): Neurotrophic effect on isolated chick embryo muscle in culture. *Science,* 178:1298–1330.

Okun, L. M. (1972): Isolated dorsal root ganglion neurons in culture: Cytological maturation and extension of electrically active processes. *J. Neurobiol.,* 3:111–151.

Okun, L. M., Ontkean, F. K., and Thomas, C. A. (1972): Removal of non-neuronal cells from suspension of dissociated embryonic dorsal root ganglia. *Exp. Cell Res.,* 73:226–229.

O'Lague, P. H., MacLeish, P. R., Nurse, C., Claude, P., Furshpan, E. J., and Potter, D. D. (1976): Physiological and morphological studies of developing sympathetic neurons in dissociated cell culture. *Cold Spring Harbor Symp. Quant. Biol. (in press).*

O'Lague, P. H., Obata, K., Claude, P., Furshpan, E. J., and Potter, D. D. (1974): Evidence for cholinergic synapses between dissociated rat sympathetic neurons in cell culture. *Proc. Natl. Acad. Sci. U.S.A.,* 71:3602–3603.

Olson, L. (1967): Outgrowth of sympathetic adrenergic neurons in mice treated with a nerve-growth factor (NGF). *Z. Zellforsch.,* 81:155–173.

Olson, L., Freedman, R., Seiger, A., and Hoffer, B. (1976): Electrophysiology and cytology of hippocampal formation transplants in the anterior chamber of the eye. I. Intrinsic organization. *Brain Res. (in press).*

Olson, L., and Seiger, A. (1972): Brain tissue transplanted to the anterior chamber of the eye. I. Fluorescence histochemistry of immature catecholamine and 5-hydroxytryptamine neurons reinnervating the rat iris. *Z. Zellforsch.,* 135:175–194.

Olson, L., and Seiger, A. (1973): Development and growth of immature neurons in rat and man in situ and following intraocular transplantation in the rat. *Brain Res.,* 62:353–360.

Olson, L., and Seiger, A. (1974): Nerve growth specificity and regulation as revealed by intraocular brain tissue transplants. In: *Dynamics of Degeneration and Growth in Neurons,* edited by K. Fuxe, L. Olson, and Y. Zotterman, pp. 499–508. Pergamon Press, New York.

Olson, L., and Seiger, A. (1975): Brain tissue transplanted to the anterior chamber of the eye. 2. Fluorescence histochemistry of immature catecholamine- and 5-hydroxytryptamine neurons innervating the rat vas deferens. *Cell Tissue Res.,* 158:141–150.

Olson, M. I., and Bunge, R. P. (1973): Anatomical observations on the specificity of synapse formation in tissue culture. *Brain Res.,* 59:19–33.

Olson, M. I., and Bunge, R. P. (1974): Spinal cord transection: results of implanting cultured embryonic spinal cord at the transection site. In: *Society of Neuroscience, 4th Annual Meeting, St. Louis,* p. 363.

Oppenheim, R. W. (1975): The role of supraspinal input in embryonic motility: A re-examination in the chick. *J. Comp. Neurol.,* 160:37–50.

Oppenheim, R. W., and Reitzel, J. (1975): The ontogeny of behavioral sensitivity to strychnine in the chick embryo: Evidence for the early onset of CNS inhibition. *Brain Behav. Evol.* 11:130–159.

Oppenheim, R. W., Chu-Wang, I-W., and Foelix, R. F. (1975): Some aspects of synaptogenesis in the spinal cord of the chick embryo: A quantitative electron microscopic study. *J. Comp. Neurol.,* 161:383–418.

Oppenheim, R. W., Reitzel, J., and Provine, R. (1972): The behavioral onset of inhibitory mechanisms in the chick embryo. In: *Society of Neuroscience, 2nd Annual Meeting, Houston, Texas,* p. 91.

Otsuka, M., and Konishi, S. (1974): Electrophysiology of mammalian spinal cord in vitro. *Nature (Lond.),* 252:733.

Otsuka, M., and Konishi, S. (1975): GABA in the spinal cord. In: *GABA in Nervous System*

Function, edited by E. Roberts, T. N. Chase, and D. Tower, pp. 197–202. Raven Press, New York.

Otsuka, M., Kravitz, E. A., and Potter, D. D. (1967): Physiologic and chemical architecture of a lobster ganglion with particular reference to gamma-amino butyrate and glutamate. *J. Neurophysiol.,* 30:725–752.

Padjen, A., Forman, D. S., and Siggins, G. R. (1975): Longterm growth and electrophysiological properties of peripheral ganglia of adult frog in vitro. In: *Society of Neuroscience, 5th Annual Meeting, New York,* p. 813.

Palacios, E., Garber, B. B., and Larramendi, L. M. H. (1975): The "reazione nera:" a tool for the analysis of neuronal aggregates reconstituted in vitro from dissociated embryonic brain cells. In: *Golgi Centennial Symposium,* edited by M. Santini, pp. 593–601. Raven Press, New York.

Pannese, E., Luciano, L., Urato, S., and Reale, E. (1971): Cholinesterase activity in ganglia neuroblasts: A histochemical study at the electron microscope. *J. Ultrastruct. Res.,* 36:46–67.

Pappas, G. D. (1966): Electron microscopy of neuronal junctions involved in transmission in the central nervous system. In: *Nerve as a Tissue,* edited by K. Rodahl and B. Issekutz, pp. 49–87. Hoeber, New York.

Pappas, G. D., Fox, G. Q., Masurovsky, E. B., Peterson, E. R., and Crain, S. M. (1975): Differentiation in neuronal growth cone relationships in the mammalian CNS. In: *Advances in Neurology, Vol. 12: Physiology and Pathology of Dendrites,* edited by G. W. Kreutzberg, pp. 163–180. Raven Press, New York.

Pappas, G. D., Peterson, E. R., Masurovsky, E. B., and Crain, S. M. (1971*a*): The fine structure of developing neuromuscular synapses in vitro. *Ann. N.Y. Acad. Sci.,* 183:33–45.

Pappas, G. D., Peterson, E. R., Masurovsky, E. B., and Crain, S. M. (1971*b*): The fine structure of developing neuromuscular synapses in vitro. *Anat. Rec.,* 169:395–396.

Paterson, P. Y. (1969): Immune processes and infectious factors in central nervous system disease. In: *Annual Review of Medicine,* edited by A. C. DeGraff, pp. 75–100. Annual Reviews, Inc., California.

Patterson, P. H., and Chun, L. L. Y. (1974): The influence of non-neuronal cells on catecholamine and acetylcholine synthesis and accumulation in cultures of dissociated sympathetic neurons. *Proc. Natl. Acad. Sci. USA,* 71:3607–3610.

Patterson, P. H., Reichardt, L. F., and Chun, L. L. Y. (1976): Biochemical studies on the development of primary sympathetic neurons in cell culture. *Cold Spring Harbor Symp. Quant. Biol. (in press).*

Peach, M. J. (1972): Stimulation of release of adrenal catecholamine by adenosine $3':5'$cyclic monophosphate and theophylline in the absence of extracellular Ca^{2+}. *Proc. Natl. Acad. Sci. U.S.A.,* 69:834–836.

Peacock, J. H., and Nelson, P. G. (1973): Chemosensitivity of mouse neuroblastoma cells in vitro. *J. Neurobiol.,* 4:363–374.

Peacock, J. H., Nelson, P. G., and Goldstone, M. W. (1973): Electrophysiologic study of cultured neurons dissociated from spinal cords and dorsal root ganglia of fetal mice. *Dev. Biol.,* 30:137–152.

Perri, V., Sacchi, O., and Casella, C. (1970): Electrical properties and synaptic connections of the sympathetic neurons in the rat and guinea pig superior cervical ganglion. *Pfluegers Arch.,* 314:40–54.

Peterson, E. R. (1950): Production of myelin sheaths in vitro by embryonic spinal ganglion cells. *Anat. Rec.,* 106:232.

Peterson, E. R., and Crain, S. M. (1970): Innervation in cultures of fetal rodent skeletal muscle by organotypic explants of spinal cord from different animals. *Z. Zellforsch.,* 106:1–21.

Peterson, E. R., and Crain, S. M. (1972): Regeneration and innervation in cultures of adult mammalian skeletal muscle coupled with fetal rodent spinal cord. *Exp. Neurol.,* 36:136–159.

Peterson, E. R., and Crain, S. M. (1973): CNS regeneration and formation of new functional connections in vitro after transfer of mature spinal cord cultures. *Anat. Rec.,* 175:411–412.

Peterson, E. R., and Crain, S. M. (1975): Selective growth of neurites from isolated fetal mouse dorsal root ganglia toward specific CNS target tissues. In: *Society of Neuroscience, 5th Annual Meeting, New York,* p. 783.

Peterson, E. R., and Murray, M. R. (1955): Myelin sheath formation in cultures of avian spinal ganglia. *Am. J. Anat.,* 96:319–356.

Peterson, E. R., Crain, S. M., and Murray, M. R. (1965): Differentiation and prolonged maintenance of bioelectrically active spinal cord cultures (rat, chick and human). *Z. Zellforsch.,* 66:130–154.

Peterson, E. R., Masurovsky, E. B., and Crain, S. M. (1974): Enhanced survival and selective 'hypertrophy' of dorsal root ganglia after exposure of fetal rodent spinal cord-ganglion explants to nerve growth factor. *J. Cell Biol.,* 63:265a.

Phillips, C. G., Powell, T. P. S., and Shepherd, G. M. (1963): Responses of mitral cells to stimulation of the lateral olfactory tract in the rabbit. *J. Physiol. (Lond.),* 168:65–88.

Phillis, J. W., and York, D. H. (1968a): An intracortical cholinergic inhibitory synapse. *Life Sci.,* 7:65–69.

Phillis, J. W., and York, D. H. (1968b): Pharmacological studies on a cholinergic inhibition in the cerebral cortex. *Brain Res.,* 10:297–306.

Politoff, A., Blitz, A. L., and Rose, S. (1975): Incorporation of acetylcholinesterase into synaptic vesicles is associated with blockade of synaptic transmission. *Nature (Lond.),* 256:324–325.

Pollack, E. D., and Crain, S. M. (1972): Development of motility in fish embryos in relation to release from early CNS inhibition. *J. Neurobiol.,* 3:381–385.

Pomerat, C. M., and Costero, I. (1956): Tissue cultures of cat cerebellum. *Am. J. Anat.,* 99:211–247.

Potter, D. D., Furshpan, E. J., and Lennox, E. S. (1966): Connections between cells of the developing squid as revealed by electrophysiological methods. *Proc. Natl. Acad. Sci. U.S.A.,* 55:328–336.

Prince, D. A., and Gutnick, M. J. (1972): Neuronal activities in epileptogenic foci of immature cortex. *Brain Res.,* 45:455–468.

Prince, W. T., Berridge, M. J., and Rasmussen, H. (1972): Role of calcium and adenosine-3':5'-cyclic monophosphate in controlling fly salivary gland secretion. *Proc. Natl. Acad. Sci. U.S.A.,* 69:553–557.

Privat, A. (1975): Dendritic growth in vitro. In: *Advances in Neurology,* Vol. 12, edited by G. W. Kreutzberg, pp. 201–216. Raven Press, New York.

Provine, R. R. (1971): Embryonic spinal cord: Synchrony and spatial distribution of polyneuronal burst discharges. *Brain Res.,* 29:155–158.

Provine, R. R. (1972): Ontogeny of bioelectric activity in the spinal cord of the chick embryo and its behavioral implications. *Brain Res.,* 41:365–378.

Provine, R. R. (1973): Neurophysiological aspects of behavior development in the chick embryo. In: *Studies on the Development of Behavior and the Nervous System, Vol. 1: Behavior Embryology,* edited by G. Gottlieb, pp. 77–102. Academic Press, New York.

Provine, R. R., Aloe, L., and Seshan, K. R. (1973): Spontaneous bioelectric activity in long term cultures of the embryonic insect central nervous system. *Brain Res.,* 56:364–370.

Provine, R. R., Sharma, S. C., Sandel, T. T., and Hamburger, V. (1970): Electrical activity in the spinal cord of the chick embryo, in situ. *Proc. Natl. Acad. Sci. U.S.A.,* 65:508–515.

Puck, T. T., Cieciura, S. J., and Robinson, A. (1958): Genetics of somatic mammalian cells. III. Long-term cultivation of euploid cells from human and animal subjects. *J. Exp. Med.,* 108:945–956.

Purpura, D. P. (1959): Nature of electrocortical potentials and synaptic organization in the cerebral and cerebellar cortex. *Int. Rev. Neurobiol.,* 1:47–163.

Purpura, D. P. (1960): Pharmacological actions of α-amino acid drugs on different cortical synaptic organizations. In: *Inhibition in the Nervous System and Gamma-Aminobutyric Acid,* edited by E. Roberts, C. F. Baxter, A. Van Harreveld, C. A. G. Wiersma, W. R. Adey, and K. F. Killam, pp. 495–514. Pergamon Press, New York.

Purpura, D. P. (1964): Relationship of seizure susceptibility to morphologic and physiologic properties of normal and abnormal immature cortex. In: *Symposium: Neurological and Electroencephalographic Correlative Studies in Infancy,* edited by P. Kellaway and I. Petersén, pp. 117–157. Grune & Stratton, New York.

Purpura, D. P. (1969): Stability and seizure susceptibility of immature brain. In: *Basic Mechanisms of the Epilepsies,* edited by H. H. Jasper, A. A. Ward, and A. Pope, pp. 481–505. Little, Brown, Boston.

Purpura, D. P. (1971): Synaptogenesis in mammalian cortex: Problems and perspectives. In: *Brain Development and Behavior,* edited by M. B. Sterman, D. J. McGinty, and A. M. Adinolfi, pp. 23–41. Academic Press, New York.

Purpura, D. P. (1972): Ontogenetic models in studies of cortical seizure activities. In: *Experimental Models of Epilepsy,* edited by D. P. Purpura, J. K. Penry, D. Tower, D. M. Woodbury, and R. Walter, pp. 531–556. Raven Press, New York.

Purpura, D. P., and Housepian, E. M. (1961): Morphological and physiological properties of chronically isolated immature neocortex. *Exp. Neurol.,* 4:377–401.

Purpura, D. P., and Reaser, G. P. (1974): *Methodological Approaches to the Study of Brain Maturation and its Abnormalities.* University Park Press, Baltimore.

Purpura, D. P., and Shofer, R. J. (1972): Excitatory action of dibutyryl cyclic adenosine monophosphate on immature cerebral cortex. *Brain Res.,* 38:179–181.

Purpura, D. P., Carmichael, M. W., and Housepian, E. M. (1960): Physiological and anatomical studies of development of superficial axodendritic synaptic pathways in neocortex. *Exp. Neurol.,* 2:324–347.

Purpura, D. P., Prélevic, S., and Santini, M. (1968): Postsynaptic potentials and spike variations in the feline hippocampus during postnatal ontogenesis. *Exp. Neurol.,* 22:408–422.

Purpura, D. P., Shofer, R. J., and Scarff, T. (1965): Properties of synaptic activities and spike potentials of neurons in immature neocortex. *J. Neurophysiol.,* 28:925–942.

Purves, R. D., Hill, C. E., Chamley, J. H., Mark, G. E., Fry, D. M., and Burnstock, G. (1974): Functional autonomic neuromuscular junctions in tissue culture. *Pfluegers Arch.,* 350:1–7.

Ramón y Cajal, S. (1928): *Degeneration and Regeneration of the Nervous System,* edited by R. M. May, pp. 616, 669. Oxford University Press, London.

Ramón y Cajal, S. (1960): *Studies on Vertebrate Neurogenesis,* translated by L. Guth. C. C Thomas, Springfield, Ill.

Ransom, B. R., and Barker, J. L. (1975): Pentobarbital modulates transmitter effects of mouse spinal neurones grown in tissue culture. *Nature (Lond.),* 254:703–705.

Ransom, B. R., and Nelson, P. G. (1975): Neuropharmacological responses from nerve cells in tissue culture. In: *Handbook of Psychopharmacology,* Vol. 2, edited by L. L. Iversen, S. D. Iversen, and S. H. Snyder, pp. 101–127. Plenum Press, New York.

Ransom, B. R., Giller, E. L., and Nelson, P. G. (1974): Chemosensitivity of mouse spinal cord neurons in cell culture. In: *Society of Neuroscience, 4th Annual Meeting, St. Louis,* p. 386.

Rasmussen, H. (1970): Cell communication, calcium ion, and cyclic adenosine monophosphate. *Science,* 170:404–412.

Rees, R., and Bunge, R. P. (1974): Morphological and cytochemical studies of synapses formed in culture between isolated rat superior cervical ganglion neurons. *J. Comp. Neurol.,* 157:1–12.

Reichelt, K. L., and Kvamme, E. (1973): Histamine-dependent formation of N-acetyl-aspartyl peptides in mouse brain. *Neurochemistry,* 21:849–859.

Reyniers, J. A. (1933): Studies in micrurgical technique. V. A moist chamber for tissue culture and cellular dissection. *Anat. Rec.,* 56:295–305.

Richelson, E. (1975): Tissue culture of the nervous system: applications in neurochemistry and psychopharmacology. In: *Handbook of Psychopharmacology,* Vol. 1, edited by L. L. Iversen, S. D. Iversen, and S. H. Snyder, pp. 101–135. Plenum Press, New York.

Ripley, K. L., and Provine, R. R. (1972): Neural correlates of embryonic motility in the chick. *Brain Res.,* 45:127–134.

Ritchie, J. M. (1970): Central nervous stimulants. II. The xanthines. In: *The Pharmacological Basis of Therapeutics,* 4th ed., edited by L. S. Goodman and A. Gilman, pp. 358–370. Macmillan, New York.

Ritter, W., and Vaughan, H. G. (1969): Averaged evoked responses in vigilance and discrimination: A reassessment. *Science,* 164:326–328.

Robbins, N., and Yonezawa, T. (1971): Physiological studies during formation and development of rat neuromuscular junctions in tissue culture. *J. Gen. Physiol.,* 58:467–481.

Roberts, E. (1972): An hypothesis suggesting that there is a defect in the GABA system in schizophrenia. *Neurosci. Res. Prog. Bull.,* 10:468–482.

Roberts, E. (1974): A model of the vertebrate nervous system based largely on disinhibition: a key role of the GABA system. In: *Advances in Behavioral Biology, Vol. 10: Neurohumoral Coding of Brain Function,* edited by R. D. Myers and R. R. Drucker-Colin, pp. 419–449. Plenum Press, New York.

Roberts, E. (1975): Disinhibition as an organizing principle in the nervous system—The role of the GABA system. In: *GABA in Nervous System Function,* edited by E. Roberts, T. N. Chase, and D. B. Tower, pp. 515–539. Raven Press, New York.

Robertson, J. D. (1966): The synapse: morphological and chemical correlates of function. I. Living synapses. In: *Neurosciences Research Symposium Summaries*, Vol. 1, edited by F. O. Schmitt and T. Melnechuk, pp. 470–476. M.I.T. Press, Cambridge, Mass.

Rodnight, R. (1975): Cyclic AMP and protein phosphorylation in the central nervous system in relation to synaptic function. In: *Metabolic Compartmentation and Neurotransmission. Relation to Brain Structure and Function*, edited by S. Berl, D. D. Clarke, and D. J. Schneider, pp. 205–228. Plenum Press, New York.

Rose, G. G., Pomerat, C. M., Shindler, T. O., and Trunnell, J. B. (1958): A cellophane-strip technique for culturing tissue in multipurpose culture chambers. *J. Biophys. Biochem. Cytol.*, 4:761–764.

Rutledge, L. T. (1969): Effect of stimulation on isolated cortex. In: *Basic Mechanisms of the Epilepsies*, edited by H. H. Jasper, A. A. Ward, and A. Pope, pp. 349–355. Little, Brown, Boston.

Sabelli, H. C., DeFoe-May, J., and Bulat, M. (1974): Selective drug effects on motor and sensory nerves: a "Dale's principle" for receptors. In: *Society of Neuroscience, 4th Annual Meeting, St. Louis*, p. 405.

Sakai, K. J., Marks, B. H., George, J. M., and Koestner, A. (1974): The isolated organ-cultured supraoptic nucleus as a neuropharmacological test system. *J. Pharmacol. Exp. Ther.*, 190:482–491.

Sato, G., editor (1973): *Tissue Culture of the Nervous System.* Plenum Press, New York.

Scharf, J. H. (1958): Sensible ganglien. In: *Handbuch der Mikroskopischen Anatomie*, edited by W. Bargmann, pp. 336–352. Springer, Berlin.

Schlapfer, W. T. (1970): Bioelectric activity of neurons in tissue culture: synaptic interactions and effects of environmental changes. Ph.D. thesis, University of California.

Schlapfer, W. T., Mamoon, A.-M., and Tobias, C. A. (1972): Spontaneous bioelectric activity of neurons in cerebellar cultures: Evidence for synaptic interactions. *Brain Res.*, 45:345–363.

Schlumpf, M., and Shoemaker, W. (1975): Synthesis and storage of catecholamines by central and peripheral neurons in vitro. In: *Society of Neuroscience, 5th Annual Meeting, New York*, p. 811.

Schmidt, R. P., Thomas, L. B., and Ward, A. A. (1959): The hyperexcitable neurone: Microelectrode studies of chronic epileptic foci in monkey. *J. Neurophysiol.*, 22:285–296.

Schrier, B. K., Wilson, S. H., and Nirenberg, M. W. (1974): Cultured cell systems and methods for neurobiology. In: *Methods in Enzymology*, Vol. 32, edited by S. Fleischer and L. Packer, pp. 765–788. Academic Press, New York.

Schwartz, I. R., Pappas, G. D., and Purpura, D. P. (1968): Fine structure in the feline hippocampus during postnatal ontogenesis. *Exp. Neurol.*, 22:394–407.

Schwartzkroin, P. A. (1975): Characteristics of CA1 neurons recorded intracellularly in the hippocampal in vitro slice preparation. *Brain Res.*, 85:423–436.

Scott, B. S., Engelberg, V. E., and Fisher, K. C. (1969): Morphological and electrophysiological characteristics of dissociated chick embryonic spinal ganglion cells in culture. *Exp. Neurol.*, 23:230–248.

Sedlacek, J. (1975): Interaction of strychnine and GABA in spontaneous motility of developing chick embryos. *Physiol. Bohemoslov.*, 24:465.

Seecof, R. L., Alleaume, N., Teplitz, R. L., and Gerson, I. (1971): Differentiation of neurons and myocytes in cell cultures made from Drosophila gastrulae. *Exp. Cell Res.*, 69:161–173.

Seecof, R. L., Donady, J. J., and Teplitz, R. L. (1973): Differentiation of Drosophila neuroblasts to form ganglion-like clusters of neurons in vitro. *Cell Differentiation*, 2:143–149.

Seecof, R. L., Teplitz, R. L., Gerson, I., Ikeda, K., and Donady, J. J. (1972): Differentiation of neuromuscular junctions in cultures of embryonic Drosophila cells. *Proc. Natl. Acad. Sci. U.S.A.*, 69:566–570.

Seeds, N. W. (1971): Biochemical differentiation in reaggregating brain cell culture. *Proc. Natl. Acad. Sci. U.S.A.*, 68:1858–1861.

Seeds, N. W. (1973): Differentiation of aggregating brain cell cultures. In: *Tissue Culture of the Nervous System*, edited by G. Sato, pp. 35–53. Plenum Press, New York.

Seeds, N. W., and Vatter, A. E. (1971): Synaptogenesis in reaggregating brain cell culture. *Proc. Natl. Acad. Sci. U.S.A.*, 68:3219–3222.

Segal, M., and Bloom, F. E. (1974): The action of norepinephrine in the rat hippocampus. I. Iontophoretic studies. *Brain Res.*, 72:79–97.

Seiger, A., and Olson, L. (1975): Brain tissue transplanted to the anterior chamber of the eye.
3. Substitution of lacking central noradrenaline input by host iris sympathetic fibers in the
isolated cerebral cortex developed in oculo. *Cell Tissue Res.*, 159:325–338.

Seiger, A., Olson, L., and Farnebo, L.-O. (1976): Brain tissue transplanted to the anterior
chamber of the eye. 4. Drug-modulated transmitter release in central monoamine nerve
terminals lacking normal postsynaptic receptors. *Cell Tissue Res.*, 165:157–170.

Seil, F. (1972): Neuronal groups and fiber patterns in cerebellar tissue cultures. *Brain Res.*,
42:33–51.

Seil, F. J., Kelly, J. M., and Leiman, A. I. (1974): Anatomical organization of cerebral neocortex in tissue culture. *Exp. Neurol.*, 45:435–450.

Seil, F. J., Smith, M. E., Leiman, A. L., and Kelly, J. M. (1975): Myelination inhibiting and
neuroelectric blocking factors in experimental allergic encephalomyelitis. *Science*, 187:951–
953.

Seshan, K. R., Provine, R. R., and Levi-Montalcini, R. (1974): Structural and electrophysiological properties of nymphal and adult insect medial neurosecretory cells: An in vitro
analysis. *Brain Res.*, 78:359–376.

Shagass, C. (1972): *Evoked Brain Potentials in Psychiatry*, pp. 66–69. Plenum Press, New
York.

Shahar, A., Grunfeld, Y., Spiegelstein, M. Y., and Monzain, R. (1975): Myelination in long-
term cultures of dissociated mammalian neurons. *Brain Res.*, 88:44–51.

Sharpless, S. K. (1964): Reorganization of function in the nervous system: Use and disuse.
Ann. Rev. Physiol., 26:357–388.

Sharpless, S. K. (1969): Isolated and deafferented neurons: disuse supersensitivity. In: *Basic
Mechanisms of the Epilepsies*, edited by H. H. Jasper, A. A. Ward, and A. Pope, pp. 329–
348. Little, Brown, Boston.

Shepherd, G. M. (1972): Synaptic organization of the mammalian olfactory bulb. *Physiol. Rev.*,
52:864–917.

Sherrington, C. S. (1951): *Man on His Nature*, 2nd ed., p. 184. Cambridge University Press,
Cambridge, England.

Shevrin, H., and Fritzler, D. E. (1968): Visual evoked response correlates of unconscious
mental processes. *Science*, 161:295–298.

Shevrin, H., Smith, W. H., and Fritzler, D. E. (1971): Average evoked response and verbal
correlates of unconscious mental processes. *Psychophysiology*, 8:149–162.

Shimada, Y., and Fischman, D. A. (1973): Morphological and physiological evidence for the
development of functional neuromuscular junctions in vitro. *Dev. Biol.*, 31:200–225.

Shimada, Y., Fischman, D. A., and Moscona, A. A. (1967): The fine structure of embryonic
chick skeletal muscle cells differentiated in vitro. *J. Cell Biol.*, 35:445–453.

Shimada, Y., Fischman, D. A., and Moscona, A. A. (1969): The development of nerve-muscle
junctions in monolayer cultures of embryonic spinal cord and skeletal muscle cells. *J. Cell
Biol.*, 43:382–387.

Shoemaker, W. J., Schlumpf, M., Forman, D. S., Siggins, G. R., and Bloom, F. E. (1974):
Primary explant cultures of rat brain regions: catecholamine production in brain stem
cultures. In: *Society of Neuroscience, 4th Annual Meeting, St. Louis*, p. 425.

Shtark, M. B., Ratushnjak, A. S., Voskresenskaja, L. V., and Olenev, S. N. (1974): Multielectrode perfusion chamber for the study of tissue culture. *Bull. Exp. Biol.*, 9:122–124.

Shtark, M. B., Stratievsky, V. I., Ratushnjak, A. S., Voskresenskaja, L. V., and Karasev,
N. P. (1976): A comparative statistical study of hippocampal neuronal spontaneous spike
activity in situ and in vitro. *J. Neurobiol. (in press)*.

Shtark, M. B., Voskresenskaja, L. W., Ratushnjak, A. S., Olenev, S. N., and Popov, J. W.
(1972): A study of the impulse activity of the hippocampal neurons in vitro. *Rep. Ac. Sci.
USSR*, 202:731–736.

Sidman, R. L., and Wessells, N. K. (1975): Control of direction of growth during the elongation
of neurites. *Exp. Neurol.*, 48:237–251.

Siggins, G. R., Hoffer, B. J., and Bloom, F. E. (1971*a*): Response to J. M. Godfraind and
R. Pumain: Cyclic adenosine monophosphate and norepinephrine: Effect on Purkinje cells
in rat cerebellar cortex. *Science*, 174:1257–1259.

Siggins, G. R., Oliver, A. P., Hoffer, B. J., and Bloom, F. E. (1971*b*): Cyclic adenosine monophosphate and norepinephrine: Effects on transmembrane properties of cerebellar Purkinje
cells. *Science*, 171:192–194.

Silberberg, D. H. (1972): Cultivation of nerve tissue. In: *Growth, Nutrition and Metabolism of Cells in Culture*, Vol. III, edited by G. H. Rothblatt and V. J. Cristolfalo, pp. 131–167. Academic Press, New York.

Silberstein, S. D., Johnson, D. G., Jacobowitz, D. M., and Kopin, I. J. (1971): Sympathetic reinnervation of the rat iris in organ culture. *Proc. Natl. Acad. Sci. U.S.A.*, 68:1121–1124.

Singer, J. J., and Goldberg, A. L. (1970): Cyclic AMP and transmission at the neuromuscular junction. In: *Role of Cyclic AMP in Cell Function*, edited by P. Greengard and E. Costa, pp. 335–348. Raven Press, New York.

Sisken, B. F., and Smith, S. D. (1975): The effects of minute direct electrical currents on cultured chick embryo trigeminal ganglia. *J. Embryol. Exp. Morphol.*, 33:29–41.

Sobkowicz, H. M., Bereman, B., and Rose, J. E. (1975): Organotypic development of the organ of Corti in culture. *J. Neurocytol.*, 4:543–572.

Sobkowicz, H. M., Bleier, R., and Monzain, R. (1974a): Cell survival and architectonic differentiation of the hypothalamic mamillary region of the newborn mouse in culture. *J. Comp. Neurol.*, 155:355–376.

Sobkowicz, H. M., Bleier, R., Bereman, B., and Monzain, R. (1974b): Axonal growth and organization of the mamillary nuclei of the newborn mouse in culture. *J. Neurocytol.*, 3:431–447.

Sobkowicz, H., Guillery, R. W., and Bornstein, M. B. (1968): Neuronal organization in long term cultures of the spinal cord of the fetal mouse. *J. Comp. Neurol.*, 132:365–396.

Sobkowicz, H. M., Hartmann, H. A., Monzain, R., and Desnoyers, P. (1973): Growth, differentiation and ribonucleic acid content of the fetal rat spinal ganglion cells in culture. *J. Comp. Neurol.*, 148:249–284.

Spencer, W. A., and Kandel, E. R. (1969): Synaptic inhibition in seizures. In: *Basic Mechanisms of the Epilepsies*, edited by H. H. Jasper, A. A. Ward, and A. Pope, pp. 575–602. Little, Brown, Boston.

Sperry, R. W. (1963): Chemoaffinity in the orderly growth of nerve fiber patterns and connections. *Proc. Natl. Acad. Sci. U.S.A.*, 50:703–710.

Sperry, R. W. (1965): Embryogenesis of behavioral nerve nets. In: *Organogenesis*, edited by R. L. DeHaan and H. Ursprung, pp. 161–186. Holt, Rinehart and Winston, New York.

Sperry, R. W. (1971): How a developing brain gets itself properly wired for adaptive function. In: *Biopsychology of Development*, edited by E. Tobach, L. R. Aronson, and E. Shaw, pp. 27–44. Academic Press, New York.

Sperry, R. W., and Hibbard, E. (1968): Regulative factors in the orderly growth of retinotectal connexions. In: *Ciba Foundation Symposium, Growth of the Nervous System*, edited by G. E. W. Wolstenholme and M. O'Connor, pp. 41–52. Churchill, London.

Stavraky, G. W. (1961): *Supersensitivity Following Lesions of the Nervous System.* University of Toronto Press, Toronto.

Stefanelli, A., Zacchei, A. M., Caravita, A., and Ieradi, D. A. (1967): New-forming retinal synapses in vitro. *Experientia*, 23:199–200.

Stenevi, U., Bjerre, B., Bjorklund, A., and Mobley, V. (1974): Effects of localized intracerebral injections of nerve growth factor on the regenerative growth of lesioned central noradrenergic neurones. *Brain Res.*, 69:217–234.

Stokes, B. T., and Bignall, K. E. (1974): The emergence of inhibition in the chick embryo spinal cord. *Brain Res.*, 77:231–242.

Stone, T. W., Taylor, D. A., and Bloom, F. E. (1975): Cyclic AMP and cyclic GMP may mediate opposite neuronal responses in the rat cerebral cortex. *Science*, 187:845–847.

Strumwasser, F. (1971): The cellular basis of behavior in Aplysia. *J. Psychiatr. Res.*, 8:237–257.

Strumwasser, F. (1974): Neuronal principles organizing periodic behaviors. In: *The Neurosciences, Third Study Program*, edited by F. O. Schmitt and F. G. Worden, pp. 459–478. M. I. T. Press, Cambridge, Mass.

Studitsky, A. N. (1963): Dynamics of the development of myogenic tissue under conditions of explantation and transplantation. In: *Cinemicrography in Cell Biology*, edited by G. G. Rose, pp. 171–200. Academic Press, New York.

Székely, G. (1966): Embryonic determination of neural connections. *Adv. Morphog.*, 5:181–219.

Székely, G., and Szentágothai, J. (1962): Experiments with "model nervous system." *Acta Biol. Hung.*, 12:253–268.

Szepsenwol, J. (1941): La participación de las neuronas del arco reflejo en la primera actividad embrionairia. *Soc. Argentina Biol. Rev.,* 17:374–384.

Szepsenwol, J. (1946): A comparison of growth, differentiation, activity and action currents of heart and skeletal muscle in tissue. *Anat. Rec.,* 95:125–146.

Szepsenwol, J. (1947): Electrical excitability and spontaneous activity in explants of skeletal and heart muscle of chick embryos. *Anat. Rec.,* 98:67–85.

Takamori, M. (1972): Caffeine, calcium and Eaton-Lambert syndrome. *Arch. Neurol.,* 27:285–291.

Tapia, R. (1974): The role of γ-aminobutyric acid metabolism in the regulation of cerebral excitability. In: *Advances in Behavioral Biology, Vol. 10: Neurohumoral Coding of Brain Function,* edited by R. D. Myers and R. R. Drucker-Colin, pp. 3–26. Plenum Press, New York.

Teichberg, S., and Holtzman, E. (1973): Axonal agranular reticulum and synaptic vesicles in cultured embryonic chick sympathetic neurons. *J. Cell Biol.,* 57:88–108.

Teichberg, S., Holtzman, E., Crain, S. M., and Peterson, E. R. (1975): Circulation and turnover of synaptic vesicle membrane in cultured fetal mammalian spinal cord neurons. *J. Cell Biol.,* 67:215–230.

Ten Cate, J. (1950): Spontaneous electrical activity of the spinal cord. *Electroencephalogr. Clin. Neurophysiol.,* 2:445–451.

Tennyson, V. M. (1970): The fine structure of the developing nervous system. In: *Developmental Neurobiology,* edited by W. A. Himwich, pp. 47–116. Charles Thomas, Springfield, Ill.

Terävänen, H. (1968): Development of the myoneural junction in the rat. *Z. Zellforsch.,* 87:249–265.

Thomas, C. A., Springer, P. A., Loeb, G. E., Berwald-Netter, Y., and Okun, L. M. (1972): A miniature microelectrode array to monitor the bio-electric activity of cultured cells. *Exp. Cell Res.,* 74:61–66.

Thompson, R. F., and Patterson, M. M. (1973): *Methods in Physiological Psychology, Vol. 1: Bioelectric Recording Techniques: Cellular Processes and Brain Potentials.* Academic Press, New York.

Tinbergen, N. (1950): The hierarchical organization of nervous mechanisms underlying instinctive behaviour. *Symp. Soc. Exp. Biol.,* 4:305–312.

Tischler, A. S., Dichter, M. A., Biales, B., DeLellis, R. A., and Wolfe, H. (1976): Neural properties of cultured human endocrine tumors of neural crest origin. *Science (in press).*

Tischner, K., and Thomas, E. (1973): Development and differentiation of fetal rat sensory ganglia and spinal cord segments in vitro. *Z. Zellforsch.,* 144:339–351.

Toran-Allerand, C. D. (1975): Sex hormone induction of preoptic/hypothalamic development in the newborn mouse in vitro. In: *Society of Neuroscience, 5th Annual Meeting, New York,* p. 775; *Brain Res. (in press).*

Torda, C. (1972): Effect of cyclic adenosine 3′,5′-monophosphate (c-AMP) on synaptic spike generation. *Adv. Cyclic Nucleotide Res.,* 1:589.

Tower, S. S. (1937a): Function and structure in the chronically isolated lumbo-sacral spinal cord of the frog. *J. Comp. Neurol.,* 67:109–131.

Tower, S. S. (1937b): Trophic control of non-nervous tissues by the nervous system: A study of muscle and bone innervated from an isolated and quiescent region of the spinal cord. *J. Comp. Neurol.,* 67:241–267.

Tweedle, C. D., Popiela, H., and Thornton, C. S. (1974): Ultrastructure of the development and subsequent breakdown of muscle in aneurogenic limbs (Ambystoma). *J. Exp. Zool.,* 190:155–166.

Van den Berg, C. J., Van Kempen, G. M. J., Schadé, J. P., and Velstia, H. (1965): Levels and intracellular localization of glutamic decarboxylase and γ-aminobutyric transaminase and other enzymes during the development of the brain. *J. Neurochem.,* 12:863–869.

Vandervael, F. (1945): Contribution à l'étude du tissu nerveux sympathique cultivé in vitro. *Arch. Biol.,* 56:383–393.

Varon, S. (1970): In vitro study of developing neural tissue and cells: past and prospective contributions. In: *The Neurosciences, Second Study Program,* edited by F. O. Schmitt, pp. 83–99. Rockefeller University Press, New York.

Varon, S. (1975): Neurons and glia in neural cultures. *Exp. Neurol.,* 48:93–134.

Varon, S., and Raiborn, C. W. (1969): Dissociation, fractionation, and culture of embryonic brain cells. *Brain Res.,* 12:180–199.

Varon, S., and Raiborn, C. (1971): Excitability and conduction in neurons of dissociated ganglionic cell cultures. *Brain Res.,* 30:83–98.

Varon, S., and Saier, M. (1975): Culture techniques and glial-neuronal interrelationships in vitro. *Exp. Neurol.,* 48:135–162.

Varon, S., Raiborn, C., and Tyszka, E. (1973): In vitro studies of dissociated cells from newborn mouse dorsal root ganglia. *Brain Res.,* 54:51–63.

Vaughn, J. E., and Grieshaber, J. A. (1973): A morphological investigation of an early reflex pathway in developing rat spinal cord. *J. Comp. Neurol.,* 148:177–210.

Vaughn, J. E., Henrikson, C. K., Chernow, C. R., Grieshaber, J. A., and Wimer, C. C. (1975): Genetically-associated variations in the development of reflex movements and synaptic junctions within an early reflex pathway of mouse spinal cord. *J. Comp. Neurol.,* 161:541–554.

Voeller, K., Pappas, G. D., and Purpura, D. P. (1963): Electron microscope study of development of cat superficial neocortex. *Exp. Neurol.,* 7:107–130.

Wagman, I. H., and Battersby, W. S. (1964): Neural limitations of visual excitability. V. Cerebral after-activity evoked by photic stimulation. *Vision Res.,* 4:193–208.

Wakerly, J. B., and Lincoln, D. W. (1971): Phasic discharge of antidromically identified units in the paraventricular nucleus of the hypothalamus. *Brain Res.,* 25:192–194.

Walker, F. D. (1975): Rhythmic neuronal activity in tissue culture. *Experientia,* 31:308–309.

Walker, F. D., and Hild, W. J. (1972): Spreading depression in tissue culture. *J. Neurobiol.,* 3:223–235.

Wall, P. D. (1964): Presynaptic control of impulses at the first central synapse in the cutaneous pathway. *Prog. Brain Res.,* 12:92–118.

Walter, W. G. (1962): Oscillatory activity in the nervous system. I. Spontaneous oscillatory systems and alterations in stability. In: *Neural Physiopathology, Progress in Neurobiology,* Vol. V, edited by R. G. Grenell, pp. 222–257. Hoeber, New York.

Ward, A. A. (1969): The epileptic neuron: chronic foci in animals and man. In: *Basic Mechanisms of the Epilepsies,* edited by H. H. Jasper, A. A. Ward, and A. Pope, pp. 263–288. Little, Brown, Boston.

Weber, A. (1968): The mechanism of the action of caffeine on sarcoplasmic reticulum. *J. Gen. Physiol.,* 52:760–772.

Weiss, P. (1934): In vitro experiments on the factors determining the course of the outgrowing nerve fiber. *J. Exp. Zool.,* 68:393–448.

Weiss, P. (1941a): Further experiments with deplanted and deranged nerve centers in amphibians. *Proc. Soc. Exp. Biol. Med.,* 46:14–15.

Weiss, P. (1941b): Self-differentiation of the basic patterns of coordination. *Comp. Psychol. Monogr.,* 17:1–96.

Weiss, P. (1950): The deplantation of fragments of nervous system in amphibians. *J. Exp. Zool.,* 113:397–461.

Weiss, P. (1955): Nervous system. In: *Analysis of Development,* edited by H. Willier, P. Weiss, and V. Hamburger, pp. 346–401. Saunders, Philadelphia.

Weiss, P. (1966): Specificity in the neurosciences. In: *Neuroscience Research Symposium Summaries,* Vol. 1, edited by F. O. Schmitt and T. Melnechuk, pp. 179–212. M. I. T. Press, Cambridge, Mass.

Weiss, P., and Wang, H. (1936): Neurofibrils in living ganglion cells of the chick, cultivated in vitro. *Anat. Rec.,* 67:105–117.

Wenzel, J., Wenzel, M., Grosse, G., and Kirsche, W. (1973): Elektroenmikroskopische Untersuchungen zur Entwicklung der Synapsen in Explantatkulturen des Hippocampus bei Rattenembryonen. *Z. mikrosk.-anat. Forsch.,* 87:195–217.

Werman, R., Davidoff, R. A., and Aprison, M. H. (1968): Inhibitory action of glycine on spinal neurons in the cat. *J. Neurophysiol.,* 31:81–95.

Wilson, D. M. (1964): The origin of the flight-motor command in grasshoppers. In: *Neuronal Theory and Modeling,* edited by R. F. Reiss, pp. 331–345. Stanford University Press, Stanford.

Wilson, D. M. (1967): An approach to the problem of control of insect locomotion. In: *In-*

vertebrate Nervous Systems, edited by C. A. G. Wiersma, pp. 219–229. Chicago University Press, Chicago.

Windle, W. F. (1934): Correlation between the development of local reflexes and reflex arcs in the spinal cord of cat embryos. *J. Comp. Neurol.,* 59:487–505.

Windle, W. F., and Baxter, R. E. (1935–1936): Development of reflex mechanism in the spinal cord of albino rat embryos: Correlations between structure and function, and comparisons with the cat and chick. *J. Comp. Neurol.,* 63:189–210.

Windle, W. F., and Orr, D. W. (1934): The development of behavior in chick embryos: Spinal cord structure correlated with early somatic motility. *J. Comp. Neurol.,* 60:287–308.

Windle, W. F., Minear, W. L., Austin, M. F., and Orr, D. W. (1935): The origin and early development of somatic behaviour in the albino rat. *Physiol. Zool.,* 8:156–185.

Wolf, M. K. (1964): Differentiation of neuronal types and synapses in myelinating cultures of mouse cerebellum. *J. Cell Biol.,* 22:259–279.

Wolf, M. K. (1970): Anatomy of cultured mouse cerebellum. II. Organotypic migration of granule cells demonstrated by silver impregnation of normal and mutant cultures. *J. Comp. Neurol.,* 140:281–298.

Wolf, M. K., and Dubois-Dalcq, M. (1970): Anatomy of cultured mouse cerebellum. I. Golgi and electron microscopic demonstration of granule cells, their afferent and efferent synapses. *J. Comp. Neurol.,* 140:261–280.

Wood, J., McLaughlin, B. J., and Vaughn, J. E. (1975): Immunocytochemical localization of GAD in electron microscopic preparations of rodent CNS. In: *GABA in Nervous System Function,* edited by E. Roberts, T. N. Chase, and D. B. Tower, pp. 133–148. Raven Press, New York.

Wooten, G. F., Thoa, N. B., Kopin, I. J., and Axelrod, J. (1973): Enhanced release of dopamine β-hydroxylase and norepinephrine from sympathetic nerves by dibutyryl cyclic adenosine 3',5'-monophosphate and theophylline. *Mol. Pharmacol.,* 9:178–183.

Yamamoto, C. (1972): Intracellular study of seizure-like afterdischarges elicited in thin hippocampal sections in vitro. *Exp. Neurol.,* 35:154–164.

Yamamoto, C. (1975): Recording of electrical activity from microscopically identified neurons of the mammalian brain. *Experientia,* 31:309–310.

Yamamoto, C., and Kawai, N. (1967): Seizure discharges evoked in vitro in thin section from guinea pig hippocampus. *Science,* 155:341–342.

Yamamoto, C., and Kawai, N. (1968): Generation of the seizure discharge in thin sections from the guinea pig brain in chloride-free medium in vitro. *Jap. J. Physiol.,* 18:620–631.

Yamamoto, C., and McIlwain, H. (1966): Electrical activities in thin sections from the mammalian brain maintained in chemically-defined media in vitro. *J. Neurochem.,* 13:1333–1343.

Yamauchi, A., Lever, J. D., and Kemp, K. W. (1973): Catecholamine loading and depletion in the rat superior cervical ganglia: A formol fluorescence and enzyme histochemical study with numerical assessments. *J. Anat.,* 114:271–282.

Young, J. Z. (1964): *A Model of the Brain,* pp. 282–284. Clarendon Press, Oxford.

Young, J. Z. (1966): *The Memory System of the Brain.* University of California Press, Berkeley.

Zipser, B., Crain, S. M., and Bornstein, M. B. (1973): Directly evoked "paroxysmal" depolarizations of mouse hippocampal neurons in synaptically organized explants in longterm culture. *Brain Res.,* 60:489–495.

Zweifler, N. J., and Robinson, J. O. (1969): Rabbit homocytotropic antibody: A unique rabbit immunoglobulin and analogous to human IgE. *J. Exp. Med.,* 130:907–929.

Subject Index

A

Acetylcholine (ACh), *see also* Cholinergic synapses
  depolarizing effects on dissociated sympathetic (but not DRG) neurons, 133-136, 139
  excitant and depressant effects on cerebral explants, 163
Acetylcholinesterase
  cholinergic synapses in neural cultures and, 164
  development in brain cell reaggregates, 150, 164
  development in spinal cord and DRG explants, 164
  localized at neuromuscular junctions in explants, 59, 62, 218, 220, 221, 232
  not found at synapses between dissociated neurons and muscle, 232
ACh, *see* Acetylcholine
Adrenal medulla chromaffin cells, action potentials, ACh depolarization, and catecholamine fluorescence of, 134
Adrenergic synapses, *see also* Noradrenergic CNS neurons
  between dissociated sympathetic ganglion cells, 137, 138
  sympathetic ganglia and cardiac muscle, 40, 41, 137
  sympathetic ganglia and smooth muscle, 41
Adult muscle cultures
  human and mouse skeletal muscle, 62-68, 219-227
  rat iris, 41
Adult neural cultures
  fish CNS, 15
  frog CNS and peripheral ganglia, 15, 16, 40
  human and rat sympathetic ganglia, 15, 41
  rat CNS, 15
  subculture of *in vitro*-matured CNS explants, 228-230
Allergic encephalomyelitis (EAE), *see also* Multiple sclerosis
  depressant effects of EAE sera on CNS explant discharges, 177-182
  experimental model of MS, 177-182
  possible role of myelin in serum depression of CNS explant discharges, 181, 182
  role of circulating serum factors, 177-182
Alpha rhythms, *see* EEG spindles
γ-Aminobutyric acid, *see* GABA
Aminophylline, *see* Cyclic AMP-PDE inhibitors
5'AMP, synaptic functions (cf. cyclic AMP), non-enhancement of, 168, 169
Antineuronal autoantibodies
  increase in serum of aging mice, 180
  related to serum γ-globulin depression of CNS explant discharges, 178-181
Aplysia ganglion explants, spike firing patterns and circadian rhythms, 129, 130
ATP, synaptic functions (cf. cyclic AMP), non-enhancement of, 168
Axoaxonic synapses, related to presynaptic inhibition, 75, 76
Axodendritic synapses, *see also* Synaptic junctions; Synaptogenesis
  abundant in all CNS explants generating complex network discharges, 49, 50, 108, 120, 143
  after maturation in spinal cord explants, 44, 45, 48-50
  characteristic mossy fiber endings on pyramidal neurons after maturation in hippocampus explants, 106, 120
  role of axodendritic inhibition, 107, 157, 158
Axon collateral sprouting
  hyperexcitability in CNS explants and isolated cerebral slabs *in situ* and, 197, 198
  possible homeostatic function of sprouting by inhibitory neurons, 197, 198
Axosomatic synapses
  dissociated DRG neurons, 38, 132

Axosomatic synapses (*contd.*)
    early formation in fetal rodent spinal
        cord and cerebral explants, 48,
        49, 101-103

B

Balanced salt solution (BSS), 13, 15, 67
Barbiturates, *see also* Xylocaine
    depression of chick embryo telencepha-
        lon slow-wave discharges, 187
    depression of fetal rat cerebellar spike
        discharges, 126
Bicuculline (and picrotoxin)
    antagonism of GABA depression of
        spike firing in cerebellum, 126,
        160, 161
    convulsive effects in ventral cord, 74-76
    depression of PADs in dorsal cord, 74,
        75, 78
    enhancement of immature cerebral ex-
        plant discharges, 97, 99, 100
    enhancement of immature network
        discharges in spinal cord *in vitro*
        and *in situ,* 46, 47, 201, 202
    excitation of cerebral and spinal cord ex-
        plants, and antagonism of GABA
        depression, 157-159
    excitation of hippocampal and olfactory
        bulb explants, 116, 118, 123, 124
    polarity reversal of positive slow-wave
        potentials, 157, 199
Blood-brain barrier
    diffusion barriers over CNS explants and,
        55, 58, 180
    possible role in EAE and MS dysfunc-
        tions, 178
"Body-space" in culture
    degree to which CNS explants maintain
        geometry based on body axes,
        233, 234
    nerve territorial fields and, 233, 234
Brain slices, freshly isolated
    cerebellum, 80 μm thick, 128
    cerebral cortex, 1, 4
    hippocampus, 119, 166
Brainstem cultures
    dissociated spinal cord and brainstem
        neurons, 142-146
    DRG-cord arrayed with explant of
        medulla at level of dorsal column
        nuclei, 83-88
    isolated DRGs presented to dorsal
        column nuclei explants, 88
    locus ceruleus explants, 89
    medulla-cerebral explant arrays, 189-194
    nonspecific connections between spinal
        cord and medulla explants, 79-83
    raphe explants, 89
    substantia nigra explants and reaggre-
        gates of dopaminergic midbrain
        cells, 89, 90

C

Caffeine, *see also* Cyclic AMP-PDE inhibitors
    depression of spike firing in cerebellar
        explants, 176
    enhancement of neuromuscular trans-
        mission during low-Ca^{++} block-
        ades, 173, 174
    excitation of spinal cord and cerebral
        explants, 166-171
    inhibition of cyclic AMP-PDE, leading to
        increased endogenous cyclic
        AMP, 166-174
    mobilization of membrane-bound cal-
        cium in nerve terminals, 173, 174
    reduction of network discharge thres-
        holds in immature CNS explants,
        99, 100, 170-172
    restoration of synaptic transmission in
        spinal cord and cerebral explants
        during low-Ca^{++} blockades, 168
Calcium ions (Ca^{++})
    critical role in synaptic transmitter re-
        lease, 167, 168, 174, 175
    depletion by chelator (EGTA), produc-
        ing synaptic blockade, 167, 168
    mediation of DRG perikaryal action
        potentials, 38, 133
    mobilization from membrane-bound
        calcium stores by cyclic AMP,
        173-176
    possible increase in intracellular levels
        during post-tetanic potentiation,
        175
    storage sites of membrane-bound calci-
        um, 175
Cardiac muscle explants
    action potentials of chick fibers, 35
    increased rate of spontaneous contrac-
        tions following sympathetic
        ganglion volley, 40, 41
Catecholaminergic fluorescence, *see also*
        Monoaminergic neurons; Noradrener-
        gic CNS neurons
    dissociated spinal cord neurons, 143
    enhancement in cord neurons growing
        on liver "feeder layer," 143
    noradrenergic sympathetic neurites in-
        nervating iris explants, 41
Cerebellar deplants *in oculo,* spontaneous
    spike firing, 120
Cerebellar slow-wave discharges, onset after
    chronic exposure of explants to
    antimitotic agents,
    126-128

Cerebellar spike firing, neonatal rat cultures
  amino acids, effects of, 126, 160, 161
  depression by inhibitors of cyclic AMP-
    PDE and noradrenalin, 176
  extracellular units in explants, 125-128
  intracellular PSPs and spikes in dissoci-
    ated neurons, 150-152
  irregular bursts blocked by Mg^{++} and
    pentobarbital, 125, 126
  propagation in dendrites, 11
  synchronization after innervation by
    brainstem explants, 126
Cerebral-evoked potentials, see also Laminar
    organization in cerebral explants
  development in fetal mouse explants,
    92-101, 108, 109
  initiated from subcortical explant or
    outgrowing neurites, 111, 163,
    170
  limits to maturation in vitro, 112, 113
  negative slow waves as summated EPSPs,
    108, 110, 111
  polarity reversal in cortical depth re-
    cordings in explants, deplants,
    and in situ, 108, 110-112
  positive slow waves as summated IPSPs,
    108, 110, 111
Cerebral hyperexcitability
  in CNS explants and in isolated cerebral
    slabs in situ, 197, 198
  compensatory axon sprouting of inhibi-
    tory interneurons, 197, 198
  role of denervation hypersensitivity,
    197, 198
Cerebral slabs in situ, 1, 3, 109, 113, 114,
    186-189, 197, 198
Chemosensitive sites on neurons
  cholinergic sites near synapses in situ,
    107
  inhibitory sites in CNS explants, 107
  iontophoretic studies of dissociated
    neurons, 133-139, 149-152
Chick embryo explants
  DRGs, 8-10, 31-39
  skeletal and cardiac muscle, 10, 35
  spinal cord and myotomes, 7, 11, 55
  sympathetic ganglia, 40-42
Chloride-free media
  enhancement of immature cerebral ex-
    plant discharges, 97-99, 105
  onset of paroxysmal discharges in CNS
    explants and freshly isolated
    brain slices, 164-166
  possible role of chloride ions in EPSPs
    of DRG terminals in spinal cord,
    166
  role of chloride ions in IPSPs of CNS
    neurons, 164, 166
Choline acetyltransferase

activity in brain cell reaggregates, 150
  development of cholinergic synapses in
    cultures and, 136, 137, 150, 164
Cholinergic synapses
  between dissociated sympathetic neu-
    rons, 134-137
  motor endplates in spinal cord muscle
    explants, 59, 62, 63, 68, 218,
    220, 221, 224
  spinal cord and sympathetic neurons,
    137-141
  sympathetic neurons and skeletal
    muscle, 40, 41, 65, 67, 136, 137,
    225-227
Chronic anesthesia during embryonic
    development
  limitations of in situ experiments, 212
  noninterference with CNS maturation
    in most studies, 212
  tissue culture models, 210-213
Chronic block of discharges in CNS
    explants
  normal development of synaptic net-
    works during Xylocaine or Mg^{++}
    blockade, 210-213
  rapid onset of complex network dis-
    charges after removal of chronic
    Xylocaine or Mg^{++}, 210-213
  spontaneous transmitter release during
    chronic block of nerve impulses,
    212
Chronic curarization of cord-muscle cul-
    tures, see also d-Tubocurarine
  formation of mature neuromuscular
    junctions during curare blockade,
    222, 224
  signs of drug tolerance, 224
Chronic electric stimulation of muscle
  possible role of contractions in mainte-
    nance of denervated muscle, 224
  reduction in spread of ACh sensitivity
    in muscle cultures, 224
Chronic recordings of CNS discharges
  chick and rat cerebral explants, 120,
    187, 188
  rodent hippocampal explants, 120
  sterile recording chambers, 25, 26, 120,
    187, 188
Cockroach CNS explants, spontaneous dis-
    charges, 128, 129
Colchicine, interference with trophic fac-
    tors regulating axon territory, 234
Collagen gel substrates, 13
Complement factor in sera
  effects on neuromuscular transmission
    in frog in situ, 180
  role in immunologic serum depression
    of CNS explant discharges,
    177-181

Conduction velocity of
    dissociated DRG neurites, 132, 133
    dorsal roots in DRG-cord explants, 132
    neurites in CNS explants, 11, 93, 95,
        175
Cortisone
    depression of muscle development in cul-
        ture and *in situ,* 218
    enhancement of CNS development in
        explants, 218
Culture media
    effects of cell "conditioning," 14, 15,
        136, 137, 143
    general types for neural explants, 13-16
    hormonal effects, 15, 40, 41, 69-72, 91,
        122, 218
    simplified for cells with yolk storage
        vesicles, 67, 68
Cuneate nucleus, *see* Dorsal column nuclei
Cyclic AMP, *see also* Caffeine
    depression of spike firing in cerebellar
        explants, 176
    enhancement of inhibitory and excita-
        tory synapses, 176, 177
    enhancement of transmitter release at
        neuromuscular junctions, 173,
        174
    excitation of cerebral and spinal cord
        explants, 168-170
    excitation of hippocampal deplants *in
        oculo,* 173
    excitation of invertebrate ganglion cells,
        173
    mobilization of membrane-bound cal-
        cium in nerve terminals, 174
    onset of convulsive activity in neonatal
        cat cerebral cortex, 172
    postsynaptic effects, 176
    presynaptic effects, 173-176
    reduction in excitation thresholds during
        synaptogenesis in CNS explants,
        170-172
    restoration of synaptic transmission in
        spinal cord and cerebral explants
        during low-Ca^{++} blockades, 168,
        169, 171, 173-175
Cyclic AMP-PDE inhibitors
    aminophylline, 176
    caffeine, 99, 100, 166-171, 174, 176
    isobutyl methyl xanthine, 173
    papaverine, 176
    SQ 65,442, 168, 174

D

Demyelination of CNS explants, restoration
        of network discharges after
        removal of demyelinating
        serum, 178

Denervated muscle atrophy
    loss of cross striations and reduced fiber
        diameters, 222, 223
    possible prevention by trophic agents,
        224-227
    rapid onset after removal of spinal cord
        neurons innervating mature mus-
        cle explants, 222, 223
    translocation of myonuclei from sub-
        sarcolemmal to central loci, 222,
        223
Deplants of CNS tissues
    amphibian larva dorsal fin, 4, 5, 200,
        226
    rat anterior eye chamber (*"in oculo"*),
        4, 5, 90, 91, 108, 120, 173
Desensitization, of spinal cord (but not
        cerebral) neurons after chronic
        glycine exposure, 149, 152
Dibutyryl cyclic AMP, *see* Cyclic AMP
Disinhibition
    analogous to selective gene depression,
        206
    learning mechanisms and, 206
    mechanism for switching on neuronal
        cell assemblies during develop-
        ment, 205
Dissociated neurons
    bioelectric functions of DRG, sympa-
        thetic, spinal cord, brainstem,
        cerebellar, and cerebral neurons,
        131-152
    cell separation and culture techniques,
        16, 17, 131, 141, 143
    monoaminergic brainstem cultures, 89,
        90
    vs. explant cultures, 2-4, 131, 141,
        231-233
Disuse muscle atrophy
    studies *in situ,* 219-221
    tissue culture models, 219-222, 224
Dopaminergic CNS neurons
    explants of substantia nigra, 89
    formation of dopaminergic reaggregates
        by dissociated midbrain cells, 89,
        90
    innervation of host iris, by deplants of
        substantia nigra *in oculo,* 90, 91
Dorsal column nuclei, medulla
    negative slow-wave potentials evoked by
        DRG stimuli, 84-88
    responses resembling primary afferent
        depolarization (PAD), 84-88
    target neurons for DRG sensory fibers,
        83, 88
Dorsal column tracts, formation between
        DRG-cord and medulla explants,
        84-88
Dorsal horn, spinal cord, *see also* Primary

afferent depolarization; Ventral
horn
negative slow-wave potentials evoked
by DRG stimuli, 73-76, 84-88
resemblance to PAD patterns, 75, 76
silver-impregnated explants, 45, 53-57
substantia gelatinosa, 45
target neurons for DRG sensory fibers,
78, 79
Dorsal root ganglia (DRGs)
chick and rodent explants, 8-10, 31-39
dissociated neurons, 17, 38, 131-133
DRG-cord-brainstem arrays, 80-88, 234
frog explants, 15
isolated DRGs presented to spinal cord
or medulla "target" explants,
77-79
spinal cord explant with attached ganglia, 14, 43, 52, 53, 60, 65, 66,
69-77, 216, 222, 223, 233
DRGs, *see* Dorsal root ganglia
Drosophila cell cultures, formation of neuromuscular junctions, 129
Drug tolerance and desensitization
chronic glycine in dissociated CNS
cultures, 149, 152
chronic *d*-tubocurarine in cord-muscle
explants, 222, 224, 232
Dual transmitter hypothesis, 137

E

EAE, *see* Allergic encephalomyelitis
EEG, *see* Electroencephalogram
EEG spindles, mimicked by oscillatory afterdischarges in CNS explants, 186,
193-197; *see also* Electroencephalogram
Electric currents and neurite growth patterns, 228
Electric recording and stimulating techniques, 19, 22-29
Electroencephalogram (EEG)
alpha rhythms, 196, 197
cerebral explant models, 108, 109,
113-116, 186-197
chronic recordings from CNS explants,
120, 187, 188
isolated cerebral slabs *in situ*, 109,
113-116, 186-189
medulla-cerebral explant arrays, 189-
194
neonatal cerebral neocortex *in situ*, 96,
97, 101
spindle activity, 186, 193-197
strychnine convulsive effects, 95-97
Embryonic motility
Coghill's theory of patterned behavioral
development and, 203-207

functional significance during development, 203-207
widespread spinal cord discharges and,
183, 184, 186, 188, 201, 204
Epileptiform discharges
cerebral neocortex explants, 109, 113,
114, 116, 189, 190, 197, 198
cord-limb deplants, 200, 226
hippocampal explants, 117-119
EPSPs, *see* Excitatory postsynaptic potentials
Eserine, enhancement of neuromuscular
transmission, 59, 62, 68
Evaporation of culture medium, techniques
for prevention, 19, 21-24
Excitation-secretion coupling, *see* Synaptic
transmitter release
Excitatory postsynaptic potentials (EPSPs)
dissociated cerebral and cerebellar
neurons, 150-152
dissociated spinal cord neurons, 142,
147-149
dissociated sympathetic ganglion cells,
134-141
DRG cells, 36-38, 132
extracellular negative slow waves and,
106, 116-119, 157, 158,
198, 199
hippocampal explants, 116-119
Exocytosis and endocytosis, of peroxidase-
labeled presynaptic vesicles in spinal
cord neurons, 58
Explants of neural tissues
CNS culture techniques, 13-15, 43, 83,
85, 92, 93
limitations in techniques, 231-233
vs. dissociated cell cultures, 2-4, 131,
141, 233, 235

F

Facilitation
of cerebral neocortex and hippocampal
discharges, 116, 118, 212, 213
of PAD potentials in dorsal cord and
medulla by DRG volleys, 75,
84, 85
role of Ca^{++} and cyclic AMP, 173, 175,
177
of spinal cord network discharges, 46,
47, 212, 214
Feeder layers, development of catecholaminergic properties in dissociated
spinal cord neurons growing on liver
monolayer, 143
Fixed action patterns
development of stereotyped CNS networks and, 209
selective disinhibition, 205

Fluorescence histochemical analyses, *see
    also* Catecholaminergic fluorescence;
    Monoaminergic neurons
  dissociated spinal cord neurons, 143
  monoaminergic brainstem neurons,
      89-91
  noradrenergic sympathetic ganglion
      neurons, 41, 42
Fluorodeoxyuridine (FdU)
  enhancement of maturation of dissocia-
      ted cerebral neurons, 16, 17, 150
  prevention of fibroblast overgrowth, 16,
      17, 138
"Forward reference"
  maturation of CNS networks in advance
      of later functions, 201, 205
  tissue culture models, 210-212
Frog explants
  adult sympathetic ganglia, 15, 16, 40
  embryonic neurulae and presumptive
      muscle, 67-69
  embryonic spinal cord and myotomes,
      6, 7, 55, 67-69
  tadpole spinal cord, 55

G

GABA (γ-aminobutyric acid)
  antagonism by bicuculline, picrotoxin,
      and penicillin, 157-162
  depolarizing effects on dissociated DRG
      and sympathetic neurons, 133,
      134
  depolarizing effects on DRG neurons,
      75-78
  depression of slow waves and spike
      firing in cerebral, cerebellar,
      and olfactory bulb explants,
      123, 157-162
  depression of spike firing in hypothala-
      mic explants, 122
  depression of ventral cord discharges,
      75, 76
  enhancement of PADs in dorsal cord
      and medulla, 74-78, 84-88
  hyperpolarizing effects on dissociated
      spinal cord and cerebral neurons,
      133, 149, 152
  perfusion vs. iontophoresis in cerebellar
      explants, 126, 161
  possible role as inhibitory transmitter,
      123, 157-161
  specificity of depressant effects *in situ*
      and in culture, 155, 159-162
GABA dipeptides, nondepressant effects
    on CNS explants and cerebral cortex
    in situ, 155
GAD, *see* Glutamate decarboxylase
"Giant" extracellular spikes

  amplitudes as high as 70 mV in DRG
      explants, 124
  blocked by GABA, and firing enhanced
      by bicuculline, in olfactory bulb
      explants, 124
Glutamate
  alterations in membrane conductance of
      dissociated spinal cord neurons,
      149
  excitation of cerebellar and hypothala-
      mic explants, 122, 126
Glutamate decarboxylase (GAD)
  dissociated brain cell reaggregates, 150
  hippocampal explants and *in situ,* 107,
      150
  labeling of GABA-ergic presynaptic
      terminals in cord *in situ,* 76
Glycine
  antagonism by strychnine, 153-156
  depression of reflexes *in situ,* 156
  depression of spinal cord explant dis-
      charges, 153, 154
  desensitization of spinal cord (but not
      cerebral) neurons after chronic
      exposure, 149, 152
  evidence for specificity of depressant
      effects, 155
  hyperpolarizing effects on dissociated
      spinal cord and cerebral neurons,
      149, 152
  ineffective on olfactory bulb explants,
      123
  possible role as inhibitory transmitter,
      155, 156
Glycyl dipeptides, nondepressant effects on
    spinal cord explants, 155
Gracilis nucleus, *see* Dorsal column nuclei

H

Heart-conditioned medium, *see* Muscle-
    conditioned media
Hexamethonium, *see also* Nicotinic-cholin-
    ergic blocking agents
  blockade of cord-evoked EPSPs of dis-
      sociated sympathetic neurons,
      139
  blockade of nicotinic synapses between
      dissociated sympathetic neurons,
      136, 137
Hippocampal deplants *in oculo*
  absence of spontaneous spikes, 120
  evoked slow-wave potentials, 108
  excitatory effects of cyclic GMP, 173
Hippocampal explants
  chronic extracellular recordings of
      complex discharges, 120
  intracellular recordings in older explants
      (EPSPs, IPSPs, and PDSs), 116-119

Hippocampal explants *(contd.)*
  morphologic development and synapto-
    genesis, 101-106, 120
  onset of synaptic functions, 96-100
Histiotypic cultures, 2, 4
Homeostatic inhibitory mechanisms
  CNS collateral sprouting and hyperex-
    citability and, 197, 198, 207
  early behavior and, 202-207
Human tissue cultures
  adult muscle explants, 62, 66-68
  adult sympathetic ganglia, 15
  embryonic spinal cord explants, 47, 51
Hyperexcitability, *see* Cerebral hyperexcitability
Hypothalamic explants
  chemically evoked spike firing in dog
    supraoptic explants, 122
  spontaneous phasic spike firing patterns
    in rat tuberal explants, 121
  testosterone growth stimulation of
    specific regions, 122

I

Immunocytochemical labeling of GAD, 76
Immunoglobulins
  serum γ-globulin depression of CNS
    explant discharges, 179-181
  thermolability, 179, 180
Information storage, *see* Memory and
  learning
Inhibition, early onset in CNS cultures,
    see also Tonic inhibition
  fetal rodent spinal cord and cerebral
    explants, 46, 47, 105-107, 201
  revealed by GABA-antagonist drugs,
    47, 98, 100, 105, 106
Inhibition, early onset in embryos
  behavioral significance, 201-207
  concomitance of inhibitory and excita-
    tory synaptic functions in fish,
    201, 202
  coordinated motor output related to
    early inhibition, 206
  role of inhibitory interneurons in regu-
    lating cell assemblies, 205
  strychnine effects on motility and spinal
    cord discharges, 201, 202
Inhibitory "phasing" mechanism, *see* Recurrent inhibition
Inhibitory postsynaptic potentials (IPSPs)
  blockade by picrotoxin and polarity
    reversal of positive slow-wave
    potentials, 157, 158
  correlated with extracellular positive
    slow-wave potentials in cerebral
    explants and *in situ,* 106, 111,
    116, 118, 119, 157, 159, 198, 199

  in dissociated cerebral and cerebellar
    neurons, 150-152
  in fetal cat spinal cord *in situ,* 200
  in hippocampal explants, 116-119
  in neonatal rat cerebral cortex and
    hippocampus *in situ,* 198, 199
  inverted by hyperpolarization of dis-
    sociated spinal cord neurons,
    142, 148, 149
Injury discharges, DRGs, 35, 37
Innate releasing mechanisms, related to
  selective disinhibition, 205
Intracellular impalement techniques, 28, 29
Invertebrate neural cultures
  Aplysia ganglion explants, 129, 130
  cockroach CNS explants, 128, 129
  dissociated *Drosophila* neurons and
    muscle cells, 129
  dissociated lobster ventral nerve cord,
    17, 18
  leech ganglion explants, 129
IPSPs, *see* Inhibitory postsynaptic potentials

L

Laminar organization in cerebral explants
  cerebral neocortex, 92-94
  polarity reversals of evoked potentials
    and, 108-112
Leech ganglion explants, action potentials
  and PSPs, 129
Limb and CNS deplants in amphibian larvae
  epileptiform movements related to
    humoral factors, 200
  excitatory effects of strychnine, 200
  innervation of limb by internuncial
    cord and medulla neurons, 226
Limbic cultures, *see* Hypothalamic explants; Olfactory bulb explants

M

Magnesium ions (Mg^{++})
  antagonism of Ca^{++}-dependent trans-
    mitter release, 166-168
  blockade of EPSPs in dissociated sym-
    pathetic neurons, 135, 136, 138,
    140, 141
  blockade of synaptic network discharges
    in CNS cultures, 46, 75, 123,
    145, 146, 164
  blockade of synaptic transmission in
    CNS cultures and *in situ,* 166-
    168
  depression of irregular spike firing in
    cerebellar explants,
    125, 126, 160,
    168

Magnesium ions (Mg^{++}) *(contd.)*
  depression of stimulus-dependent up-
      take of peroxidase in presynaptic
      terminals, 55, 57
Maximow slide chamber, vs. larger culture
      dishes, 13-15
Mecamylamine, *see* Nicotinic-cholinergic
      blocking agents
Medulla, *see* Brainstem cultures
Medulla-cerebral explant discharges
  excitatory and inhibitory interactions,
      189-193
  pacemaker neurons in medulla, 190-193
Memory and learning, tissue culture models,
      193-197, 205, 206, 212-215
Methylazoxymethanol acetate (MAM)
  inhibition of mitosis of granule cells in
      cerebellar explants, 126
  onset of synchronized slow-wave dis-
      charges in cerebellar explants
      after chronic MAM exposure,
      126-128
Microelectrodes
  extracellular glass microsaltbridges, 19,
      22, 23, 26, 27
  intracellular pipettes, 28, 29
  metal types, 25, 27, 187, 188
Micromanipulators
  large conventional types, 19-21
  miniaturized magnetic types, 22-25
Micrurgical techniques
  definition, 18
  open chamber with inverted micro-
      scope, 21
  open chamber with upright microscope,
      18-21
  sealed chamber with miniature micro-
      manipulators, 22-25
Miniature synaptic potentials
  in dissociated spinal cord neurons, 142,
      148
  in dissociated sympathetic ganglion
      cells innervated by spinal cord,
      138, 139
  possibly involved in early tonic inhibi-
      tion, 107
  probable generation in CNS explants
      during chronic anesthesia, 212
Mitotic inhibitors
  prevention of cerebellar granule cell
      multiplication, 126, 128
  prevention of fibroblast overgrowth,
      16, 17, 138, 147, 150
Monoaminergic neurons, *see also* Catechol-
      aminergic fluorescence; Noradren-
      ergic CNS neurons
  brainstem cultures, 89-91
  sympathetic ganglion explants,
      41, 42

Motor endplate, *see* Neuromuscular junc-
      tions
MS, *see* Multiple sclerosis
Multiple sclerosis (MS), *see also* Allergic
      encephalomyelitis
  depressant effects of MS sera on rodent
      CNS explants and frog spinal
      cord *in situ,* 177-179
  role of circulating serum factors, 177-
      182
Muscle-conditioned media
  enhancement of ACh synthesis and
      cholinergic synapses in dissocia-
      ted sympathetic ganglion cultures
      by cardiac factor, 136, 137
  enhancement of choline acetyltransfer-
      ase in dissociated spinal cord
      neurons by co-culture with
      skeletal muscle, 143
Muscle contractions, *see* Skeletal muscle
      cultures; Cardiac muscle explants
Myelin inhibition, *see also* Demyelination
      of CNS explants
  development of synaptic networks in
      myelin-inhibited spinal cord ex-
      plants, 181, 182, 232
  myelination of CNS explants prevented
      during chronic exposure to EAE
      serum, 181, 182, 232
Myelination, development in neural ex-
      plants, 2, 9, 11
Myotome explants, innervation by spinal
      cord neurons, 59; *see also* Chick
      embryo explants; Frog explants

N

Negative slow-wave potentials, extracellular
      recordings of summated EPSPs, 47,
      106, 108, 111, 116-119, 157-159,
      198, 199; *see also* Excitatory post-
      synaptic potentials
Nerve growth factor (NGF), stimulation of
      brainstem monoaminergic neurons *in
      situ,* 91
  chick embryo DRGs *in ovo,* 71, 72
  dissociated chick DRG and sympathetic
      neurons, 71, 218
  fetal rodent DRG explants, 69-71
  sympathetic ganglion explants, fetal and
      adult, rodent and frog, 15, 40,
      41, 218, 225
Neurite growth between explants, *see also*
      Patterned neuritic arborizations in
      CNS explants
  "dorsal column" fascicles toward dorsal
      column nuclei in medulla ex-
      plants, 85, 87, 88,
      234

Neurite growth between explants, *see also*
    Patterned neuritic arborizations in
    CNS explants *(contd.)*
    DRG fascicles toward dorsal and away
        from ventral regions of spinal
        cord explants, 77-79
    motor axon deviation around DRG
        toward muscle, 60, 61
    nonspecific neuritic bridges between
        cord and brainstem explants,
        79-83
    role of meninges and Schwann cells,
        78, 79, 83, 85
Neurite outgrowth, *see also* Patterned
    neuritic arborizations
    embryonic chick and rodent DRG
        explants, 9, 35, 36, 38, 39
    embryonic frog spinal cord explants,
        Harrison's pioneering experi-
        ments, 5-7
    fetal rodent cerebral neocortex ex-
        plants, 92, 93
    fetal rodent spinal cord explants, 43,
        216
Neuroblastoma cell cultures
    action potentials and chemosensitivity,
        131
    cholinergic synapses of hybrid cells
        with muscle, 131
Neuromuscular junctions
    cholinesterase localization, 59, 62, 218,
        220, 221, 232
    infoldings of postsynaptic membrane in
        mature endplates, 62, 63, 220,
        232
    motor axon tracts and terminals in
        muscle, 60-63, 216, 217, 220
    terminal Schwann cells, 61, 63, 220,
        221, 232
    ultrastructural features, 62-64, 220
Neuromuscular transmission, *see also* Limb
    and CNS deplants in amphibian
    larvae; Neuromuscular junctions;
    Skeletal muscle cultures
    deplants of CNS and limbs, 200, 226
    dissociated neuroblastoma hybrid cells
        and skeletal muscle, 131
    dissociated spinal cord neurons and
        skeletal muscle, 142
    explants of spinal cord and skeletal
        muscle, 58-69, 216, 220, 221,
        224
    sympathetic ganglia and cardiac muscle,
        40, 41, 137
    sympathetic ganglia and skeletal muscle,
        40, 136, 137, 225, 226
    sympathetic ganglia and smooth muscle,
        41
Neuronal specificity

DRG and target neurons in spinal cord
    and medulla explants, 73-79,
    83-89
phenotypic and locus specificity con-
    cepts, 234
possible locus specificity in arrays of
    DRG and CNS neurons, 234
Neuropil, formation over spinal cord and
    cerebral explants, 43, 92, 111
Neurotrophic effects on muscle mainte-
    nance, *see also* Trophic control of
    regeneration of skeletal muscle
    explants
    major role of spinal cord neurons, 62,
        64, 65, 216-222
    secondary role of DRG neurons, 222
    substitution of sympathetic ganglia for
        spinal cord neurons in culture
        and *in situ*, 65, 225, 226
    surgical denervation in culture, 222,
        223, 225, 226
    trophic effects of sympathetic ganglion
        extract and cyclic AMP on
        smooth muscle, 225
Neurotrophic factors
    definition, 215
    development and maintenance of synap-
        ses and, 215
    effects on muscle, 215-226
    role of glial cells, 215
Nicotine, excitatory effects on hypotha-
    lamic explants, 122
Nicotinic-cholinergic blocking agents
    hexamethonium, 136, 137, 139
    mecamylamine, 137
    d-tubocurarine, 59, 62, 65, 67, 136,
        139, 162-164, 222, 224
Nomarski interference microscopy, visual-
    ization of synaptic boutons in living
    cultures, 148
Noradrenalin (norepinephrine)
    depression of spike firing in hypothalam-
        ic explants, 122
    depression of spike firing in Purkinje
        cells in cerebellar explants, 176
    ineffective on dissociated sympathetic
        ganglion cells, 137
    released by dissociated sympathetic
        ganglion cells in high K^+, 137
    selective accumulation in some neurons
        in brainstem explants, 89
Noradrenergic CNS neurons, *see also*
    Catecholaminergic fluorescence
    deplants of locus ceruleus *in oculo* in-
        nervating host iris, 90, 91
    dissociated sympathetic ganglion cells
        releasing noradrenalin, 137
    explants of locus ceruleus,
        89

Noradrenergic CNS neurons, *see also*
 Catecholaminergic fluorescence
 (contd.)
 sympathetic neurites growing into
  cardiac and iris muscle explants,
  41
Norepinephrine, *see* Noradrenalin

O

Olfactory bulb explants, fetal mouse
 GABA-ergic inhibition of spike and
  slow-wave discharges, 123, 124
 giant extracellular spikes, 124
 granule-to-mitral cell synapses, 124
 slow waves blocked by Mg^{++} and
  GABA, but not by glycine, 123
 slow waves enhanced by GABA antagonists, but not by strychnine, 123
 spontaneous unit firing of mitral cells
  in vitro and *in situ*, 123, 124
Onset of action potentials, in dissociated
  DRG neurons, 132, 133
Onset of spinal reflex activity
 in 15- to 16-day fetal rodents *in utero,*
  49, 69, 201
 related to onset of synaptic network
  discharges in fetal spinal cord-
  DRG explants, 49, 69, 201
Onset of synaptic functions
 dissociated fetal cerebral cortex neurons,
  143, 146, 149, 150
 dissociated fetal spinal cord neurons,
  143, 146, 147
 fetal rodent cerebral neocortex and
  hippocampus explants, 95-101,
  105, 106, 109
 fetal rodent olfactory bulb explants,
  123, 124
 fetal rodent spinal cord explants, 45-47,
  49, 201
 neonatal rodent cerebral neocortex *in
  situ,* 100, 101
Organotypic cultures, 1-12, 231-235
Oscillatory CNS afterdischarges
 cerebral neocortex explants, 95, 96,
  98-100, 109, 116
 cerebral slabs *in situ,* 109, 113, 114,
  186, 197, 198
 dissociated cerebral cortex reaggregates,
  146, 149, 150
 hippocampus explants, 98-100, 116-119
 mimicry of spindle-like alpha activity,
  196, 197
 neuronally isolated dog spinal cord *in
  situ,* 186
 relevance to mechanisms in perception
  and information storage,
  195-197

resemblance to sensory-evoked cerebral
  afterdischarge *in situ,* 193-197
spinal cord and medulla explants, 47,
  50, 51, 183, 184, 186

P

Pacemaker neurons
 in medulla-cerebral explant arrays,
  189-193
 spontaneous spike firing, leading to network discharges in CNS explants,
  62, 69, 81, 83, 126-129, 183,
  186-190
PAD, *see* Primary afferent depolarization
Papaverine, *see* Caffeine; Cyclic AMP-PDE
  inhibitors
Paroxysmal depolarizing shift (PDS)
 dissociated cerebellar neurons, 151, 152
 hippocampal explants, 117-119
Patterned nerve cell migrations, of DRG
  perikarya away from spinal cord
  region of explant, 14, 52, 53, 60-66,
  70, 71, 80, 222, 223, 233
Patterned neuritic arborizations in CNS
  explants
 dorsal and ventral root fascicles in spinal
  cord-DRG explants, 14, 52, 53,
  60, 66, 70, 71, 80, 222, 223,
  233
 dorsal column tracts between DRG-cord
  and medulla explants, 83-89,
  234
 mechanisms of development *in vitro,*
  233-234
 organized axon tracts within CNS explants, 45, 51-54, 71, 78-80,
  86-88, 92, 94, 104, 121, 122,
  128
PDE inhibitors, *see* Phosphodiesterase
  inhibitors
PDS, *see* Paroxysmal depolarizing shift
Penicillin
 antagonism to GABA depressant effects,
  162
 convulsive effects on cerebral explants,
  162
Perception, culture models of cerebral sensory afterdischarges, 193-197
Perfusion vs. iontophoresis of drugs, advantages of each mode, 156, 160,
  161
Peroxidase labeling of presynaptic vesicles
 stimulus-dependent uptake at spinal
  cord synapses, 55, 57, 58
 tests on motor-nerve terminals, 57
pH regulation of cultures, 19, 232
Phenotypic variance of CNS networks
 CNS plasticity and, 209, 210

Phenotypic variance of CNS networks
  (contd.)
  role of small interneurons, 210
  tissue culture models, 209-215
Phosphodiesterase (PDE) inhibitors, *see*
  Cyclic AMP-PDE inhibitors; Caffeine
Picrotoxin, *see* Bicuculline
Plasticity in CNS
  alteration of synaptic efficacy and/or
    structure, 210
  cultures for studies of conditioning,
    learning, and memory, 213-215
  functional shaping, 210
  increased excitability of CNS explants
    following repetitive stimulation,
    116, 212-214
  response decrement during repetitive
    stimulation of CNS explants,
    214
  tissue culture models, 210-215
Positive slow-wave potentials, extracellular
    recordings of summated IPSPs, 47,
    106, 108, 111, 116-119, 157-159,
    198, 199; *see also* IPSPs
Postsynaptic potentials (PSPs), *see* Excita-
    tory postsynaptic potentials; Inhibi-
    tory postsynaptic potentials
Post-tetanic potentiation, *see also* Facili-
    tation
  possible role of cyclic AMP, 173, 177
  role of intracellular Ca^{++}, 175
Presynaptic inhibition
  CNS *in situ*, 76, 77
  spinal cord explants, 76, 77
Primary afferent depolarization (PAD)
  CNS *in situ*, 75, 76
  medulla explants, 84-88
  spinal cord explants, 73-76, 78
Procaine, selective blockade of slow-wave
    discharges in cerebral explants,
    167, 170; *see also* Xylocaine
PSPs, *see* Postsynaptic potentials

R

Reaggregates of dissociated embryonic
    CNS neurons
  brainstem, 16, 89, 90, 142-147
  cerebral cortex and cerebellum, 16, 17,
    149-151
  spinal cord, 16, 17, 141-147
Recurrent collaterals
  cerebral explants, 197, 198
  DRG cells, 38, 39
  hippocampus explants, 119
  spinal cord explants, 54
Recurrent inhibition
  medulla-cerebral explants, 190-
    192

rhythmic oscillatory CNS discharges
    and, 197, 198
Refractory period
  cerebral neocortex neurons, 95, 96
  DRG cells, 31
  olfactory bulb mitral cells, 124
  spinal cord neurons, 44-46
Regeneration in CNS
  formation of functional connections
    between subcultured mature
    spinal cord explants, 228, 229
  possible enhancement of adult CNS
    regeneration by fetal CNS
    transplants, 229, 230
  subcultures of mature CNS explants as
    model system, 228-230
Repetitive spike activity, *see also* Spontan-
    eous spike firing
  brainstem neurons, 80, 81, 83, 183,
    189-194
  cerebral neurons, 96, 114-118, 120
  DRG cells, 31, 35-38
  spinal cord neurons, 44-47, 50, 59,
    65, 67, 73-75, 183, 186
Repetitive stimulation
  enhancement of peroxidase uptake in
    presynaptic terminals in spinal
    cord explants, 55, 56
  facilitation of PADs in spinal cord and
    medulla by DRG volleys, 75,
    84, 85
  spike generation at 10–300/sec, in con-
    trast to frequent failure of slow
    waves at 1–10/sec, 31, 36, 37,
    46
  sustained excitation of hippocampal
    explants, freshly isolated slices,
    and *in situ*, 116, 118
Response latency
  conduction time and synaptic delays,
    31, 33, 35, 46, 50, 59, 65, 67,
    68, 73, 74, 79-83, 175, 190, 191
  marked increase in synaptic delays dur-
    ing Ca^{++} deficits, 167, 169, 170,
    175, 176
Retrograde transport, of labeled synaptic
    vesicle components in spinal cord
    explants, 57, 58
Rhythmic network discharges, *see*
    Oscillatory CNS afterdischarges;
    Spontaneous CNS network dis-
    charges

S

Satellite cells
  latent myoblasts associated
    with skeletal muscle fibers,
    219

Satellite cells *(contd.)*
  specialized Schwann cells surrounding
    peripheral ganglion perikarya, 8
Sensory-evoked CNS networks, *see* Primary
    afferent depolarization; Dorsal col-
    umn nuclei; Dorsal horn
Serotonergic CNS neurons, *see also* Mono-
    aminergic neurons
  explants of brainstem raphe, 89
  innervation of host iris by deplants of
    brainstem raphe *in oculo,* 90, 91
Serum depressant factors
  complement dependence, 177-181
  depressant effects of sera and γ-globulins
    on discharges of CNS explants,
    177-181
  greater depressant potency of γ-globulin
    from EAE sera, 181
  present in normal animals and humans,
    as well as in EAE and MS, 177-
    182
  thermolability, 177-180
Skeletal muscle atrophy
  factors controlling muscle maturation
    in uninnervated cultures, 218,
    219
  prevention or reversal by innervation *in
    vitro* and *in situ,* 62-65, 216-226
  role of overt muscle contractions, 219-
    222, 224
Skeletal muscle cultures, *see also* Neuromus-
    cular junctions; Neuromuscular
    transmission
  action potentials of chick fibers, 10, 35
  cord-evoked potentials and contractions
    in fetal rodent fibers, 58, 59, 62
  cord-evoked responses in adult rodent
    and human fibers, 62-68
  cross-striated properties, 62-68, 219-227
  culture techniques, 58-62, 215-220,
    222, 225
  myonuclei, 60, 61, 64, 216, 217, 220-
    224
Sliding microscope scanning technique, 20,
    21
Smooth muscle
  enhancement of isolated muscle growth
    by ganglion extract and cyclic
    AMP, 225
  innervation by sympathetic ganglia, 41
Spinal reflexes, onset in fetal rodents *in
    utero,* 49, 69, 201
Spontaneous CNS network discharges, *see
    also* Electroencephalogram; Oscilla-
    tory CNS afterdischarges
  chick embryo brain explants, 120, 187,
    188
  chick embryo spinal cord *in ovo,* 184,
    186

frog embryo cord-muscle explants, 68,
    69
frog larval cord-limb deplants, 200
mouse fetal hippocampal explants, 116-
    120
relation to embryonic motility, 183,
    184, 186, 201-204
rodent and human fetal spinal cord and
    medulla explants, 51, 59, 62, 67,
    79-83, 183-186, 190-194, 220-
    222
rodent fetal cerebral cortex explants and
    in situ, 95-100, 109, 113-115,
    186, 188, 190-194
Spontaneous spike firing, *see also* Repetitive
    spike activity
  Aplysia ganglion explants, 129, 130
  cerebellar explants and deplants, 120,
    125-128
  cockroach CNS explants, 129
  hippocampal explants, 116-120
  hypothalamic explants, 121, 122
  medulla-cerebral explants, 190-193
  olfactory bulb explants, 123, 124
  spinal cord explants, 59, 62, 67, 183-186
"Staggered" neural explants, *see also* "Sub-
    cultures" of CNS explants
  fetal spinal cord-DRGs added to mature
    medulla cultures, 87, 229
  fetal sympathetic ganglia added to
    spinal cord-muscle cultures, 225
Stimulus current, control tests for non-
    neural spread in culture, 82, 83
Stimulus-response latency, *see* Response
    latency
Stimulus-secretion coupling, *see* Synaptic
    transmitter release
Strychnine, *see also* Glycine
  convulsive effects in spinal cord-muscle
    explants, 59, 62, 184
  enhancement of immature cerebral ex-
    plant discharges, 95-100
  epileptiform movements of cord-limb
    deplants, 200
  excitation of brainstem explants, 81, 83
  excitation of reaggregates of dissociated
    spinal cord and cerebral neurons,
    143, 145, 146
  excitation of spinal cord and cerebral
    explants, 44-47, 74, 153-156,
    168, 169, 171, 172, 177, 183,
    184, 187-191
  excitatory effects on limb motility in
    early chick embryo, 201, 202
  ineffective on olfactory bulb explants,
    123
  precocious swimming of fish embryos in,
    201, 202

Strychnine, *see also* Glycine *(contd.)*
  prevention of glycine depression of
    spinal cord explant discharges,
    153-156
  selective inhibitory antagonism *in situ*
    and in culture, 153-156, 198,
    199
"Subcultures" of CNS explants
  model for studies of CNS regeneration,
    229, 230
  transfer of portion of *in vitro*-matured
    CNS explant to new culture,
    228, 229
Sympathetic ganglia
  co-cultured with muscle, 40-42, 136,
    137, 225-227
  dissociated fetal neurons, 134-141
  fetal and adult explants, 15, 16, 40-42
  innervated by spinal cord neurons,
    138-141
Synaptic junctions, *see* Adrenergic synap-
    ses; Axoaxonic synapses; Axoso-
    matic synapses; Cholinergic synap-
    ses; Neuromuscular junctions;
    Peroxidase labeling of presynaptic
    vesicles; Synaptogenesis
Synaptic network fatigability, during early
    development of CNS explants, 46,
    99
Synaptic transmitter release
  noradrenalin released by dissociated
    sympathetic ganglion cells in
    high K^+, 137
  regulation by Ca^{++}, 166-176
  role of cyclic AMP, 168-176
  stimulus-dependent peroxidase-labeling
    of presynaptic vesicles in spinal
    cord explants, 55, 57, 58
Synaptogenesis, ultrastructural data, *see
    also* Onset of synaptic functions
  dissociated spinal cord and cerebral
    neurons, 141-143, 148
  explants of fetal and neonatal rodent
    cerebral neocortex and hippo-
    campus, 101-106
  fetal rodent spinal cord explants, 44,
    45, 48-50
  neonatal rodent cerebrum *in situ,* 101-
    105
Synchronized CNS discharges, *see also*
    Oscillatory CNS afterdischarges
  medulla and cerebral explant arrays,
    189-194
  occurrence in CNS explants correlated
    with maturation of synaptic net-
    works, 47, 50, 95, 98-100, 109-
    116
  spinal cord and brainstem explant
    arrays, 79-83

T

Taurine
  depression of cerebral explants, 159,
    160
  possible role as inhibitory transmitter,
    159, 160
Temperature regulation of cultures, 18, 19
Testosterone, growth stimulation of ex-
    plants of specific hypothalamic
    regions, 122
Tetrodotoxin (TTX), blockade of
  axonal but not perikaryal DRG action
    potentials, 38, 133, 134
  skeletal muscle fibers, 224
  spinal cord perikaryal and axonal spikes,
    46, 142, 148
  sympathetic ganglion cell spikes, 134
Tissue cultures, contrasted with
  cell cultures, 4, 131, 233
  freshly isolated tissues, 3, 4
Tonic inhibition, *see also* Embryonic motil-
    ity; Inhibition, early onset in CNS
    cultures; Inhibition, early onset in
    embryos
  antagonism by strychnine and picro-
    toxin in amphibian larvae *in
    situ* and in deplants of spinal
    cord-innervated limbs, leading
    to convulsive movements, 200
  precocious swimming of fish embryos
    in strychnine, 201, 202
  related to restraints on early embryonic
    motility and CNS explant models,
    201-207
Transplants of CNS tissues
  fetal tissues into adult CNS, 229, 230
  vs. deplants, 5
Trophic control of regeneration of skeletal
    muscle explants, *see also* Neuro-
    trophic effects on muscle mainte-
    nance; Neurotrophic factors
  mediation by nonspecific fetal tissue
    factors, 219, 222
  requirement of specific neurotrophic
    factors for long-term maintenance
    of mature muscle, 220-226
d-Tubocurarine
  antagonized by ACh and eserine, 162-
    164
  blockade of neuromuscular transmission,
    7, 59, 62, 65, 67, 68, 222, 224
  blockade of nicotinic synapses between
    dissociated sympathetic ganglion
    cells, 136, 162
  blockade of spinal cord-evoked EPSPs
    of dissociated sympathetic
    ganglion cells,
    139

d-Tubocurarine (*contd.*)
  depression of some components of
      cerebral networks, 163, 164
  formation of neuromuscular junctions
      during chronic blockade, 222,
      224
  paroxysmal discharges in cerebral
      cortex explants and *in situ*, 110,
      111, 162, 163
  possible depression of cholinergic or
      GABA-ergic inhibitory synapses,
      162-164

V

Ventral horn, spinal cord, *see also* Dorsal
    horn
  depression of ventral cord discharges by
      glycine and GABA, and glycine
      antagonism by strychnine, 73-
      76, 153-155, 158
  histologic analyses of silver-impregnated
      explants, 45, 53-62

  identification of motoneurons in ex-
      plants, 43, 45, 54, 56, 57, 59-63

X

Xylocaine, *see also* Procaine
  anesthetic effects, 167, 168
  antagonism of Ca^{++}-dependent trans-
      mitter release, 167, 168
  blockade of network discharges in spinal
      cord and cerebral explants, 55,
      170, 210
  normal development of synaptic net-
      works during chronic blockade
      of nerve impulses, 210-213

Y

Yolk storage vesicles
  development of neuromuscular explants
      in simple saline media, 67, 68
  endogenous nutrients in early frog
      neurula cells, 67, 68